Study Guide to Accompany

Fundamental Nursing Skills and Concepts

EIGHTH EDITION

Study Guide to Accompany

Fundamental Nursing Skills and Concepts

EIGHTH EDITION

BARBARA R. STRIGHT, PH.D, R.N.
Associate Professor
Division of Nursing Education
University of the Virgin Islands
St. Thomas U. S. Virgin Islands

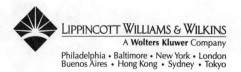
LIPPINCOTT WILLIAMS & WILKINS
A **Wolters Kluwer** Company

Philadelphia • Baltimore • New York • London
Buenos Aires • Hong Kong • Sydney • Tokyo

Ancillary Editor: Doris S. Wray
Senior Production Manager: Helen Ewan
Composition: LWW
Printer/Binder: Victor Graphics

8th Edition

ISBN: 0-7817-5349-X

The material contained in this volume was submitted as previously unpublished
material, except in the instances in which credit has been given to the source from
which some of the illustrative material was derived.

Any procedure or practice described in this book should be applied by the health
care practitioner under appropriate supervision in accordance with professional
standards of care used with regard to the unique circumstances that apply in each
practice situation. Care has been taken to confirm the accuracy of information
presented and to describe generally accepted practices. However, the authors, editors,
and publisher cannot accept any responsibility for errors or omissions or for any
consequences from application of the information in this book and make no
warranty express or implied, with respect to the contents of the book.

The authors and publisher have exerted every effort to ensure that drug selection
and dosage set forth in this text are in accordance with current recommendations
and practice at the time of publication. However, in view of ongoing research,
changes in government regulations, and the constant flow of information relating to
drug therapy and drug reactions, the reader is urged to check the package insert for
each drug for any change in indications and dosage and for added warnings and
precautions. This is particularly important when the recommended agent is a new or
infrequently employed drug.

9 8 7 6 5 4 3 2

Dedication

This work is dedicated to my two newest children, my daughter-in-law Tricia and my son-in-law Kris, who have joined our family circle and brought with them even more love and joy. I am thankful that they chose us.

I would also like to remember my friend and partner, Lee-Olive Harrison, with whom this work actually started many years ago.

Preface

This study guide has been prepared in conjunction with the textbook *Fundamental Nursing Skills and Concepts,* eighth edition. The two books are correlated chapter by chapter. The study guide is ideally suited to be used with the textbook. However, it also can be used with other texts, or it can be used by anyone interested in examining his or her knowledge of basic skills in client care without reference to a specific text.

The primary purpose of this study guide is to offer tools so that the student can evaluate fundamental knowledge and skills that are considered important in the practice of nursing. Each chapter begins with a summary statement of learning objectives. These are followed by examination items and other exercises designed to test the objectives.

Attempting to test everything related to a particular body of knowledge is an impractical and impossible goal. As is true of all evaluation tools, those in this study guide sample relevant material. If the reader believes certain material was omitted that should have been included, the study guide can be used as a guide to develop similar tools for particular situations.

This study guide contains matching, multiple choice, true or false, short answer questions, performance checklists, and critical thinking exercises. Samples of alternative format questions that might appear on the National Council Licensure Examination (NCLEX) in the future are also included to provide practice in answering these kinds of questions.

Answers to the multiple choice, true or false, matching, short answer, and alternative format questions are provided at the end of the study guide. The correct answer and rationale are given for each item. Answers are not provided for the critical thinking exercises since these questions are mainly subjective and for discussion and expansion purposes.

The performance checklists offer an opportunity for students to examine their techniques when providing care. Students may complete the forms themselves, or they may select an observer to complete the form for them. There is space provided for comments where notes can be made about what further practice is indicated, what errors were made, or suggestions that will help improve performance. It is intended that these forms be completed during or immediately after care is given. However, many could be used in laboratory situations when students are practicing skills before giving care to clients. There are no correct answers to these forms because they apply to specific care.

The chapters in Units I through III deal with basic information that nurses use whenever they care for people, regardless of each person's specific needs. Units IV through XII present nursing skills required in specific areas of client care, that is, health maintenance and promotion, changing levels of wellness, health restoration, and death and dying.

The pages of this study guide are perforated. The examinations may be removed if this proves convenient. Instructors may wish to remove the correct answers and rationales and then return them for each chapter as students complete their self-testing. The performance checklists may be removed for review and discussion.

The primary objective of this study guide will have been met when the student is able to use basic nursing skills with confidence.

To the Student

The primary purpose of this study guide is to offer tools for you to evaluate your mastery of the fundamental knowledge and skills that are considered important in the practice of nursing. The study guide is correlated chapter by chapter with *Fundamental Nursing Skills and Concepts,* eighth edition.

Each chapter begins with a summary of the content of the relevant text chapter and a list of learning objectives. These are followed by examination items and other exercises designed to test your achievement of these objectives.

Included are multiple choice, true or false, and short answer questions, as well as matching and discussion questions and performance checklists. In addition, the National Council Licensure Examination (NCLEX) changes periodically. To prepare you for the most recent change in this examination, sample alternative format questions have been included in this text. Some of these questions may ask you to fill in a blank left in the question or place a mark on a drawing. Other questions may ask you to select, from the options given, all that are correct. Lastly, given a situation, you may be asked to place all of the options presented in the order of occurrence or in order of priority.

Answers to multiple choice, true or false, matching, short answer, and alternative format questions are provided in the Answers and Rationale section at the end of the book. Answers are not provided for the critical thinking exercises, since these are mainly subjective and are for discussion and expansion purposes.

You will have defeated part of the reason for using this study guide, however, if you look at the answers prior to working through the examinations. Also, avoid searching for clues to the correct answer among the items in each question or in subsequent questions.

Sometimes it may be relatively quick and easy to rule out one or two choices as incorrect. Then concentrate on the remaining choices. Narrowing your options sharpens your thinking by placing attention on choices you believe are reasonably correct.

Be sure to read each item carefully. Watch for key words such as *best, least, rarely, primarily,* and *contraindicated.* When key words are overlooked, there is often no basis for selecting a correct answer.

Use only the information you are given. Do not attempt to read additional information into an item or make assumptions about it.

Pace yourself occasionally. Select a certain number of items and plan to spend an average of about one minute on each item. If you are doing well, slow your speed; if you are falling behind, try to work faster. This type of practice helps prepare you for timed examinations such as the state licensing examinations.

After learning which items you have answered incorrectly, go back and study them again. Also study the items you answered correctly to see whether you understand the information on which it was based, Concentrate on *understanding* the information, rather than memorizing it.

The examinations do not have a passing or failing score. If all or nearly all items are answered correctly, you probably have mastered the chapter's content. If you fail to give correct answers to at least 80% to 90% of the items, review is suggested. You should seriously question whether you have mastered the content of a chapter if you fail to answer at least 80% of the items correctly.

The performance checklists contain directions concerning their use. You may examine your own nursing practice, or you may wish to ask another person to evaluate you. After the forms are completed, you should know which skills you have mastered and what further study is indicated.

Acknowledgments

The author wishes to thank the following people for their assistance in preparing this study guide:

- Doris Wray for her continued support of my writing efforts
- Elizabeth A. Nieginski, Senior Acquisitions Editor
- Megan Klim, Associate Development Editor
- Josh Levandoski, Editorial Assistant
- Nursing students who have used this text for their suggestions and assistance in identifying omissions and errors

Contents

Nursing Foundations

■ Summary

Nursing is one of the youngest professions but one of the oldest arts. It evolved from the familial roles of nurturing and caretaking. Early responsibilities included assisting women during childbirth, suckling healthy newborns, and ministering to the ill, aged, and helpless within the household and surrounding community. Its hallmark was caring more than curing.

Chapter 1 traces the historical development of nursing from its unorganized beginning to current practice. Ironically, nursing is returning to the community-based practice from which it originated.

■ Matching Questions

Directions: For items 1 through 4, match the theorists in Part B with the theories in Part A.

PART A

1. _C_ The Adaptation Theory

2. _A_ The Environmental Theory

3. _d_ The Self-Care Theory

4. _b_ The Basic Needs Theory

PART B

a. Florence Nightingale

b. Virginia Henderson

c. Sister Callista Roy

d. Dorothea Orem

Directions: For items 5 through 8, match the definitions in Part B with the skills in Part A.

PART A

5. _d_ Assessment skills

6. _C_ Caring skills

7. _A_ Comforting skills

8. _b_ Counseling skills

PART B

a. Those skills that convey security and stability during a health-related crisis

b. Those skills that involve both talking and listening

c. Those skills that restore or maintain an individual's health

d. Those skills used for interviewing, observing, and examining a client

Directions: For items 9 through 16, match the definitions in Part B with the terms in Part A.

PART A

9. _e_ Art

10. _f_ Active listening

11. _d_ Caring

12. _a_ Empathy

13. _G_ Nursing

14. _C_ Theory

15. _h_ Science

16. _J_ Sympathy

PART B

a. Intuitive awareness of what the client is experiencing

b. A personal view of oneself

c. An opinion, belief, or view that explains a process

d. The concern and attachment that occur from the close relationship of one human being with another

e. The ability to perform an act skillfully

f. The diagnosis and treatment of human responses to actual or potential health problems

g. Care intended primarily to maintain or restore physical function immediately upon admission

h. A body of knowledge unique to a particular subject

i. Hearing the content of what the client says as well as the unspoken message

j. Feeling as emotionally distraught as the client

■ Multiple-Choice Questions

Directions: For items 1 through 12, circle the letter that corresponds to the best answer for each question.

1. The service of caring for the sick changed drastically as a result of the split between King Henry VIII of England and the Catholic church. These changes were caused by which of the following:

   a. The administration of English hospitals became a duty of the state

   b. The state started hiring the ranks of criminals, widows, and orphans

   c. Nuns and priests were exiled to Western Europe

   d. The Catholic Church of England was forced to change client care

2. Which of the following statements *best* describes how funding became available for the first school for nurses:

   a. Servicemen and their families showed their appreciation of Florence Nightingale by donating funds because of her work in Scutari

   b. Servicemen and their families supplied funding for new schools of nursing being established in the United States

   c. Florence Nightingale and her 38 volunteers proved that they could lower the infection and death rates

   d. The first Nightingale school at St. Thomas Hospital in England obtained sufficient funding to set up models for others in Europe and the United States

3. Virginia Henderson proposed which of the following definitions about nursing:

   a. Nursing is the "diagnosis and treatment of human responses to actual or potential health problems"

   b. Nursing involves a special relationship and service between the nurse and the client

   c. Nursing is a human service that assists individuals to progressively maximize their self-care potential

d. Nurses modify unhealthy aspects of the environment to put the client in the best possible condition for nature to act

4. Which of the following theorists proposed the associate's degree program in nursing:

   a. Virginia Henderson

   b. Dorothea Orem

   c. Sister Callista Roy

   d. Mildred Montag

5. The Environmental Theory was developed by:

   a. Florence Nightingale

   b. Dorothea Orem

   c. Virginia Henderson

   d. Sister Callista Roy

6. Dorothea Orem's theory, as it relates to people, states that a human being is:

   a. An individual whose natural defenses are influenced by a healthy or unhealthy environment

   b. An individual with human needs that have meaning and value unique to each person

   c. An individual who utilizes self-care to sustain life and health, recover from disease or injury, or cope with its effects

   d. A social, mental, spiritual, and physical being who is affected by stimuli within his or her internal and external environment

7. When the nurse is using assessment skills, the primary source of information is:

   a. The client

   b. The medical record

   c. Other health practitioners

   d. Data collected

8. The primary focus of nursing, no matter what level of care is provided for the client, is:

   a. To give all clients "tender loving care"

   b. To give clients exactly what the doctor prescribes

   c. To be able to use complex devices and equipment

   d. To assist the client to eventually become self-reliant

9. Nursing skills that would be used to assist the client in becoming an active participant in decision making are:
   a. Caring skills
   b. Counseling skills
   c. Comforting skills
   d. Assessment skills

10. Of the following, which must be understood before the nurse will be able to apply assessment skills to predict which nursing interventions are most appropriate for producing the desired outcome:
    a. Nursing science
    b. Nursing arts
    c. Nursing diagnoses
    d. Nursing theories

11. The most recent definition of nursing was developed by:
    a. The International Council of Nurses
    b. The American Nurses Association
    c. The National League for Nursing
    d. The National Association for Practical Nurse Education and Service

12. Attendance at a workshop that discusses food fads and myths best illustrates an example of:
    a. Lifetime commitment
    b. Required education
    c. Nursing accountability
    d. Continuing education

■ Alternative Format Questions

1. Arrange the following theories in order of their appearance in nursing:
   1. Basic Needs Theory
   2. Adaptation Theory
   3. Environmental Theory
   4. Self-Care Theory
   5. Reformation Theory

   ENV.
   ADAP.
   BASIC
   Self care
   Reformation

2. How many years of study would a hospital-based diploma program in nursing education usually require?

   2 (3)

3. The Nurse Reinvestment Act (2002) authorizes funding for which of the following activities in order to address the shortage of nurses? Select all that apply:
   1. Loan repayment for nursing students
   2. Funding for public service announcements about nursing
   3. Training for advanced practice roles in nursing
   4. Cross-training for non-nursing jobs in health care
   5. Career ladder programs to facilitate advancement to higher levels of nursing practice
   6. Grants to incorporate gerontology into the curricula of nursing programs

■ True or False Questions

Directions: For items 1 through 7, decide if the statement is true or false and mark T or F in the space provided.

1. __T__ Nursing is one of the youngest professions yet one of the oldest arts.

2. __F__ Florence Nightingale was called into nursing after hospitals began to show evidence of improving health care.

3. __T__ Planned, consistent, and formal education was the priority of Nightingale schools, while the training of American nurses was more of an unsubsidized apprenticeship.

4. __T__ The associate's degree graduates are not expected to work in management positions.

5. __F__ The definition of nursing has finally stabilized after many changes.

6. __T__ Giving an abundance of "tender loving care" may delay the client from resuming the normal activities of daily living.

7. __F__ Nurses should give advice to their clients.

■ Short Answer Questions

Directions: Read each of the following statements and supply the word(s) necessary in the space provided.

1. The Union government appointed Dorothea Dix, a social worker, to select and organize women volunteers to care for its Civil War troops. List four of the criteria used to select these applicants.

   a. _____

   _____

   b. _____

   _____

   c. _____

   _____

   d. _____

   _____

2. Describe five of the rationales for acquiring continuing education.

   a. _____

   _____

   b. _____

   _____

   c. _____

   _____

   d. _____

   _____

   e. _____

   _____

3. List five of the factors affecting the choice of nursing educational programs.

   a. _____

   _____

   b. _____

   _____

   c. _____

   _____

   d. _____

   _____

   e. _____

   _____

4. List the three factors that delayed the decision to make baccalaureate education the entry level into nursing practice.

   a. _____

   _____

   b. _____

   _____

   c. _____

   _____

5. Compare the level of responsibility among practical/vocational, associate's degree, and baccalaureate degree nurses for each step of the nursing process:

   _____

   _____

   _____

   _____

■ Critical Thinking Exercises

1. Explain the factors that influenced your decision to choose the nursing program in which you are enrolled.

2. Describe the philosophy of your nursing program.

3. Based on your school's philosophy, construct a working model of nursing.

CHAPTER 2

Nursing Process

■ Summary

As nursing practice takes on a more independent role, nurses are being held responsible and accountable for providing appropriate nursing interventions that reflect current acceptable standards for nursing practice.

This chapter discusses the five parts of the nursing process: assessment, nursing diagnosis, planning, implementation, and evaluation. Simply stated, assessment is gathering appropriate and accurate data. Nursing diagnosis is the problem statement derived from accurate analysis of the data. The problem identified may be actual, possible, or potential. Planning involves putting the needs in order of priority, setting short- and long-term goals, and identifying possible options. Implementation is actually carrying out the nursing orders. Evaluation determines how effective the nursing interventions were and the degree to which each goal was met. Evaluation is an ongoing part of the nursing process and may indicate a need to revise the plan of care. When nursing practice reflects the nursing process, clients receive quality care in minimal time with maximum efficiency.

■ Matching Questions

Directions: Match the steps of the problem-solving process in Part B with the steps of the nursing process in Part A.

PART A

1. ____ Assessment

2. ____ Nursing diagnosis

3. ____ Planning

4. ____ Implementation

5. ____ Evaluation

PART B

a. The identification of desired outcomes

b. The review of the entire process

c. The collection of information

d. Carrying out the plan

e. The identification of the exact nature of the problem

Directions: Match the terms in Part B with the signs and symptoms in Part A. Each of the terms in Part B must be used more than once.

PART A

6. ____ Pulse 140 beats/minute

7. ____ Cloudy urine

8. ____ Burning with urination

9. ____ Feeling warm

10. ____ Emesis—green liquid

11. ____ Pain in left groin

PART B

a. Subjective

b. Objective

■ Multiple-Choice Questions

Directions: For items 1 through 15, circle the letter that corresponds to the best answer for each question.

1. A change in the practice of nursing as it is today was brought about by:

   a. Nurses now directing client care more dependably

   b. The development and use of the nursing process for providing appropriate care according to priorities of need

   c. Nurses being held accountable and responsible for providing appropriate care according to accepted standards

   d. The knowledge that nurses should continue to work interdependently with other health care professionals

2. The primary goal of the nursing process is:

   a. To set into action the process of obtaining objectives

   b. To facilitate a united effort between the client and the nursing team to achieve the desired outcome

c. To learn to use the steps so that nursing will be organized and more efficient

d. To give client care within a minimum amount of time with maximum efficiency

3. Subjective data are *best* described as:

   a. Information that is measurable and observable

   b. Information that only the client describes

   c. Information that is lengthy and comprehensive

   d. Information that is detailed and specific

4. The step in the nursing process involved with problem identification is:

   a. Assessment

   b. Planning

   c. Diagnosis

   d. Implementation

5. Which of the following *best* supports the concept that the nursing process is dynamic:

   a. Each client is the unique product of physical, emotional, social, and spiritual components

   b. The health status of any client is constantly changing; the nursing process acts like a continuous loop

   c. It is important that the client and the nurse understand the final expected outcomes and work together

   d. The nurse practice acts are expanding to describe nursing in terms of more independent roles

6. Which of the following *best* supports the concept that the nursing process is client centered:

   a. The nursing process facilitates a plan of care for each client as a unique individual

   b. The health status of a client changes constantly, and one problem is often related to another

   c. It is important that the client and nurse work together toward the expected outcome

   d. All clients have needs that must be met in order of priority, as directed by the hierarchy

7. The *best* definition of assessment is:

   a. The process of measuring how well a goal or objective is reached

   b. An expected outcome or desired end result toward which the nurse works

   c. The action of collecting and organizing client information

   d. The acquisition of skills required to meet the needs of the client

8. Certain physiologic problems that nurses monitor to detect onset of illness or change in status but are beyond the scope of independent nursing practice are referred to as:

   a. Actual problems

   b. Collaborative problems

   c. Potential problems

   d. Possible problems

9. Which of the following indicates the three parts of a nursing diagnostic statement:

   a. Problem, etiology, and signs and symptoms

   b. Risk, dysfunction, and impairment

   c. Possibility, problem, and purpose

   d. Physiology, etiology, and collaboration

10. The etiology named in the nursing diagnosis is:

    a. The problem according to the client

    b. The cause of the problem

    c. The information relating to the problem

    d. The physician's diagnosis

11. The most commonly used method for determining priorities is:

    a. For the nurse to think in terms of Maslow's Hierarchy of Needs

    b. For the nurse to evaluate which problems can be solved or reduced in a short time

    c. For the nurse to analyze which problem, if changed, would result in change in others

    d. For the nurse to consult with the client concerning his or her wishes

12. The *best* example of a goal statement is:

    a. Mr. J. would like to walk 10 steps without assistance today

    b. Mrs. B. will be discharged in a wheelchair on Sunday afternoon

c. Mrs. S. would like to have family visitors in the evening

d. Johnny will walk to the playroom unassisted by May 5

13. The *best* example of a nursing order is:

a. Give 2 ounces of clear fluids every 2 hours until 10 p.m.

b. Give clear fluids of choice when awake until 10 p.m.

c. Change the client's position and give him or her a back rub frequently

d. Encourage the client to breathe deeply and cough to bring up sputum

14. In terms of the nursing process, evaluation provides:

a. Information on the degree to which the nursing assessment was correct

b. Information on the degree to which the nursing diagnosis was correct

c. Information on the degree to which a goal is being met through the use of specific nursing measures

d. Information on the degree to which the client has agreed with the plan of nursing care to be given

15. Which of the following is carried out when the results of the nursing evaluation show that the goal has not been met:

a. The plan of care is discarded and a new plan is written

b. The nursing orders to accomplish the goal are discontinued

c. The nursing orders described in the plan are continued

d. The plan of care is revised, and activities may be changed

■ Alternative Format Questions

1. The nurse has gathered the following assessment data. Which data are subjective? Select all that apply:

1. Client-rated pain 8 on a scale of 0 to 10 with 10 being the most pain ever experienced

2. Heart rate 78, irregular

3. Client is experiencing hunger

4. Incisional scar on the right lower quadrant of the abdomen

5. Blood pressure 165/86

6. Denial of need to void

2. Which of the following contribute to the database assessment? Select all that apply:

1. Review of systems

2. Admission vital signs

3. Drug and food allergies

4. Reason for seeking care

5. Preoperative laboratory reports

6. Daily weight

3. Prioritize the following nursing diagnoses:

1. Spiritual Distress

2. Caregiver Role Strain

3. Impaired Swallowing

4. Parental Role Conflict

5. Anxiety

6. Powerlessness

TRUE OR FALSE QUESTIONS

Directions: For items 1 through 10, decide if the statement is true or false and mark T or F in the space provided.

1. _____ Assessment data should be gathered only from the client's record.

2. _____ A nursing diagnosis closely resembles a medical diagnosis.

3. _____ The North American Nursing Diagnosis Association uses the word *potential* when making a nursing diagnosis about a problem for which the client is at risk.

4. _____ When setting priorities for the client's problems, the nurse should always list them according to the Hierarchy of Needs.

5. _____ The terms *goals* and *outcomes* may be used synonymously.

6. _____ A limited collection of a few, specific, related facts is known as a focus assessment.

7. ____ Validation is the process of measuring how well a goal has been reached.

8. ____ A potential health problem that would require the cooperative care of the nurse and the physician is known as a collaborative problem.

9. ____ Objective data consist of information that only the client can describe.

10. ____ The nursing process is within the legal scope of nursing practice.

■ Short Answer Questions

Directions: Read the following nursing diagnosis: Impaired Skin Integrity related to immobility.

1. Write the words below that pertain to the etiology.

   _____

   _____

2. Write the words below that pertain to the problem.

   _____

   _____

■ Critical Thinking Exercises

1. Assessment is composed of data from many sources. List four sources of data. State several examples of data you might collect from each source. Decide whether the data are subjective or objective. Explain your choices.

2. Read the short case study that follows. Underline the cues that represent a data cluster implying a nursing diagnosis. Write the diagnosis first as a two-part statement. Expand your diagnosis to a three-part statement. Ask your instructor to review and evaluate your work.

Mrs. S., age 93, has lived alone since the death of her husband 20 years ago. Until recently, she has been able to manage her own care and medications. Her son and his family live next door and provide her with transportation and socialization.

About 4 months ago, Mrs. S. decided she could no longer get out of bed. She began forgetting to eat, bathe, and take her medications. Her short-term memory began to fail, and she lost track of time. She now spends approximately 20 hours per day in bed. She requires assistance to get up and walks with a walker; her son and his wife must bring her meals to her and administer her medications. Several times a day she says, "I'm worried about what will become of me. I'm too old. I feel so helpless. I want to go to a rest home."

Two months later, she is a resident in a nursing home. She gets up to a chair with assistance, is incontinent of bowel and bladder, and is unable to swallow. Most of the time she is not aware of time or place.

CHAPTER 3

Laws and Ethics

■ Summary

In the United States, laws are designed to empower federal, state, and local governments to ensure the health and safety of citizens, protect the public welfare, and uphold individual rights and freedom. In this chapter, the student will find a brief overview of laws as they apply to nursing. Common crimes and torts, as well as laws that affect nursing practices, are discussed. The role of the state board of nursing as the regulatory agency for managing the education, licensure, and clinical practice of nurses in the state is briefly described.

■ Matching Questions

Directions: For items 1 through 6, match the definitions in Part B with the terms in Part A.

PART A

1. ____ Libel

2. ____ Assault

3. ____ Duty

4. ____ Battery

5. ____ Slander

6. ____ Malpractice

PART B

a. An untruthful oral statement about a person that subjects him or her to ridicule or contempt

b. A threat or an attempt to make bodily contact with another person without the person's consent

c. Alleged professional negligence

d. An untruthful written statement about a person that subjects him or her to ridicule or contempt

e. An expected action based on moral or legal obligations

f. Bodily contact with another person without the person's consent

Directions: For items 7 through 12, match the descriptions in Part B with the types of law in Part A.

PART A

7. ____ Administrative laws

8. ____ Nurse practice acts

9. ____ Criminal laws

10. ____ Civil laws

11. ____ Statutes of limitation

12. ____ Laws

PART B

a. Provide rules of conduct

b. Protect personal rights and freedom

c. Protect the public's welfare

d. Establish a time frame for filing a lawsuit

e. Give state and federal governments legal authority

f. Define the unique role of the nurse

■ Multiple-Choice Questions

Directions: For items 1 through 10, circle the letter that corresponds to the best answer for each question.

1. A tort is defined as:

   a. A legal action involving an act or its omission that harms someone

   b. An untruthful written statement about a person that subjects him or her to ridicule or contempt

   c. A threat or an attempt to make bodily contact with another person without the person's consent

   d. An illegal act that violates the right of a person to avoid public attention

2. The "Patient's Bill of Rights" was prepared by:
   a. The American Nurses Association
   b. The American Medical Association
   c. The National Federation of Licensed Practical Nurses
   d. The American Hospital Association

3. An incident report is best described as:
   a. A personal written account of an event
   b. A written account of an unusual event that may cause harm
   c. A contract between a person and a company willing to provide legal service
   d. A lawsuit alleging that a professional's failure to act responsibly caused harm

4. A situation that results in an injury although the person did not intend to cause harm is called:
   a. Negligence
   b. False imprisonment
   c. Defamation
   d. Unintentional tort

5. Which of the following is true regarding Good Samaritan laws:
   a. They provide nurses with absolute exemption from prosecution
   b. They establish a designated time frame within which a lawsuit can be filed
   c. They provide legal immunity for persons who give first aid at the scene of an accident
   d. They provide protection when nurses fail to leave people and their property alone

6. Ethics is best defined as:
   a. A list of written statements describing ideal behavior for members of a particular group
   b. A rule of conduct established and enforced by the government of a society
   c. A set of laws passed by each state that protect the public from persons considered unfit to practice nursing
   d. A system of moral or philosophical principles that directs actions as being either right or wrong

7. Which of the following best defines a code of ethics:
   a. A system of moral or philosophical principles that directs actions as being either right or wrong
   b. A system identifying the rights of individuals and respecting those rights
   c. A list of rights that arise from social customs and religious traditions
   d. A list of written statements describing ideal behavior for a group of individuals

8. The nurse practice acts are identified and published by:
   a. The state legislatures
   b. The federal government
   c. The National League for Nursing
   d. The American Nurses Association

9. Of the following statements, which best relates to the characteristic that nursing practice is self-regulated:
   a. Most states appoint nurses to boards that evaluate nursing educational programs
   b. Nurses now hold membership in various organizations that are dedicated to improving the quality of nursing practice
   c. Because nursing is a lifetime commitment, nurses are devoting more interest and energy to its advancement
   d. Nurse practice acts generally authorize a board of nursing to oversee nursing practice

10. Which statement best describes deontology:
    a. Ethical study based on moral obligation
    b. A choice between two undesirable outcomes
    c. A proposal that all clients be told the truth
    d. An ethical theory based on final outcome

■ Alternative Format Questions

1. In acute care hospitals, medical orders for restraints must be renewed every _____ hours.

2. Which of the following activities communicate a caring and compassionate attitude to the client? Select all that apply:

   1. Explaining procedures and routines
   2. Informing visitors where rest rooms are
   3. Socializing with the client at mealtime
   4. Placing medications on the bedside stand and telling the client to take them
   5. Going to lunch
   6. Answering the call light in person

3. The nurse receives a change-of-shift report for a 76-year-old client who had a total hip replacement. The client is not oriented to time, place, or person and is attempting to get out of bed and pull out an IV line that's supplying hydration and antibiotics. The client has a vest restraint and bilateral, soft wrist restraints. Which of the following actions by the nurse would be appropriate? Select all that apply:

   1. Assess and document the behavior that requires continued use of restraints
   2. Tie the restraints in quick-release knots
   3. Tie the restraints to the side rails of the bed
   4. Ask the client if he or she needs to go to the bathroom and provide range-of-motion exercises every 2 hours
   5. Position the vest restraints so that the straps are crossed in the back

■ True or False Questions

Directions: For items 1 through 10, decide if the statement is true or false and mark T or F in the space provided.

1. ____ The law that gives certain persons legal protection when they give aid to someone in an emergency is referred to as the Good Samaritan law.

2. ____ Invasion of privacy is interference with a person's freedom to move about at will without proper authority to do so.

3. ____ The prolongation of life with various types of equipment may cause the nurse to face an ethical dilemma.

4. ____ According to the "Patient's Bill of Rights," an individual has the right to refuse treatment.

5. ____ The advice to "follow your conscience" is one of the guidelines given for dealing with ethical decisions.

6. ____ The nurse is responsible for giving the client information concerning his or her medical treatment as prescribed by the physician.

7. ____ Advance directives are considered legal in all 50 states.

8. ____ There are nurse practice acts in all 50 states, but the laws vary considerably.

9. ____ The person accused of breaking the law is called the plaintiff.

10. ____ Even though health agencies carry liability insurance, it is suggested that student nurses carry their own insurance also.

■ Short Answer Questions

Directions: Read each of the following statements and supply the word(s) necessary in the space provided.

1. List the four elements that must be proven in a negligence or malpractice case.

   a. _____

   _____

   b. _____

   _____

   c. _____

   _____

   d. _____

   _____

2. List five common ethical issues that nurses encounter in everyday practice.

a. _____

_____

b. _____

_____

c. _____

_____

d. _____

_____

e. _____

_____

■ Critical Thinking Exercises

1. A client with end-stage renal disease says she wants to die and asks for assistance. Describe how two nurses with differing ideas of what is morally right and wrong might respond.

2. Explain how a professional code of ethics differs from a personal sense of what is morally right and wrong.

3. Interview a nurse who is a member of a hospital ethics committee. Describe the nurse's role on this committee. Does it differ from the role(s) of other members of this same committee?

CHAPTER 4

Health and Illness

■ Summary

Health is a goal to which nursing is committed. However, it is a predictable characteristic of human nature that there will be changes in health. One cannot expect to stay healthy forever. In this context, nurses are committed to helping individuals prevent illness and restore or improve their health.

In this discussion, health is defined recognizing individual differences and values. Spiritual, emotional, social, and physical well-being are described within the scope of the individual's rights and obligations for health promotion and maintenance. Most Americans believe that health is a resource, a right, and a personal responsibility. Because of its dynamic state, health is depicted as a continuum from high-level wellness to death. The individual functions within a wide range of variations at any given time. The concept of a hierarchy of human needs that motivate behavior is introduced. Nurses use this hierarchy to assist in identifying the area of priority requiring nursing intervention. The needs on the lowest tier must be met first.

■ Matching Questions

Directions: For items 1 through 12, match Maslow's Hierarchy of Needs in Part B with the human needs in Part A. (Note: The choices in Part B may be used more than once.)

PART A

1. _C_ Love
2. _A_ Rest
3. _b_ Safety
4. _b_ Protection
5. _d_ Esteem
6. _e_ Exploration
7. _A_ Food
8. _b,c_ Closeness

9. _A_ Sex
10. _A_ Air
11. _A_ Activity
12. _A_ Water

PART B

a. Physiologic
b. Safety and security
c. Love and belonging
d. Self-esteem
e. Self-actualization

■ Multiple-Choice Questions

Directions: For items 1 through 10, circle the letter that corresponds to the best answer for each question.

1. The term *health* is best described as:
   a. A generally accepted right belonging to everyone
   b. An acceptable quality of life as defined by the individual who is experiencing the problem
   c. A state of complete physical, mental, and social well-being and not merely the absence of disease
   d. A state of being that cannot always be maintained and acquired alone

2. The term *morbidity* refers to:
   a. The incidence of a specific disease
   b. The number of deaths per unit of population
   c. A state of discomfort caused by impaired health
   d. The disappearance of signs and symptoms

3. Which of the following are true concerning the state of wellness:

   a. A state in which body organs function normally

   b. A state in which one feels safe

   c. A state of discomfort in which one's health is impaired as a result of injury, stress, disease, or accident

   d. A state in which one feels a balanced integration of physical, emotional, social, and spiritual health

4. Which of the following statements best describes acute illness:

   a. One that comes on slowly and lasts a long time

   b. One in which there is no potential for cure

   c. One that comes on suddenly and is of short duration

   d. One that has developed independently of other diseases

5. An idiopathic illness is best described as:

   a. One that is acquired from the parents' genetic codes

   b. One that is present at birth

   c. One for which there is no known cause

   d. One that results from permanent organ damage

6. The method of nursing care in which each nurse on a client unit is assigned specific tasks is known as:

   a. Primary nursing

   b. Functional nursing

   c. Team nursing

   d. Nurse-managed care

7. Providing nursing care by the case method involves:

   a. Assigning specific tasks to each nurse on the client unit

   b. Assigning one nurse to administer all the care a client needs for the shift

   c. Assigning one nurse the responsibility of the client's care for a designated time

   d. Assigning many nursing staff members to care for a group of clients until all the work is complete

8. Of the following, which best describes the concept of team nursing:

   a. The client's total 24-hour care is the responsibility of one nurse

   b. Each of the nurses on a client unit is assigned a specific task

   c. Many nursing staff members divide client care and all the work until it is completed

   d. The head nurse plans client care, and then all of the nurses work until it is completed

9. Nursing care that is similar to the principles practiced by a successful business is:

   a. Primary nursing

   b. Nurse-managed care

   c. Team nursing

   d. Functional nursing

10. The term *continuity of care* refers to:

    a. A continuum of health care

    b. A method of providing care

    c. A network of health care services

    d. A group of health care specialists

■ Alternative Format Questions

1. The nurse is assessing a newly admitted client. When filling out the family assessment, who should the nurse consider to be a part of the client's family? Select all that apply:

   1. People related by blood or marriage

   2. All the people whom the client views as family

   3. People who live in the same house

   4. People whom the nurse thinks are important to the client

   5. People who live in the same house with the same racial background as the client

   6. People who provide for the physical and emotional needs of the client

2. The nurse is caring for a 45-year-old married woman who has undergone a hemicolectomy for colon cancer. The woman has two children. Which of the following concepts about families should the nurse keep in mind when providing care for this client? Select all that apply:

   1. Illness in one family member can affect all members.

   2. Family roles don't change because of illness.

   3. A family member may have more than one role at a time in a family.

   4. Children typically aren't affected by adult illness.

   5. The effects of an illness on a family depend on the stage of the family's life cycle.

   6. Changes in sleeping and eating patterns may be signs of stress in a family.

3. A nurse is working with the family of a client who has Alzheimer's disease. The nurse notes that the client's spouse is too exhausted to continue providing care all alone. The adult children live too far away to provide relief on a weekly basis. Which nursing interventions would be most helpful? Select all that apply:

   1. Calling a family meeting to tell the absent children that they must participate in helping the client

   2. Suggesting the spouse seek psychological counseling to help cope with exhaustion

   3. Recommending community resources for adult day care and respite care

   4. Encouraging the spouse to talk about the difficulties involved in caring for a loved one with Alzheimer's disease

   5. Asking whether friends or church members can help with errands or provide short periods of relief

   6. Recommending that the client be placed in a long-term care facility

4. Medicare is a federal program that finances health care costs for people age ____ and older.

■ True or False Questions

Directions: For items 1 through 10, decide if the statement is true or false and mark T or F in the space provided.

1. ____ A chronic illness is one that comes on slowly and lasts a relatively short time.

2. ____ Functional nursing is one of the most-practiced methods of nursing.

3. ____ Health is a state in which the body organs function normally.

4. ____ Remission is the term used to describe the period during an illness when the symptoms subside.

5. ____ Wellness is more than just the absence of physical symptoms.

6. ____ A state in which one feels safe, well liked, and productive is known as spiritual well-being.

7. ____ The primary nurse is accountable for the client's care even though he or she may be off duty.

8. ____ Health could be measured by the client's physical, emotional, social, and spiritual well-being.

9. ____ Because health is an intangible substance, it is not considered a resource.

10. ____ Functional nursing tends to focus more on the tasks to be completed than on the client's needs.

■ Critical Thinking Exercises

Research each of the following methods of administering client care, and do the following:

Primary nursing

Team nursing

Functional nursing

Nurse-managed care

a. List the characteristics of the method

b. Identify the individual who is responsible and accountable

c. State one advantage and one disadvantage of the method

d. Give an example of the type of health care facility in which this method could be used

CHAPTER 5

Homeostasis, Adaptation, and Stress

■ Summary

Health is a tenuous state. To sustain it, the body continuously adapts to changes that have the potential for disturbing equilibrium. As long as the stressors are minor, the response is negligible, occurring quite unnoticed. However, when a stressor is intense or when multiple stressors occur at the same time, the effort to restore balance may result in uncomfortable signs and symptoms many call "stress." If stress is prolonged, stress-related disorders and even death may occur. This chapter explores the nature of homeostasis, adaptive mechanisms for homeostatic regulation, the effect of stress, and nursing interventions that promote and restore health.

■ MATCHING QUESTIONS

Directions: For items 1 through 6, match the descriptions given in Part B with the terms in Part A.

PART A

1. _d_ Holism
2. _f_ Stress
3. _C_ Adaptation
4. _e_ Coping mechanism
5. _B_ Homeostasis
6. _A_ Stress management

PART B

a. Therapeutic activities used to reestablish physiologic balance

b. A stable state of physiologic equilibrium

c. The manner in which an organism responds to change

d. A term that implies multiple entities contributing to the whole person

e. Unconscious tactics used to protect the psyche

f. A term that describes reactions that occur when equilibrium is disturbed

Directions: For items 7 through 12, match the categories given in Part B with the stressors in Part A. (Note: Each answer may be used more than once.)

PART A

7. _d_ Guilt
8. _C_ Gender
9. _A_ Aging
10. _d_ Hopelessness
11. _b_ Bitterness
12. _C_ Poverty

PART B

a. Physiologic
b. Psychologic
c. Social
d. Spiritual

table 5.2 pg 57
(TABLE 5.3 pg 58)
PG 62

Directions: For items 13 through 20, match the examples given in Part B with the coping mechanisms in Part A.

PART A

13. _C_ Suppression
14. _F_ Rationalization
15. _A_ Somatization
16. _G_ Reaction formation
17. _B_ Identification
18. _E_ Displacement
19. _h_ Denial
20. _d_ Sublimation

Alarm stage
— body prepares for action

Resistance —

Exhaustion

d, G

PART B

a. Developing diarrhea to stay home from work

b. Imitating the way your boss dresses and talks

c. "Sleeping on the problem"

d. Becoming a sports announcer when you can't be an athlete

e. Kicking the wastebasket after your boss reprimands you

f. Blaming failure on a test on how it was constructed

g. Being extremely nice to someone you really dislike

h. Refusing to believe your best friend has terminal cancer

■ Multiple-Choice Questions

Directions: For items 1 through 8, circle the letter that corresponds to the best answer for each question.

1. The term *homeostasis* refers to:

   a. Negligible responses that come about unnoticed

   b. The relationship between the mind and the body

   c. A relatively stable state of physiologic equilibrium

   d. A philosophic concept of interrelatedness in humans

2. The autonomic nervous system is composed of:

   a. The reticular activating system near the cortex

   b. Peripheral nerves that affect physiologic function

   c. The structures in the midbrain and the brain stem

   d. A collective group of glands located throughout the body

3. The function of the parasympathetic nervous system is to:

   a. Accelerate physiologic functions necessary for "fight or flight"

   b. Regulate and maintain physiologic activities that promote survival

   c. Allow for abstract thought, use of language, and decision making

   d. Inhibit physiologic stimulation resulting from "fight or flight"

4. Behaving in a manner that is characteristic of a younger age best describes which of the following coping mechanisms?

   a. Displacement

   b. Regression

   c. Rationalization

   d. Repression

5. The general adaptation syndrome refers to:

   a. The collective physiologic processes that take place in response to a stressor

   b. The collection of diseases and disorders that result from prolonged exposure to stress

   c. The collection of techniques available to promote physiologic comfort and well-being

   d. The collection of potential stressors that particularly affect clients in the hospital

6. The Social Readjustment Rating Scale was developed by:

   a. Holmes and Watson

   b. Abraham Maslow

   c. Dorothea Orem

   d. Holmes and Rahe

7. Powerlessness is an example of which of the following categories of stressors:

   a. Physiologic

   b. Psychologic

   c. Social

   d. Spiritual

8. Rapid heart rate, rapid breathing, and dry mouth are examples of which of the following categories of signs and symptoms of stress:

   a. Physical

   b. Emotional

   c. Cognitive

   d. Affective

■ Alternative Format Questions

1. The nurse is caring for a client who is about to undergo a bronchoscopy. Which of the following are expected sympathetic effects of stress? Select all that apply:

   1. Constricted pupils
   2. Increased heart rate
   3. Increased salivation
   4. Increased perspiration
   5. Flushed appearance
   6. Increased blood glucose

2. Nurses must be aware of potential and actual stressors affecting their clients. When a person is experiencing stress, all of the following are appropriate interventions. Place them in the order of priority.

   1. Identify the stressor
   2. Assist in maintaining a network of social support
   3. Prevent additional stressors
   4. Support the client's psychologic coping strategies
   5. Assess the client's response to stress

3. Which of the following are examples of spiritual stressors? Select all that apply:

   1. Fear
   2. Isolation
   3. Guilt
   4. Abandonment
   5. Doubt
   6. Hopelessness

■ True or False Questions

Directions: For items 1 through 10, decide if the statement is true or false and mark T or F in the space provided.

1. _____ When internal or external changes overwhelm homeostatic adaptation, stress results.

2. _____ Forgetfulness is a physical sign of increased stress. *Cognitive*

3. _____ Coping mechanisms enable individuals to maintain their mental equilibrium.

4. _____ The general adaptation syndrome describes the pathologic effects of the overuse of stress reduction techniques.

5. _____ Responses to stress may be mediated by interactions that manipulate sensory stimuli.

6. _____ An individual's attitudes and values may affect his or her response to stressors.

7. _____ Irritability, withdrawal, and depression are common physical signs and symptoms of increased stress. *emotional*

8. _____ Gastritis and irritable bowel syndrome are examples of stress-related disorders.

9. _____ Bruxism is a synonym for snoring.

10. _____ Accusing a person of a race different from your own of being prejudiced is an example of regression.

■ Short Answer Questions

Directions: Read each of the following statements and supply the word(s) necessary in the space provided.

1. List the stages of the general adaptation syndrome.
   a. *Alarm*
   b. *Resistance*
   c. *Exhaustion*

2. Describe the reticular activating system.

3. List and describe three levels of prevention related to stressors.

   Level: Description:
   a. _____   _____
        _____   _____
   b. _____   _____
        _____   _____
   c. _____   _____

■ Critical Thinking Exercises

Investigate one stress management technique that is available in your area. Prepare a brief report that includes the following:

  a. Time required to learn and use the activity

  b. The cost

  c. How many complete the program

  d. The target population

Include an analysis of the effectiveness of the technique. _____

_____

_____

_____

CHAPTER 6

Culture and Ethnicity

■ Summary

No two clients are ever exactly alike. Nurses have always cared for clients with various kinds of differences. These variations include, but are not limited to, age, gender, race, health status, religion, education, occupation, and income. Culture and ethnicity, the focus of this chapter, are other ways clients may vary. Despite the existence of these characteristics, the tendency has been to treat all clients alike. This type of care, acultural nursing, may be politically popular, but it may not be in the best interest of promoting, maintaining, or restoring health.

The time has come to promote "transcultural nursing," a term conceived in the 1970s to describe nursing within the context of another's culture. This kind of nursing care requires acceptance of each person as an individual, knowledge of health problems that affect particular cultural groups, planning of health care within the client's belief system, and respect for alternative health practices.

■ Matching Questions

Directions: For items 1 through 5, match the definitions in Part B with the terms in Part A.

PART A

1. ____ Culture

2. ____ Race

3. ____ Ethnicity

4. ____ Stereotype

5. ____ Minority

PART B

a. A unique cultural group that coexists within a dominant group

b. Values, beliefs, and practices of a particular group

c. A fixed attitude toward a particular group

d. Refers to biologic variations

e. A bond of kinship with a country

Directions: For items 6 through 10, match the corresponding health beliefs in Part B with the subcultures in Part A.

PART A

6. ____ Anglo American

7. ____ African American

8. ____ Asian American

9. ____ Latino

10. ____ Native American

PART B

a. Illness results when equilibrium is disturbed

b. Illness occurs when Mother Earth is disturbed

c. Illness is caused by microorganisms

d. Illness occurs as a punishment from God

e. Illness is caused by supernatural forces

■ Multiple-Choice Questions

Directions: For items 1 through 9, circle the letter that corresponds to the best answer for each question.

1. The term *transcultural nursing* refers to:

   a. The confusion one experiences when exposed to culturally atypical behavior

   b. The ability to provide care within the context of another's culture and beliefs

   c. The ability to speak a second language as part of one's culture

   d. The belief that one's own ethnicity is superior to all others

2. Of the remaining tribes of Native Americans present in the United States today, which of the following is the largest:

   a. The Navajos

   b. The Sioux

   c. The Eskimos

   d. The Aleuts

3. Several drugs may precipitate the anemic response G-6-PD in African Americans. From the following list, select the name of one of these drugs:
   a. Calcium
   b. Probenecid
   c. Acetic acid
   d. Lactase

4. The drug referred to in question 3 is used to treat which of the following health problems:
   a. Malaria
   b. Urinary infections
   c. Gout
   d. Respiratory infections

5. A lactase deficiency is exhibited as intolerance for which of the following products:
   a. Dairy products
   b. Alcohol
   c. Artificial sweeteners
   d. Kosher foods

6. From the following, choose the phrase(s) that is/are true regarding the way in which an individual demonstrates pride in one's ethnicity:
   a. Placing value on specific physical characteristics
   b. Giving one's children ethnic names
   c. Wearing special items of clothing
   d. All of the above are true statements

7. Which of the following represent four leading causes of death across all subcultures in the United States:
   a. HIV infection, diabetes, cancer, suicide
   b. Pneumonia, diabetes, heart disease, suicide
   c. Heart disease, cancer, stroke, accidents
   d. Influenza, pneumonia, stroke, injuries

8. The belief that illness occurs when the harmony of nature is disturbed is common among which of the following U.S. subcultures:
   a. Native Americans
   b. Latinos
   c. African Americans
   d. Asian Americans

9. Those methods of disease treatment or prevention that are outside conventional practices are called:
   a. Castigo de Dios
   b. Yin and yang
   c. Shaman
   d. Folk medicine

■ Alternative Format Questions

1. The nurse is caring for a client whose cultural background is different from her own. Which of the following actions are appropriate? Select all that apply:
   1. Consider that nonverbal cues, such as eye contact, may have a different meaning in a different culture
   2. Respect the client's cultural beliefs
   3. Ask the client if he or she has cultural or religious requirements that should be considered in his or her care
   4. Explain her or his beliefs so that the client will understand the difference
   5. Understand that all cultures experience pain in the same way

2. Which of the following statements are *true* regarding a client's culture? Select all that apply:
   1. Culture is passed from one generation to the next
   2. Culture is learned at school
   3. Culture is influenced by environment, technology, and resources
   4. Culture is dynamic
   5. Culture is based on genetic inheritance

3. The nurse in the labor and delivery unit is caring for a laboring, Caucasian woman whose stated religious preference is Roman Catholic. After 12 hours of labor, the woman gives birth to a stillborn, female infant. A culturally sensitive nurse would anticipate which of the following interventions for this infant and her family? Select all that apply:
   1. The infant is to be baptized
   2. Kosher dietary laws must be followed
   3. Religious laws require that the body not be left alone

4. A religious medal may be pinned to the infant's blanket

5. Burial must be accomplished within 24 hours

6. Photographs of the infant are forbidden

■ True or False Questions

Directions: For items 1 through 10, decide if the statement is true or false and mark T or F in the space provided.

1. ____ It is appropriate to assume that everyone who affiliates with a particular group behaves exactly alike.

2. ____ Cultural attitudes are learned by example and are passed on from one generation to the next.

3. ____ Eskimos and Aleuts are included among the native tribes of North America.

4. ____ Daily bathing, use of deodorant, and shaving are standard hygiene practices in the United States.

5. ____ Acupuncture, acupressure, and herbs are used by many Asian Americans to restore health and balance.

6. ____ If a translator is required, the nurse should choose one who is male and older than the client to be certain the client feels secure.

7. ____ If a client of a subculture different from the nurse's appears confused by a question, the nurse should repeat the question using simple words and shorter sentences.

8. ____ As a whole, Americans are time oriented and schedule their activities according to clock hours.

9. ____ Praying and doing penance, relying on spiritual healers, and eating foods that are "hot" or "cold" are common health practices among Asian Americans.

10. ____ Facilitating rituals by whomever the client identifies as a healer within his or her belief system is a means of demonstrating culturally sensitive nursing care.

■ Short Answer Questions

Directions: Read each of the following statements and supply the word(s) necessary in the space provided.

1. List five characteristics of United States culture.

   a. _____

   b. _____

   c. _____

   d. _____

   e. _____

2. As discussed in the text, list three ways of demonstrating cultural sensitivity.

   a. _____

   b. _____

   c. _____

■ Critical Thinking Exercises

1. A new postpartum Samoan woman is wearing a large kerchief (a scarf-like wrap) around her abdomen. Discuss how it would be best to inquire about this practice from a culturally sensitive perspective.

2. Discuss how an Anglo-American nurse and her Asian-American client might experience culture shock during a health care encounter.

3. Research ways your community is culturally diverse. How are the health care needs of the population being met? How can health care be improved?

CHAPTER 7

The Nurse–Client Relationship

■ Summary

Nurses provide services, or skills, that assist individuals, called clients, to resolve health problems that are beyond their own capabilities or to cope with those that will not improve. There are several differences between the services that nurses provide and those provided by other caring people.

An intangible factor that helps place nurses in high regard is the relationship that develops between nurses and their clients. One of the primary keys to establishing and maintaining a positive nurse–client relationship is the manner and style of a nurse's communication.

■ Matching Questions

Directions: For items 1 through 6, match the examples in Part B with the communication techniques in Part A.

PART A

1. _____ Informing

2. _____ Open-ended questioning

3. _____ Reflecting

4. _____ Clarifying

5. _____ Confronting

6. _____ Summarizing

PART B

a. Client: "I'm miserable." Nurse: "Miserable?"

b. "You want to go home but you haven't been doing your exercises."

c. "How does your pain feel?"

d. "We've talked about health and exercise. Would you like to join a health club?"

e. "Your physician will be in at 9:30 this morning."

f. Client: "I can't deal with it anymore." Nurse: "Tell me what it is that you are unable to deal with."

Directions: For items 7 through 12, match the examples in Part B with the nontherapeutic communication techniques in Part A.

PART A

7. _____ False reassurance

8. _____ Clichés

9. _____ Belittling

10. _____ Patronizing

11. _____ Disagreeing

12. _____ Approval

PART B

a. Nurse: "I'm glad you're exercising so regularly."

b. Nurse: "Are we ready to take our medicine now?"

c. Nurse: "Where did you get an idea like that?"

d. Nurse: "You can do it; you're a tough old bird."

e. Nurse: "Lots of people learn to do this."

f. Nurse: "Everything will be just fine."

■ Multiple-Choice Questions

Directions: For items 1 through 10, circle the letter that corresponds to the best answer for each question.

1. The example that best relates to the concept that nurses promote independence is:

   a. The nurse gives Miss H. a syringe, a needle, and an orange and tells her to practice injections

   b. The nurse selects the appropriate foods from Miss H.'s menu for her diabetic diet

   c. The nurse uses communication skills to assist Miss H. with her fears about diabetes

   d. The nurse demonstrates to Miss H. the procedures for preparing an insulin injection

2. When developing a therapeutic nurse–client relationship, a desired outcome is:
   a. Developing a friendship
   b. Making the client comfortable
   c. Moving toward restoring health
   d. Learning to know oneself

3. Of the following situations, which relates to the introductory phase of the nurse–client relationship:
   a. The nurse uses communication skills to learn about Mr. J.'s health problems during the admission procedure
   b. The nurse explains to Mr. J. that he will have to assist with some of his care while he is in the hospital
   c. The nurse shares her information about Mr. J. with the other nursing personnel that will be caring for him
   d. The nurse plans and follows through with discharge teaching when it is time for Mr. J. to go home

4. An example of verbal communication is:
   a. Moaning
   b. Laughing
   c. Writing
   d. Crying

5. An example of nonverbal communication is:
   a. Speaking
   b. Moaning
   c. Reading
   d. Writing

6. An obstacle to effective communication would be:
   a. Using the principles of touch by giving the client a back rub
   b. Accepting what the client says while being alert to what he or she is not saying
   c. Asking the client if he or she feels lonely or sad
   d. Interrupting the client when he or she seems to be deep in thought

7. When the nurse stops in during the evening, Mrs. D. states that she is very worried about her operation tomorrow. Of the following responses, which would be the most appropriate:
   a. "That is very understandable, Mrs. D., would you like to talk about your operation?"
   b. "Don't worry—everything is going to be okay."
   c. "That's just a routine operation that you are having. No need to worry about it."
   d. "You'll be okay—your doctor and our operating room staff do these procedures every day."

8. The term *kinesics* refers to:
   a. Vocal sounds that are not actually words
   b. The use of space to communicate
   c. The use of body language to communicate
   d. The use of tactile stimuli to communicate

9. Which of the following statements best describes task-oriented touch:
   a. The personal contact required to perform nursing procedures
   b. The personal contact used to demonstrate concern for another
   c. The personal contact required to maintain safety for older adults
   d. The personal contact used to demonstrate affection for another

10. It is suggested that the nurse sit in a relaxed position at eye level with the client when communicating with him or her because:
    a. This indicates that the nurse is fully involved in what is being communicated
    b. If the client feels rushed, he or she may interpret this to be disinterest by the nurse
    c. Responses to stress are manifested through active listening on the part of the nurse
    d. People have less control over nonverbal communication than they do over verbal communication

■ Alternative Format Questions

1. Nursing responsibilities within the nurse–client relationship include which of the following? Select all that apply:
   1. Possessing current knowledge
   2. Performing technical skills safely
   3. Complying with the plan of care
   4. Describing desired outcomes
   5. Promoting independence
   6. Providing adequate historical data

2. Interviewing and physical assessment of a client is carried out in the individual's personal space. Personal space is a distance of _____ inches to _____ feet.

3. The nurse is performing a nursing assessment on a 72-year-old client admitted with end-stage renal failure. The nurse asks the client if he has prepared an advance directive. The client states he doesn't know what an advance directive is. The nurse explains that an advance directive is a legal document that provides instruction for his care and names a durable power of attorney for health care if the client becomes unable to act on his own behalf. Which of the following aspects of the therapeutic nurse–client relationship has the nurse observed? Select all that apply:
   1. Treating the client as a unique individual
   2. Promoting the client's physical, emotional, and spiritual well-being
   3. Communicating using terms the client understands
   4. Focusing on nursing tasks related to admission procedures
   5. Being open and flexible and compliant with health care
   6. Implementing health care techniques compatible with the client's values

■ True or False Questions

Directions: For items 1 through 10, decide if the statement is true or false and mark T or F in the space provided.

1. ____ Intimate space is reserved for sharing conversations that are not intended to be private.

2. ____ One of the most important nursing skills is the promotion of the client's independent ability to meet his or her own health needs.

3. ____ It is okay to use the titles "gramps" or "granny" to develop a therapeutic relationship with an elderly client.

4. ____ Nursing acts are prompted by observing an individual in distress.

5. ____ Identifying the problem, describing desired outcomes, and answering questions honestly are nursing responsibilities within the nurse–client relationship.

6. ____ For older adults, touching may be more important than talking.

7. ____ A therapeutic nurse–client relationship is more likely to develop when the nurse accepts that the client has the potential for growth and change.

8. ____ The introductory phase of the nurse–client relationship involves mutually planning the client's care.

9. ____ No relationship can exist without verbal and nonverbal communication.

10. ____ Therapeutic communication refers to using words and gestures to accomplish an objective.

■ Short Answer Questions

Directions: Read each of the following statements and supply the word(s) necessary in the space provided.

1. List three therapeutic uses of silence.

   a. _____

   _____

   b. _____

   _____

   c. _____

   _____

2. List the principles that provide the basis for a therapeutic nurse–client relationship.

a. _____

b. _____

c. _____

d. _____

e. _____

3. Explain the difference between task-related touch and affective touch.

_____

_____

■ Critical Thinking Exercises

1. Work with another student and attempt to express each of the following without using verbal communication:

a. Pain

b. Fear of discomfort

c. An uncaring attitude

d. Genuine concern for your client

2. Describe communication techniques that the nurse might use to communicate with an unconscious client in a critical care unit.

3. Discuss principles of communication appropriate to older adults.

CHAPTER 8

Client Teaching

■ Summary

One of the many means by which nurses apply communication skills is through the role of teacher. Health teaching promotes the client's independent ability to meet his or her own health needs. As client advocates, nurses help individuals use health information to make informed decisions about their health care. Health teaching is no longer an optional nursing activity; many state nurse practice acts require it. Client teaching is a requirement of acceptable nursing care according to ANA Standards of Nursing Practice. Health care records must show what has been taught and present evidence that learning did indeed take place. Limited hospitalization demands that health teaching begin as soon after admission as possible.

■ Matching Questions

Directions: For items 1 through 17, match the categories of the learner in Part B with the characteristics in Part A. (Note: Categories may be used more than once.)

PART A

1. ____ Compulsory learner

2. ____ Active leaner

3. ____ Needs structure

4. ____ Motivated by own interest

5. ____ Learning is problem-centered

6. ____ Short attention span

7. ____ Practical thinker

8. ____ Motivated by need

9. ____ Rote learner

10. ____ Goal oriented

11. ____ Concrete thinker

12. ____ Needs frequent feedback

13. ____ Responds to family encouragement

14. ____ Task oriented

15. ____ Passive

16. ____ Subject centered

17. ____ Crisis learner

PART B

a. Pedagogic learner

b. Androgogic learner

c. Gerogogic learner

Directions: For items 18 through 27, match the domains in Part B with the behaviors in Part A. (Note: The domains may be used more than once.)

PART A

18. ____ Remove

19. ____ Promote

20. ____ List

21. ____ Empty

22. ____ Locate

23. ____ Identify

24. ____ Assemble

25. ____ Advocate

26. ____ Change

27. ____ Label

PART B

a. Cognitive domain

b. Psychomotor domain

c. Affective domain

■ Multiple-Choice Questions

Directions: For items 1 through 15, circle the letter that corresponds to the best answer for each question.

1. An example of cognitive learning is:
   a. A demonstration of correct injection technique
   b. Successful completion of a test about anatomy
   c. Understanding one's anger over having cancer
   d. Expressing excitement over learning to give an injection.

2. Which of the following would be an example of learning in the psychomotor domain:
   a. Reciting the alphabet
   b. Identifying leaves from various trees
   c. Refusing to talk to strangers
   d. Assembling a puzzle

3. For the visually impaired client, it is easier to read:
   a. Large print in black ink on white paper
   b. Small print in black ink on white paper
   c. Large print in blue ink on off-white glossy paper
   d. Small print in blue ink on off-white glossy paper

4. For the hearing impaired client, the nurse can facilitate communication by:
   a. Talking louder, using simple words, and lowering voice pitch
   b. Sitting or standing beside the client's "bad" ear when talking
   c. Selecting words that do not begin with the letters F, S, or K
   d. Raising the voice pitch, talking softly, and repeating the words

5. When instructing an older adult, it is important to:
   a. Reduce noise and distraction
   b. Sit at eye level beside the client
   c. Speak rapidly and distinctly
   d. Use sentences with 12 words or less

6. Which of the following statements is true of pedagogic learners:
   a. Learning is outcome oriented
   b. Learning is self-centered
   c. Learning requires structure and encouragement
   d. Learning is motivated by reward or punishment

7. The term literacy refers to:
   a. The ability to process information
   b. Below-average intellectual capacity
   c. The ability to read and write
   d. The consequences of a learning disability

8. Scheduling a return demonstration with a client who has just been taught self-injection is an example of which step of the nursing process:
   a. Assessment
   b. Planning
   c. Implementation
   d. Evaluation

9. Of the following learning activities, which is the most effective for increasing learner retention:
   a. Reading
   b. Listening
   c. Demonstrating
   d. Observing

10. Informal teaching refers to situations in which:
    a. Teaching is unplanned and spontaneous
    b. Lessons are planned and scheduled
    c. Teaching is haphazard and occurs when the client asks
    d. Lessons have set guidelines and follow a model

11. An appropriate time for teaching the client would be:
    a. At the time the nurse is doing the admission interview
    b. At the time the nurse is giving medication for pain
    c. When the client needs fluids to lower his high fever
    d. When the client is physically and psychologically ready

12. Learning a neuromuscular skill is:
    a. In the cognitive domain
    b. In the psychomotor domain
    c. In the affective domain
    d. In the neurological domain

13. Select the cognitive domain behavior from the following list:
    a. Advocate
    b. Identify
    c. Assemble
    d. Remove

14. Which of the following is an example of informal teaching:
    a. Discussing the importance of good hygiene during the client's bath
    b. Discussing prenatal diet principles during a class for young couples
    c. Explaining hospital policies during the admission procedure
    d. Teaching only when the client requests information

15. Optimum learning takes place when the individual has:
    a. A command of the English language
    b. A purpose for acquiring new information
    c. The desire to please others
    d. The opportunity to attend formal classes

■ Alternative Format Questions

1. The nurse is preparing a teaching plan on self-administration of insulin for a diabetic client who is also hearing impaired. Which of the following nursing interventions will help to ensure an optimum learning experience for this client? Select all that apply:
    1. Use a magic slate or flash cards to communicate
    2. Speak in a normal tone of voice
    3. Avoid words that begin with "f," "s," "k," or "sh" when possible
    4. Turn on the ceiling lights
    5. Rephrase statements that the client does not understand
    6. Stand in front of the client

2. The nurse is preparing a teaching plan for a client who was prescribed enalapril maleate (Vasotec) for treatment of hypertension. Which of the following should the nurse include in the teaching plan? Select all that apply:
    1. Tell the client to avoid salt substitutes
    2. Tell the client that light-headedness is a common adverse effect that need not be reported
    3. Inform the client that he or she may have a sore throat for the first few days of therapy
    4. Advise the client to report facial swelling or difficulty breathing immediately
    5. Tell the client that blood tests will be necessary every 3 weeks for 2 months and periodically after that
    6. Advise the client not to change position suddenly to minimize orthostatic hypotension

3. A client is prescribed lisinopril (Zestril) for treatment of hypertension. He asks the nurse about possible adverse effects. The nurse should teach him about which of the following common adverse effects of ACE inhibitors? Select all that apply:
    1. Constipation
    2. Dizziness
    3. Headache
    4. Hyperglycemia
    5. Hypotension
    6. Impotence

■ True or False Questions

Directions: For items 1 through 10, decide if the statement is true or false and mark T or F in the space provided.

1. ____ Teaching is more effective when the client is included in the planning.

2. ____ The client's level of literacy is not difficult to assess.

3. ____ Learning objectives provide the basis for evaluating whether learning has taken place.

4. ____ Health teaching is an optional nursing activity.

5. ____ A thorough assessment of the client and the factors affecting learning helps to identify learning needs accurately.

6. ____ Ceiling lights tend to diffuse light, making it easier for a visually impaired client to see.

7. ____ Knowledge of the communication process is necessary for effective client teaching.

8. ____ An acceptable motivation for learning is to "avoid criticism."

9. ____ Nurse–teachers must be able to communicate effectively with individuals and small groups.

10. ____ Culture and ethnicity have no effect on how health teaching needs are met.

■ Short Answer Questions

Directions: Read each of the following statements and supply the word(s) necessary in the space provided.

1. List at least three characteristics that are unique to gerogogic learners.

   a. _____

   _____

   b. _____

   _____

   c. _____

2. Identify four factors that are assessed before teaching can begin.

   a. _____

   _____

   b. _____

   _____

   c. _____

   _____

   d. _____

■ Critical Thinking Exercises

1. What teaching strategies from the cognitive, affective, and psychomotor domains would be required to teach a 10-year-old how to inject his own insulin? How would you alter your teaching strategies for an older adult?

2. Give examples of how to determine if the information was actually learned for each of the situations described in Question 1.

3. Refer to Questions 1 and 2. What would be appropriate documentation for the client's record to indicate that both teaching and learning had occurred?

CHAPTER 9

Recording and Reporting

■ Summary

When the client requires care from health practitioners, a legal document called a health record will be kept. Sharing information pertinent to a client's care is an important function among health care providers. In this chapter, various methods of organizing and recording this information are presented.

■ Matching Questions

Directions: For items 1 through 10, match the meanings in Part B with the abbreviations in Part A.

PART A

1. _____ BRP
2. _____ NKA
3. _____ NPO
4. _____ OD
5. _____ OS
6. _____ PO
7. _____ WC
8. _____ s̄
9. _____ c̄
10. _____ dc

PART B

a. Without
b. Left eye
c. Discontinue
d. No known allergies
e. Nothing by mouth
f. Bathroom privileges
g. By mouth
h. Right eye
i. Wheelchair
j. With

■ Multiple-Choice Questions

Directions: For items 1 through 11, circle the letter that corresponds to the best answer for each question.

1. On the client's record, entries are dated and written in chronological order because:
   a. They provide a permanent accounting of a client's health care
   b. They provide a method for keeping health personnel informed
   c. They ensure safety and continuity in the client's care
   d. They provide a method for the collection of data for research

2. Client care information is shared in order to:
   a. Provide a permanent accounting of a client's health care
   b. Provide a method for keeping health personnel informed
   c. Ensure safety and continuity in the client's care
   d. Provide a method for the collection of data for research

3. Entries on the client's record should be objective, accurate, and legible because:
   a. The client records are used by all health personnel in the health agency
   b. The client records are the property of the health agency and must be kept neat
   c. The client has a right to read his or her chart; therefore, it must be legible and accurate
   d. The client records are admissible as evidence in courts of law in this country

4. A characteristic of a traditional record is:
   a. It allows only physicians and nurses to enter information
   b. It is organized according to the source of the information

c. It is organized according to the client's specific problems

d. It allows health care personnel to record on the same form

5. A characteristic of the problem-oriented record is:

a. It allows only physicians and nurses to enter information

b. It is organized according to the source of the information

c. It is organized according to the client's specific problems

d. Its organization leads to fragmentation of the client's care

6. Which of the following are the four major parts of the problem-oriented record?

a. Database, physician's order, problem list, and progress notes

b. Database, problem list, nurse's notes, and progress notes

c. Physician's orders, problem list, initial plan, and progress notes

d. Database, problem list, initial plan, and progress notes

7. A disadvantage of narrative charting is:

a. Every member of the health care team writes entries on the same form

b. The client's problems may be entered once on the nursing care plan

c. It requires the institution to develop comprehensive documents describing norms and standards

d. It tends to produce bulky, fragmented information with each health care person writing on separate forms

8. The method of charting in which the assessments are documented on a separate form is called:

a. SOAP charting

b. PIE charting

c. Narrative charting

d. Focus charting

9. Which of the following statements best relates to the client's right to obtain information from his or her records?

a. The client has the right to read his or her record at any time

b. Each agency has a policy about clients reading their records

c. The client must obtain a court order to view his or her records

d. The record cannot be seen without permission from the physician

10. Convert 3:30 p.m. to military time:

a. 1530

b. 1330

c. 3030

d. 0330

11. The best reason for writing or printing clearly when making an entry on a client's record is:

a. Illegible entries become questionable information in a court of law

b. Errors and omissions are likely when information is gathered by many individuals

c. The charting legibly verifies that the medical and nursing plan was carried out

d. Correcting an error must be done so that the words first recorded can be clearly read

■ Alternative Format Questions

1. The nurse receives a change-of-shift report for a 76-year-old client who had a total hip replacement. The client is not oriented to time, place, or person and is attempting to get out of bed and pull out an IV line that's supplying hydration and antibiotics. The client has a vest restraint and bilateral soft wrist restraints. Which of the following actions by the nurse would be appropriate? Select all that apply:

1. Assess and document the behavior that requires continued use of restraints

2. Tie the restraints in quick-release knots

3. Tie the restraints to the side rails of the bed

4. Ask the client if he needs to go to the bathroom and provide range-of-motion exercises every 2 hours

5. Position the vest restraints so that the straps are crossed in the back

2. A 62-year-old client has just been diagnosed with terminal cancer and is being transferred to home hospice care. The client's daughter tells the nurse, "I don't know what to say to my mother if she asks me if she is going to die." Which of the following responses by the nurse would be appropriate? Select all that apply:

1. "Don't worry; your mother still has some time left."
2. "Let's talk about your mother's illness and how it will progress."
3. "You sound like you have some questions about your mother dying. Let's talk about that."
4. "Don't worry; hospice will take care of your mother."
5. "Tell me how you're feeling about your mother dying."

3. While providing care to a 26-year-old, married female, the nurse notes multiple ecchymotic areas on her arms and trunk. The color of the ecchymotic areas ranges from blue to purple to yellow. When asked by the nurse how she got these bruises, the client responds, "Oh, I tripped." How should the nurse respond? Select all that apply:

1. Document the client's statement and complete a body map indicating the size, color, shape, location, and type of injuries
2. Report suspicions of abuse to the local authorities
3. Assist the client in developing a safety plan for times of increased violence
4. Call the client's husband to discuss the situation
5. Tell the client that she needs to leave the abusive situation as soon as possible
6. Provide the client with telephone numbers of local shelters and safe houses

■ True or False Questions

Directions: For items 1 through 12, decide if the statement is true or false and mark T or F in the space provided.

1. ____ Specific requirements on the frequency for charting vary from agency to agency.

2. ____ Entries on a client's record should only be made by the physician and the nurses responsible for care.

3. ____ The traditional record is organized according to a client's specific health problems.

4. ____ All health practitioners contribute to the problem list when a problem-oriented record format is used by a health agency.

5. ____ The initial plan of the client's overall care needs does not have to include the client's input.

6. ____ The PIE method of charting is the same as SOAP charting.

7. ____ Charting by exception is a method of checklist charting.

8. ____ The Patient's Bill of Rights states that the client has the right to read his or her chart.

9. ____ One of the difficulties with computerized charting is client confidentiality.

10. ____ The need to label time as A.M. or P.M. is eliminated by the use of military time.

11. ____ The nursing care plan is considered part of the client's permanent record and is therefore a legal document.

12. ____ Information included on the Kardex should be written in ink.

■ Short Answer Questions

Directions: Read each of the following statements and supply the word(s) necessary in the space provided.

1. The problem identification section in the documentation style used for problem-oriented records is called

_____

2. The section that states the effectiveness of the intervention in the documentation style used for problem-oriented records is called

_____

3. The information reported by the client in the documentation style used in problem-oriented records is labeled

   _____

4. The section of the problem-oriented chart that shows the changes that will be made in the original plan is called

   _____

5. The section of the problem-oriented chart that gives the observations made by health personnel is called

   _____

■ Critical Thinking Exercises

1. What types of records are used in the health agency where you work or study?

   a. _____ Traditional records

   b. _____ Problem-oriented records

   Briefly describe the differences between traditional records and problem-oriented records.

2. Refer to the sample nursing care plan (Figure 9–7) in the Timby text. Identify the data you would expect to find in SOAP charting based on this plan of care.

CHAPTER 10

Admission, Discharge, Transfer, and Referrals

■ Summary

At some point in time, most of us experience changes in health. Some become ill suddenly; some become injured; others may have felt ill for a while. All may need some form of care and treatment for their illnesses. To receive this treatment, we may be required to enter a health care agency such as a hospital or nursing home. The nurse faces a challenge to carry out agency policies for admission, transfer, referral, or discharge while helping the individual maintain his or her dignity and sense of control.

The information in this chapter is intended to assist the nursing student to understand and respond to the typical reactions that occur when a person is admitted to a hospital. Skill procedures that describe the general routines for admission and discharge of clients are also included. Methods for adapting these procedures to specific client situations are discussed.

■ Matching Questions

Directions: For items 1 through 7, match the services listed in Part B with the organizations in Part A.

PART A

1. ____ Hospice

2. ____ Home health aide

3. ____ Respite care

4. ____ Adult protective services

5. ____ Commission on aging

6. ____ Homemaker services

7. ____Visiting nurse associations

PART B

a. Assists elderly with transportation to medical appointments, outpatient therapy, and community meal sites

b. Supports the family and terminally ill individuals who choose to stay at home

c. Offers intermittent nursing care to homebound persons

d. Sends adults to the home to assist in shopping, meal preparation, and light housekeeping

e. Assists with bathing, hygiene, and medication supervision

f. Makes social, legal, and accounting services available to incompetent adults who may be victimized by others

g. Provides short-term, temporary relief to full-time caregivers of homebound persons

■ Multiple-Choice Questions

Directions: For items 1 through 10, circle the letter that corresponds to the best answer for each question.

1. An extended care facility licensed to provide skilled care is allowed to:

   a. Have nursing assistants give most of the care

   b. Give wound care, tube feedings, and intravenous fluids

   c. Arrange for room and board and carry out daily supervision

   d. Arrange social and recreational activities

2. Mr. J. was admitted through the emergency room after suffering a heart attack while on an out-of-town business trip. He asks the nurse to take his wallet for safekeeping. The best method of carrying out Mr. J.'s request is:

   a. Count the money with him and then tell him that you are placing his wallet in a locked drawer at the nurse's station.

   b. Count the money in front of him, have him sign a statement, and then place the statement on his chart.

   c. Tell him you will have someone from security come to collect his valuables and place them in the hospital safe.

   d. Tell him that the hospital cannot be responsible for that much money and he will have to hide it.

3. The primary concern to the nurse when referring a client is:

   a. Arranging transportation for the client

   b. Notifying the agency that will receive the client

   c. Communicating the information to the client

   d. Getting everything organized so there is continuity of care

4. Discharge planning for the hospitalized client begins:

   a. When the client's physician gives the discharge order

   b. When the client is admitted to the health care agency

   c. When the client begins to ask about his discharge plans

   d. When all of the specific needs of the client have been identified

5. When a rational adult wishes to leave the hospital against medical advice, which of the following is true:

   a. He may not leave until the physician examines him

   b. He may leave only after he has signed a special form

   c. He may leave because he cannot be forcefully detained

   d. He may leave after his attorney obtains permission

6. The nurse's responsibility when a client wishes to leave the hospital against medical advice is:

   a. The nurse should explain to the client that he or she might leave after being seen by his or her physician

   b. The nurse responsible for the client's care should be sure the physician is notified and aware of the client's wishes

   c. The nurse should note the request on the client's record and have the client sign a special form

   d. The hospital administrator or the supervising nurse should notify the physician that his or her client has left the agency

7. Ordinarily the procedure after the client has been discharged is:

   a. The nurse should clean and sterilize all of the equipment in the room

   b. The nurse should notify the housekeeping department that the client has been discharged

   c. The nurse should notify the sterile supply personnel so that they may clean the used equipment

   d. The nurse should notify the administration office so the room will be cleaned properly

8. The term *continuity of care* means:

   a. Care provided in the home by home health aides after discharge

   b. Care that is not interrupted by a change in caregivers

   c. Care provided in a skilled, intermediate, or basic care facility

   d. Care that does not require the services offered in a nursing home

9. The process that occurs when a client leaves a health care agency is called:

   a. Discharge

   b. Transfer

   c. Referral

   d. Admission

10. Which of the following statements best describes an intermediate care facility?

a. An institution that provides health care for persons unable to care for themselves but who do not require hospitalization

b. An institution that provides health services to persons who, because of mental or physical conditions, require care

c. An institution that provides custodial care in a group setting to persons who can perform their own activities of daily living

d. An institution that provides 24-hour nursing care under the direction of a registered nurse

■ Alternative Format Questions

1. To facilitate a physical examination, the client must undress. If the client cannot undress without the nurse's help, which of the following would the nurse do to help? Select all that apply.

1. Close the door or pull the curtain around the bed

2. Have the client stand while being assisted to undress

3. Release fasteners, zippers, and buttons

4. Ask the client to "kick off" his or her shoes

5. Ask the client to lift his or her hips to remove slacks or pants

6. Place a hospital gown on and cover the client with a blanket

2. The nurse is planning discharge instructions for his or her client. The client is a diabetic who has experienced a below-the-knee amputation of her right leg. Which of the following items would be important to include in this client's discharge instructions. Select all that apply.

1. A review of the client's technique for self-administration of insulin

2. A referral to a physical therapist for rehabilitation services

3. Signs and symptoms related to her amputation that should be reported to the physician

4. A demonstration of how to walk with the use of a cane

5. Tips on how to select a nursing home

6. Self-care required by the surgical site on her right leg

3. While performing an admission physical assessment, the nurse observes a rash on the client's chest and upper arms. Which of the following questions should the nurse ask in order to gain further information about the client's rash? Select all that apply.

1. When did the rash start?

2. Are you allergic to medications, foods, or pollen?

3. How old are you?

4. What have you been using to treat the rash?

5. Have you traveled outside the country?

6. Do you smoke cigarettes or drink alcohol?

■ True or False Questions

Directions: For items 1 through 10, decide if the statement is true or false and mark T or F in the space provided.

1. _____ It is the nurse's responsibility to maintain the individual's sense of control and dignity during admission, transfer, referral, and discharge.

2. _____ Home health care services can be used to prevent hospital admission.

3. ____ Preparing an identification bracelet for the client is one of the least important components of the admission process.

4. ____ The nurse should wait until the client arrives on the unit before checking to make sure the room is prepared.

5. ____ One of the most important steps of the admission procedure is to make the client feel welcome.

6. ____ Most hospital admission departments supply the client with a policy booklet so that it is not necessary for the nurse to do the orientation.

7. ____ Losing personal items belonging to a client can have serious implications unless there has been a signed and witnessed inventory that was taken at the time of admission.

8. ____ The transfer of a client from one hospital unit to another should be handled in the same manner as discharging him or her from the one unit and admitting him or her to another.

9. ____ A step-down unit is often used for those clients who need long-term care or are terminally ill.

10. ____ A client may be referred by a nurse in a hospital to outside organizations.

■ Short Answer Question

Instructions: List six of the guidelines for transferring a client suggested in this chapter.

a. _____

_____

b. _____

_____

c. _____

_____

d. _____

_____

e. _____

_____

f. _____

■ Critical Thinking Exercises

1. Describe adjustments made in relation to admission and discharge:
   a. When the client is an infant or child
   b. When the client is elderly

2. Plan a teaching program for the client(s) for whom you are caring and complete the following form.

Topics for Teaching	Points to Cover in the Teaching Plan
The hospital environment	
Preparation for discharge	

PERFORMANCE CHECKLIST

A. This section allows you to examine your techniques for assisting the client with admission to a health care agency.

1. Place a check mark in the "S" ("satisfactory") column if you used the recommended technique.
2. Place a check mark in the "NI" ("needs improvement") column if you used some but not all of each recommended technique.
3. Place a check mark in the "U" ("unsatisfactory") column if you forgot to include that particular recommended technique.
4. Note whether further practice is indicated, what errors you made, suggestions that will improve your skills, and so on in the section for comments.

RECOMMENDED TECHNIQUE	S	NI	U	COMMENTS
Check the client's identification and greet him or her courteously	☐	☐	☐	_____
Provide privacy to allow for undressing	☐	☐	☐	_____
Assist the client with undressing as indicated	☐	☐	☐	_____
Care for clothing and valuables according to agency policy	☐	☐	☐	_____
Explain hospital routines and policies	☐	☐	☐	_____
Place a signal device for the convenience of the client	☐	☐	☐	_____
Begin indicated care and document procedure	☐	☐	☐	_____

B. Examine your techniques when discharging a client from a health agency and complete the following form.

RECOMMENDED TECHNIQUE	S	NI	U	COMMENTS
Note that the client has an order to be discharged	☐	☐	☐	_____
Ensure that the client or a family member has discharge instructions	☐	☐	☐	_____
See to it that the client has necessary supplies and equipment for care	☐	☐	☐	_____
Check to see that proper financial arrangements have been made	☐	☐	☐	_____
Help the client dress and ensure that transportation is available	☐	☐	☐	_____
Document appropriately	☐	☐	☐	_____

C. Examine your techniques after referring a client to another health agency and complete the following form.

RECOMMENDED TECHNIQUE	S	NI	U	COMMENTS
Note that the client has an order for referral	☐	☐	☐	_____
Note that the client's identifying information is complete	☐	☐	☐	_____
State the client's diagnosis	☐	☐	☐	_____
Describe the client's disabilities, if any	☐	☐	☐	_____
List the client's diet and medications and include a medication schedule	☐	☐	☐	_____
List the client's allergies	☐	☐	☐	_____
Include recent laboratory reports, if any	☐	☐	☐	_____
Suggest appropriate exercise and activities	☐	☐	☐	_____
State how the client is to get to the agency and when he or she is to arrive	☐	☐	☐	_____
Notify the agency of the client's expected time of arrival	☐	☐	☐	_____
Give a copy of this information to the client or family member	☐	☐	☐	_____
Direct the client or family member to the appropriate person for help with financial arrangements	☐	☐	☐	_____
Assist the client to his transportation if appropriate	☐	☐	☐	_____
Document appropriately	☐	☐	☐	_____

CHAPTER 11

Vital Signs

■ Summary

Vital signs (body temperature, pulse rate, respiratory rate, and blood pressure) are objective data that indicate how well or poorly the body is functioning. Vital signs are sensitive to alterations in physiology; therefore, they are measured at regular intervals to monitor a client's health status. This chapter describes how to assess each component of the vital signs and explains what the measurements indicate.

■ Matching Questions

Directions: For items 1 through 5, match the definitions in Part B with the terms in Part A.

PART A

1. ____ Sustained fever

2. ____ Remittent fever

3. ____ Intermittent fever

4. ____ Invasion phase

5. ____ Defervescence phase

PART B

a. Return of an elevated body temperature to normal

b. A fever that continues, remains elevated, and fluctuates little

c. A gradual return of an elevated body temperature to normal

d. A fever broken by periods of normal or subnormal temperature

e. The period when a fever begins

f. A fever that fluctuates several degrees but does not reach normal between fluctuations

Directions: For items 6 through 10, match the approximate average normal pulse rates per minute in Part B with the ages in Part A.

PART A

6. ____ Newborn

7. ____ 1 month to 12 months

8. ____ 3 years to 6 years

9. ____ 7 years to 12 years

10. ____ Adolescence

PART B

a. 95

b. 110

c. 140

d. 80

e. 100

f. 120

Directions: For items 11 through 14, match the description in Part B with the number and definition of the pulse volumes in Part A.

PART A

11. ____ 0 Absent pulse

12. ____ 1+ Thready pulse

13. ____ 2+ Weak pulse

14. ____ 4+ Bounding pulse

PART B

a. It is stronger than a thready pulse; light pressure causes it to disappear

b. The pulsation is strong and does not disappear with moderate pressure

c. Pulsation is easily felt and takes moderate pressure to cause it to disappear

d. Pulsation is not easily felt, and slight pressure causes it to disappear

e. No pulsation is felt despite extreme pressure

Directions: For items 15 through 24, match the definitions in Part B with the terms related to respirations in Part A.

PART A

15. ____ Apnea

16. ____ Bradypnea

17. ____ Cheyne-Stokes respiration

18. ____ Dyspnea

19. ____ Hyperventilation

20. ____ Hypoventilation

21. ____ Orthopnea

22. ____ Stertorous

23. ____ Stridor

24. ____ Tachypnea

PART B

a. A condition in which breathing is easier when the client is in a sitting or standing position

b. A respiratory rate that is more rapid than normal

c. Difficult and labored breathing

d. A period in which there is no breathing

e. Respirations performed primarily by the diaphragm

f. A below-average or slow respiratory rate

g. A general term referring to noisy breathing

h. A gradual increase and then a gradual decrease in depth of respirations, followed by a period of apnea

i. The process of exchanging oxygen and carbon dioxide between the blood and the body

j. A condition in which a reduced amount of air enters the lungs

k. A high-pitched sound that occurs repeatedly during breathing as air is forced through narrowed respiratory passages

l. The process of exchanging oxygen and carbon dioxide between the lungs and the blood

m. A grating sound caused by friction as two structures move against one another

n. A harsh, high-pitched sound heard on inspiration in the presence of an obstruction in larger airways, such as the larynx

o. Abnormally prolonged, rapid, and deep respirations

■ Multiple-Choice Questions

Directions: For items 1 through 24, circle the letter that corresponds to the best *answer for each question.*

1. In which area of the brain is the body's temperature-regulating center located:
   a. Cerebellum
   b. Spinal cord
   c. Hypothalamus
   d. Medulla oblongata

2. Which of the following is true about the Fahrenheit scale:
   a. Water freezes at 0° and boils at 100°
   b. Water freezes at 32° and boils at 212°
   c. Water freezes at 32° and boils at 100°
   d. Water freezes at 0° and boils at 212°

3. At which of the time periods listed below would an individual's temperature normally be lowest:
   a. Between 4 a.m. and 5 a.m.
   b. Between 12 noon and 2 p.m.
   c. Between 6 p.m. and 8 p.m.
   d. Between 12 midnight and dawn

4. A client's temperature is 38.8°C. The Fahrenheit equivalent is:
   a. 99.8°
   b. 100.0°
   c. 101.8°
   d. 103.2°

5. Of the following individuals, which one is most likely to have a higher-than-average temperature?
   a. The person experiencing apathy and depression
   b. The person experiencing an average day
   c. The person experiencing anxiety and nervousness
   d. The person routinely working the night shift

6. A client is considered to be in danger when his temperature reaches beyond:
   a. 38°C (100.4°F)
   b. 40°C (104.0°F)
   c. 41°C (105.8°F)
   d. 43.3°C (110°F)

7. The condition in which the body temperature is below the average normal is called:
   a. Febrile
   b. Hypothermia
   c. Hyperthermia
   d. Pyrexia

8. Death usually occurs when the temperature falls below approximately:
   a. 30°C (89.6°F)
   b. 32°C (91.4°F)
   c. 28.8°C (84°F)
   d. 35°C (95.0°F)

9. The best method of assessing temperature for a client who has experienced extreme levels of hypothermia or hyperthermia would be to use a:
   a. Tympanic thermometer
   b. Disposable, single-use thermometer
   c. Heat-sensitive patch or tape
   d. Continuous monitoring device

10. Of the following individuals, which would most likely have the slower pulse rate?
    a. A man who is 6-feet, 2-inches tall and weighs 160 pounds
    b. A man who is 5-feet, 9-inches tall and weighs 155 pounds
    c. A woman who is 5-feet, 7-inches tall and weighs 126 pounds
    d. A woman who is 5-feet, 1-inch tall and weighs 130 pounds

11. The correct term for a rapid pulse rate is:
    a. Palpitation
    b. Bradycardia
    c. Arrhythmia
    d. Tachycardia

12. The correct term for an irregular pattern of heartbeats is:
    a. Palpitation
    b. Bradycardia
    c. Arrhythmia
    d. Tachycardia

13. The condition in which a person is aware of his or her own heart contraction without having to feel the pulse is called:
    a. Arrhythmia
    b. Pulse rhythm
    c. Dysrhythmia
    d. Palpitation

14. The term commonly used to identify a feeble and weak pulse:
    a. Failing
    b. Hypoxic
    c. Febrile
    d. Thready

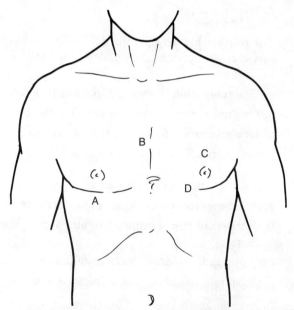

15. From the sketch above, select the best site for obtaining the apical pulse on an adult:
    a. Site A
    b. Site B
    c. Site C
    d. Site D

16. Which of the following best defines pulse deficit:
    a. The difference between the apical and radial pulse rates
    b. The difference between the radial and femoral pulse rates
    c. The difference between the brachial and radial pulse rates
    d. The difference between the temporal and the femoral pulse rates

17. Which of the following best defines *internal respiration*:
    a. The act of breathing in
    b. The act of breathing out
    c. The process of exchanging oxygen and carbon dioxide between the blood and body cells
    d. The process of exchanging oxygen and carbon dioxide between the lungs and the blood

18. The area that is very sensitive to the amount of carbon dioxide in the blood is the:
    a. Spinal cord
    b. Medulla
    c. Cerebellum
    d. Hypothalamus

19. The relationship between the pulse and respiratory rates is represented by which of the following ratios:
    a. One respiration to two or three heartbeats
    b. One respiration to three or four heartbeats
    c. One respiration to four or five heartbeats
    d. One respiration to five or six heartbeats

20. Hypoventilation is best defined as:
    a. An above-average or rapid respiratory rate
    b. A less-than-normal amount of air entering the lungs
    c. Prolonged, rapid, and deep respirations
    d. A below-average or slow respiratory rate

21. Which of the following best defines *systolic pressure*:
    a. The phase during which the heart is working
    b. The phase during which the heart is resting
    c. The pressure within the arteries while the heart is resting
    d. The pressure within the arteries while the heart contracts

22. The normal difference in systolic pressure when lying and standing tends to be no greater than:
    a. 10 mm Hg lower than it was in a reclining position
    b. 10 mm Hg higher than it was in a reclining position
    c. 15 mm Hg lower than it was in a reclining position
    d. 15 mm Hg higher than it was in a reclining position

23. When the blood pressure is 142/100, the pulse pressure is:
    a. 42
    b. 100
    c. 142
    d. 242

24. A falsely high blood pressure reading is most likely to occur when:
    a. Using a blood pressure cuff that is too wide
    b. Using a blood pressure cuff that is too narrow
    c. Applying the blood pressure cuff too tightly
    d. Applying the blood pressure cuff too low on the arm

■ Alternative Format Questions

1. The client's pulse is weak and thready, resulting in difficulty counting a radial pulse. The nurse determines that an apical pulse is required. Identify the area where the nurse should place the stethoscope to best hear the client's apical pulse.

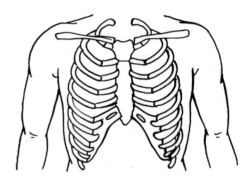

2. Auscultation of a client's blood pressure reveals a succession of sounds. Arrange the sounds in the sequence in which they would most likely have occurred.
   1. A change from tapping sounds to swishing sounds
   2. A change to loud distinct sounds
   3. The point at which the last sound is heard
   4. A faint but clear tapping sound that follows a period of silence
   5. Muffled sounds that have a blowing quality

3. The client's temperature is 101°F. Convert this Fahrenheit temperature to the Centigrade equivalent temperature.

■ True or False Questions

Directions: For items 1 through 12, decide if the statement is true or false and mark T or F in the space provided.

1. ____ In order to obtain an apical–radial pulse rate, the nurse should take the apical pulse for 1 full minute and then the radial pulse for 1 full minute.

2. ____ Infants and young children use the diaphragm when breathing.

3. ____ Women usually have a lower blood pressure on the average than men of the same age.

4. ____ As a rule, the blood pressure is lower when the individual is lying down.

5. ____ A systolic pressure of 140 mm Hg or greater in adults 18 years or older and a diastolic pressure of 90 mm Hg or greater is considered to be an abnormally high blood pressure.

6. ____ The client should be lying down for at least 10 minutes before the nurse assesses him or her for differences in lying and upright blood pressure.

7. ____ The aneroid type of sphygmomanometer uses a mercury gauge.

8. ____ The systolic pressure cannot be measured when the palpation method is utilized.

9. ____ Accuracy is improved when the probe of an electronic thermometer is placed beneath the tongue on either side of the mouth.

10. ____ Except when necessary, the nurse should avoid obtaining the vital signs when a client is experiencing strong emotions.

11. ____ The nurse should wait at least 30 minutes before taking an oral temperature if the client has been chewing gum.

12. ____ Obtaining a rectal temperature when a client has had diarrhea is contraindicated.

■ Short Answer Questions

Directions: Read each of the following statements and supply the word(s) necessary in the space provided.

1. State three circumstances in which the nurse must use judgment and double-check the client's vital signs.

   a. _____

   _____

   b. _____

   _____

   c. _____

   _____

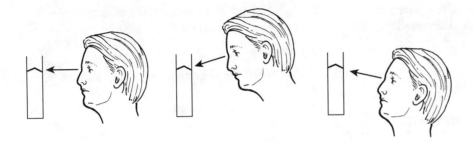

2. Study the figures shown above and answer the following questions.

   a. Describe the situation shown in the first sketch.

   _____

   _____

   b. Describe the situation shown in the second sketch. _____

   _____

   c. Describe the situation shown in the third sketch. _____

   _____

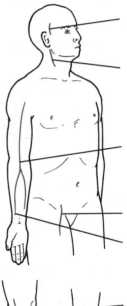

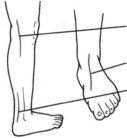

3. Study the figure shown above and label the sites for the peripheral pulses.

   _____

Performance Checklist

This section allows you to examine your techniques for obtaining the client's vital signs.

1. Place a check mark in the "S" ("satisfactory") column if you used the recommended technique.
2. Place a check mark in the "NI" ("needs improvement") column if you used some but not all of each recommended technique.
3. Place a check mark in the "U" ("unsatisfactory") column if you forgot to include that particular recommended technique.
4. Note when further practice is indicated, what errors you made, suggestions that will improve your skills, and so on in the section for comments.

RECOMMENDED TECHNIQUE	S	NI	U	Comments

Obtaining an Oral Temperature With a Glass Thermometer

	S	NI	U	
Rinse thermometer that is stored in a chemical solution	☐	☐	☐	_____
Wipe the thermometer while moving tissue from the bulb toward your fingers	☐	☐	☐	_____
Shake thermometer down and read it at eye level to check that it is at its lowest marking	☐	☐	☐	_____
Place the thermometer at the base and under the client's tongue	☐	☐	☐	_____
Leave the thermometer in place preferably 3 to 5 minutes—but no less than 3 minutes	☐	☐	☐	_____
Remove the thermometer and wipe it clean while moving tissue from your fingers toward the bulb	☐	☐	☐	_____
Hold the thermometer at eye level, read it, and then shake it down	☐	☐	☐	_____
Follow agency policy to clean and store the thermometer	☐	☐	☐	_____

Obtaining a Rectal Temperature with a Glass Thermometer

	S	NI	U	
Rinse a thermometer that is stored in a chemical solution	☐	☐	☐	_____
Wipe thermometer while moving tissue from the bulb toward the fingers	☐	☐	☐	_____
Shake the thermometer and read it at eye level to check that it is at its lowest marking	☐	☐	☐	_____
Lubricate the bulb and about 2.5 cm (1 inch) of the thermometer stem, and fold back bed linens to expose the anus	☐	☐	☐	_____
Separate buttocks, insert the thermometer about 3.8 cm (1.5 inches), and allow the buttocks to fall into place	☐	☐	☐	_____

(continued)

RECOMMENDED TECHNIQUE	S	NI	U	Comments

Obtaining a Rectal Temperature with a Glass Thermometer *(Continued)*

	S	NI	U	
Hold the thermometer in place for 2 to 3 minutes	☐	☐	☐	_____
Remove the thermometer and wipe it clean while moving tissue from your fingers toward the bulb	☐	☐	☐	_____
Hold the thermometer at eye level, read it, and shake it	☐	☐	☐	_____
Follow agency policy to clean and store the thermometer	☐	☐	☐	_____

Obtaining an Axillary Temperature With a Glass Thermometer

	S	NI	U	
Rinse a thermometer that is stored in a chemical solution	☐	☐	☐	_____
Wipe the thermometer while moving the tissue from the bulb toward your fingers	☐	☐	☐	_____
Shake the thermometer and read it at eye level to check that it is at its lowest marking	☐	☐	☐	_____
Place the thermometer well into the axillary region, with the bulb directed toward the client's head	☐	☐	☐	_____
Bring the client's arm down close to the body and place his or her forearm over his or her chest toward the opposite shoulder	☐	☐	☐	_____
Leave the thermometer in place for 10 minutes	☐	☐	☐	_____
Remove the thermometer and wipe it clean while moving tissue from your fingers toward the bulb	☐	☐	☐	_____
Hold the thermometer at eye level, read it, and then shake it	☐	☐	☐	_____
Follow agency policy to clean and store the thermometer	☐	☐	☐	_____

Obtaining the Radial Pulse Rate

	S	NI	U	
If the client is lying down, place the client's arm alongside his or her body, with the wrist extended and the palm of the hand downward	☐	☐	☐	_____
If the client is sitting, place his or her forearm at about a 90° angle to his or her body, with the forearm extended and the palm of hand downward	☐	☐	☐	_____
Place three fingertips along the radial artery while the thumb rests on the back of the client's wrist	☐	☐	☐	_____
Press gently to close the artery and then slowly release pressure until the pulse can be felt	☐	☐	☐	_____

RECOMMENDED TECHNIQUE	S	NI	U	Comments
While using a watch with a sweep second hand, count the pulse for 1/2 minute and multiply by 2	☐	☐	☐	_____
If pulse is abnormal, count the pulse for at least 1 full minute, longer if necessary for accuracy	☐	☐	☐	_____

Obtaining the Respiratory Rate

	S	NI	U	Comments
While the fingertips are in place after counting the pulse rate, observe the client's respirations	☐	☐	☐	_____
Note each rise and fall of the client's chest wall as she breathes	☐	☐	☐	_____
While using a watch with a sweep second hand, count the respiratory rate for 1/2 minute and multiply by 2	☐	☐	☐	_____
If respirations are abnormal, count the respirations for at least 1 minute, longer if necessary for accuracy				

Obtaining the Blood Pressure with a Mercury Manometer at the Brachial Artery

	S	NI	U	Comments
Delay taking the blood pressure, except in an emergency, if the client is upset, is in pain, or has just exercised	☐	☐	☐	_____
Make the client comfortable, with the forearm supported at the level of the heart, palm upward, and upper arm extended	☐	☐	☐	_____
Seat the client so that the meniscus of mercury can be read at eye level and no more than 3 feet away from the manometer	☐	☐	☐	_____
Place a cuff of appropriate size so that the inflatable bladder is centered over the brachial artery	☐	☐	☐	_____
Place the lower edge of the cuff about 2.5 to 5 cm (1 to 2 inches) above the inner aspect of the elbow	☐	☐	☐	_____
Ensure the rubber tubing leaving the cuff is at the edge nearer to the client's elbow				
Wrap cuff smoothly and snugly and secure it in place	☐	☐	☐	_____
Feel for the brachial artery after placing the stethoscope earpieces in your ears				
Place the stethoscope bell over the artery where the pulse was felt, away from clothes and the cuff	☐	☐	☐	_____
Pump air into the cuff to an amount of about 30 mm Hg above the point where the radial pulse disappears	☐	☐	☐	_____

(continued)

RECOMMENDED TECHNIQUE	S	NI	U	Comments

Obtaining the Blood Pressure with a Mercury Manometer at the Brachial Artery *(Continued)*

	S	NI	U	Comments
Release air gradually with the valve on the bulb, 2 to 3 mm Hg per second	☐	☐	☐	_____
Note the reading on the manometer when the first two consecutive heartbeats are heard; note this as systolic pressure	☐	☐	☐	_____
Continue releasing air; note when a distinct, soft, muffling sound is heard; and note this as diastolic pressure	☐	☐	☐	_____
Observe when all sounds disappear and note this as the third reading; this may occur at the same time as diastole	☐	☐	☐	_____
Allow remaining air to escape from the cuff quickly and remove the cuff from the client's arm	☐	☐	☐	_____
Clean and store equipment according to agency policy	☐	☐	☐	_____

Obtaining the Radial–Apical Pulse

	S	NI	U	Comments
While working with a second nurse, expose the client's left chest wall	☐	☐	☐	_____
First nurse: Place stethoscope diaphragm over the apical area of the heart and listen for the pulse beat	☐	☐	☐	_____
Second nurse: Place fingertips over the radial artery and feel for the pulse beat	☐	☐	☐	_____
Second nurse: Hold watch with a sweep second hand so that both nurses can read it	☐	☐	☐	_____
Select a starting time and have both nurses count pulse beats for 1 minute, longer if necessary for accuracy	☐	☐	☐	_____

CHAPTER 12

Physical Assessment

■ Summary

The examination of a client performed by the nurse is referred to as a physical assessment. Although the physical assessment focuses on the systems of the body, the nurse also uses this opportunity to gather information about the client's mood, mental ability, and social interaction. All nurses should be familiar with the methods of gathering information during a physical assessment even though the nurse's responsibility for its depth varies with the health agency and the level of practice.

■ Matching Questions

Directions: For items 1 through 7, match the criteria for physical assessment by a nurse generalist in Part B with the physical systems in Part A.

PART A

1. _____ Sensory–perceptual

2. _____ Skin

3. _____ Respiratory

4. _____ Cardiovascular

5. _____ Neurological

6. _____ Gastrointestinal

7. _____ Genitourinary

PART B

a. Pulses, blood pressure, mucous membranes, nail beds

b. Muscle tone, strength, gait, stability, range of motion

c. Lesions, presence of retention

d. Vision and appearance of eyes, hearing, touch, taste, smell

e. Mouth, gums, teeth and tongue, gag reflex, bowel sounds, distention, impaction, hemorrhoids

f. Turgor, lesions, edema, hair distribution

g. Pupillary reactions, orientation, level of consciousness, grasp strength

h. Rate, character, breath sounds, cough

Directions: For items 8 through 13, match the descriptions of common color variations of the skin in Part B with the terms in Part A.

PART A

8. _____ Flushed

9. _____ Erythema

10. _____ Jaundice

11. _____ Pallor

12. _____ Ecchymosis

13. _____ Cyanosis

PART B

a. A yellowish coloring of the skin

b. A bluish coloring of the skin

c. A brown coloring of the skin

d. A reddish-pink coloring of the skin

e. A paleness of the skin coloring

f. A reddish coloring to areas of the skin

g. A purplish coloring within areas of skin

■ Multiple-Choice Questions

Directions: For items 1 through 10, circle the letter that corresponds to the best answer for each question.

1. The synonym for rales is:
   a. Rhonchi
   b. Wheezes
   c. Gurgles
   d. Crackles

2. The technique of inspection is best described as one that uses:
   a. Tapping on a particular part of the body to produce sounds
   b. The sense of touch to feel or press on the body
   c. Many senses of the examiner to scan the client
   d. The sense of hearing to listen for sounds

3. Which of the following best describes the technique of palpation:
   a. The use of tapping on a particular part of the body to produce sounds
   b. The sense of touch to feel or press on the body
   c. The use of many senses of the examiner to scan the client
   d. The use of the sense of hearing to listen for sounds

4. The technique of percussion is most often used to examine:
   a. The entire body
   b. The abdomen and the back
   c. The lungs and the back
   d. The lungs and the abdomen

5. For breast self-examinations, female clients should be instructed to use the techniques of:
   a. Auscultation and percussion
   b. Palpation and percussion
   c. Inspection and palpation
   d. Palpation and auscultation

6. When auscultating lung sounds, the nurse would expect to hear which of the following sounds directly over the trachea:
   a. Sounds that are harsh and loud
   b. Sounds that are soft and rustling
   c. Sounds that are loud and coarse
   d. Sounds that are soft and faint

7. Normal bronchovesicular lung sounds are:
   a. Equal in length during inspiration and expiration with a short pause
   b. Short on inspiration with a slight pause before a lengthier expiration
   c. Equal in length during inspiration and expiration with no noticeable pause
   d. Long on inspiration, leading into a shorter sound during expiration with no pause between the two

8. Which of the following skin lesions is elevated, has an irregular shape, and has no free fluid?
   a. Macule
   b. Vesicle
   c. Wheal
   d. Cyst

9. A wart is an example of which of the following types of skin lesions:
   a. Macule
   b. Papule
   c. Vesicle
   d. Pustule

10. When using percussion to examine a client, an empty, moderately loud, resonant sound is a normal finding for:
   a. Lungs
   b. Muscle
   c. Liver
   d. Bone

■ Alternative Format Questions

1. While assessing a client's spine for abnormal curvatures, the nurse notes lordosis. Identify the area of the spine that is affected by lordosis.

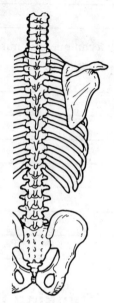

2. The nurse is performing an otoscopic examination of a client with ear pain. The nurse notes that the tympanic membrane is bulging and red. Identify the structure that the nurse is assessing.

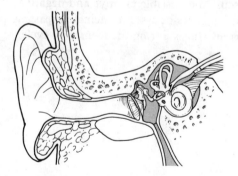

3. The nurse is performing a cardiac assessment. Identify where the nurse places the stethoscope to best auscultate the pulmonic value.

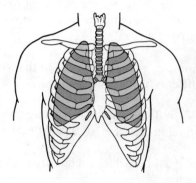

4. A young female client is being taught breast self-examination. Place the following steps in the most likely sequence in which they would be performed.

   1. Lie down, placing a folded towel under the shoulder, on the same side as the breast to be examined

   2. Stand in front of a mirror and look at both breasts

   3. Determine the appropriate time for breast self-exam

   4. Squeeze the nipple

   5. In the shower, palpate each breast in a circular fashion, beginning and ending at 12 o'clock

   6. Feel upward toward the axilla of each arm

■ True or False Questions

Directions: For items 1 through 10, decide if the statement is true or false and mark T or F in the space provided.

1. ____ Edema is the term used to describe excessive fluid trapped in tissues.

2. ____ If the nurse is present when the physician obtains a client's medical history, it is not necessary to obtain a nursing assessment because they are similar in content.

3. ____ If the client has weighed himself at home, it is not necessary to obtain his weight before the nurse starts the examination.

4. ____ Cerumen is commonly found within the ear canal.

5. ____ A diseased area of the skin is generally referred to as a fissure.

6. ____ Female clients should be taught to do breast self-examinations at least once a month.

7. ____ Jaundice is easily detected in the whites of the eyes.

8. ____ When doing a visual assessment, the nurse should check the 10 cardinal positions.

9. ____ Normal bronchial sounds are loud and coarse.

10. ____ Children may normally have an extra heart sound that comes after the "dub" sound.

■ Short Answer Questions

Directions: Read each of the following statements and supply the word(s) necessary in the space provided.

1. List six of the recommended techniques given in this chapter to obtain a client's height and weight.

a. _____

_____

b. _____

_____

c. _____

_____

d. _____

_____

e. _____

_____

f. _____

_____

2. List two of the purposes of a physical assessment as suggested in this chapter.

a. _____

_____

b. _____

_____

3. Identify four techniques the nurse uses to assess touch, taste, and smell.

a. _____

_____

b. _____

_____

c. _____

_____

d. _____

_____

■ Critical Thinking Exercise

1. Discuss the logic of conducting neurological and musculoskeletal assessments together.

2. Discuss the possible positive and negative consequences of assessing female breast tissue at various stages during the menstrual cycle.

Performance Checklist

This section allows you to examine your techniques for performing a physical assessment.

1. Place a check mark in the "S" ("satisfactory") column if you used the recommended technique.
2. Place a check mark in the "NI" ("needs improvement") column if you used some but not all of each recommended technique.
3. Place a check mark in the "U" ("unsatisfactory") column if you forgot to include that particular recommended technique.
4. Note when further practice is indicated, what errors you made, suggestions that will improve your skills, and so on in the section for comments.

RECOMMENDED TECHNIQUE	S	NI	U	Comments
Identify the client	☐	☐	☐	_____
Explain what is planned	☐	☐	☐	_____
Assemble the equipment needed	☐	☐	☐	_____
Provide privacy during the examination	☐	☐	☐	_____
Wash your hands before beginning the examination	☐	☐	☐	_____
Have the client empty his or her bladder before beginning the examination	☐	☐	☐	_____
Assist the client in putting on an examining gown	☐	☐	☐	_____
Provide a cover for other exposed areas				_____
Explain that all information will be kept confidential	☐	☐	☐	_____
Protect the client from injury	☐	☐	☐	_____
Follow the health agency's policy for the examination	☐	☐	☐	_____
Explain each technique before it is performed	☐	☐	☐	_____
Proceed through the examination in an organized manner	☐	☐	☐	_____
Review your data	☐	☐	☐	_____
Assist the client as needed upon completion of the examination	☐	☐	☐	_____
Make sure that all equipment is cleaned or replaced	☐	☐	☐	_____
Record the assessment information	☐	☐	☐	_____
Communicate any significant information to the appropriate nursing or medical personnel	☐	☐	☐	_____

CHAPTER 13

Special Examinations and Tests

■ Summary

This chapter gives a general overview of nursing responsibilities associated with examination and special test assistance. These tests are performed by various health care personnel to determine how the body is functioning. Often the nurse is required to prepare the client both physically and emotionally for the test or examination, assist with the procedure itself, and care for the client and equipment afterward. In addition, several possible nursing diagnoses are suggested for clients undergoing tests and examinations. An example of the nursing process as it relates to one of these diagnoses is included in the nursing care plan.

■ Matching Questions

Directions: For items 1 through 5, match the descriptions of the common positions for examinations and tests in Part B with the names of the positions in Part A.

PART A

1. _____ Modified standing

2. _____ Dorsal recumbent

3. _____ Lithotomy

4. _____ Sims

5. _____ Genupectoral

PART B

a. The client is lying on his or her back with the feet in stirrups and the buttocks at the edge of the table end

b. The client assumes the normal standing position with arms relaxed at the sides

c. The client rests on his or her knees and chest. The head is turned to one side, and the arms are above the head.

d. The client is lying on his or her back, with the legs separated and the knees bent so the feet are flat against the table or bed

e. The client is lying on his or her side

f. The buttocks are firmly on the edge of the bed. Most of the thighs are supported, and the feet are on the floor or on a footrest.

g. The client is standing in front of and facing the examination table, leaning forward from the waist

Directions: For items 6 through 13, match the descriptions of the tests or examinations in Part B with the names of the tests in Part A.

PART A

6. _____ Radiography

7. _____ Magnetic resonance

8. _____ Computed tomography

9. _____ Electromyography

10. _____ Ultrasonography

11. _____ Positron emission tomography

12. _____ Endoscopy

13. _____ Biopsy

PART B

a. Uses sound waves to produce images on a screen

b. Uses x-rays to produce images

c. Uses x-rays plus contrast medium to identify variations in tissue density

d. Involves removing a piece of tissue for examination

e. Uses electrical impulses from skeletal muscles to produce wave patterns

f. Scans magnetic forces with radio-frequency signals

g. Combines radionuclide scanning and layered tomography

h. Uses an instrument for visual examination of an internal structure

■ Multiple-Choice Questions

Directions: For items 1 through 12, circle the letter that corresponds to the best answer for each question.

1. The suffix "gram" refers to which of the following:
   a. An examination in which body structures are visualized by the eye
   b. The procedure in which an image of a particular body part is produced
   c. The instrument used to visualize a particular part of the body
   d. The actual image or results of the test that may be held in the hand

2. The suffix "centesis" refers to which of the following:
   a. When a procedure involves puncturing a body cavity
   b. When a procedure involves producing an image of a body part
   c. When a procedure involves visualizing an area within the body
   d. When a procedure involves the production of a paper strip of waves

3. Paracentesis is best described as:
   a. The removal of fluid from the lungs, bronchi, and trachea via the introduction of a bronchoscope
   b. The removal of fluid or air from the pleural cavity by entering the thorax through the chest wall
   c. The removal of secretions from the stomach after the insertion of a nasogastric tube
   d. The removal of body fluid by puncturing the skin and subsequently the abdominal cavity

4. The reason for a Queckenstedt's test is:
   a. To determine if there is an obstruction in the spinal canal
   b. To determine if there is an infection in the spinal canal
   c. To determine the amount of fluid in the spinal canal
   d. To determine the amount of pressure in the spinal canal

5. Of the following, which is used to determine the activity of the brain:
   a. Electrocardiography
   b. Electromyography
   c. Electroencephalography
   d. Echocardiography

6. The dorsal recumbent position is most often used to examine:
   a. The heart and lungs
   b. The rectum and vagina
   c. The rectum and colon
   d. The bladder and uterus

7. The lithotomy position is most often used to examine:
   a. The heart and lungs
   b. The rectum and vagina
   c. The rectum and colon
   d. The bladder and uterus

8. Which of the following are the three essential elements of informed consent:
   a. Capacity, consent, comprehension
   b. Ability, coercion, risks
   c. Rationality, explanation, alternatives
   d. Capacity, comprehension, voluntariness

9. A cystoscopy refers to an examination that involves:
   a. Inspection of the bronchi
   b. Inspection of the abdominal cavity
   c. Inspection of the colon
   d. Inspection of the urinary bladder

10. The modified standing position is most commonly used to:
    a. Insert a suppository
    b. Complete a cystoscopic examination
    c. Examine the prostate gland
    d. Collect a Pap smear

11. On the cellular portion of the Pap smear, a Class III result would indicate:
    a. The result is negative with no abnormal cells
    b. The result is suggestive of cancer cells; it is not definite

c. The result is strongly suggestive of cancer cells

d. The result is definitely cancerous cells

12. On the identifiable microorganisms portion of the Pap smear, a #1 result would indicate:

a. Normal microorganisms

b. Scanty microorganisms

c. *Trichomonas vaginalis*

d. *Monilia*

■ Alternative Format Questions

1. The nurse is caring for a client who is having a paracentesis. Which of the following nursing interventions are appropriate? Select all that apply:

1. Ensure that the client has signed the consent form

2. Measure and record weight, blood pressure, respiratory rate, and abdominal girth

3. Have client empty his or her bladder

4. Place the client in a side-lying position

5. Discard the fluid withdrawn

6. Measure blood pressure and respiratory rate periodically during the procedure

2. The client is preparing to test his blood glucose level with a Glucometer. Place the following activities in the most likely sequence in which they would occur:

1. Turn the Glucometer on; observe that the code number on the strip vial matches the code number on the Glucometer

2. Select an appropriate nontraumatized site

3. Gather test strips, meter, lancet, and lancing device

4. Place the strip containing the sample in the Glucometer and wait for the meter to beep

5. Pierce site and collect sample on test strip

6. Wash hands with soap and warm water and towel dry

3. At what age might a woman elect to cease cervical cancer screenings, provided the results of three prior Pap tests over the last 10 years were normal?

■ True or False Questions

Directions: For items 1 through 15, decide if the statement is true or false and mark T or F in the space provided.

1. _____ The physician is responsible for explaining an invasive procedure.

2. _____ It is important that the nurse memorize all the special requirements for the various tests and examinations that are performed.

3. _____ The nurse is usually responsible for obtaining the necessary equipment when special diagnostic examinations and tests are performed on the nursing unit.

4. _____ Draping is done prior to an examination to prevent the client from becoming chilled.

5. _____ All clients should be asked about allergies prior to tests and examinations that use contrast media.

6. _____ When iodine is altered in such a way that it gives off radiation, it is referred to as a gamma ray.

7. _____ Ultrasonography can be used to examine moving structures, such as the heart or a fetus.

8. _____ A spinal tap is a procedure in which a needle is inserted between lumbar vertebrae in the spine but below the spinal cord itself in order to obtain spinal fluid.

9. _____ Examinations using x-rays or radionuclides should not be performed on pregnant or breast-feeding women.

10. _____ Alcohol is the best cleaning agent for cleansing the skin when preparing the area for a blood glucose test.

11. _____ To produce an accurate blood glucose test, the test strip pad must be completely covered and saturated with blood.

12. _____ A preliminary diagnosis may be obtained from a throat culture in 10 minutes.

13. ____ Glucose and insulin are hormones that regulate carbohydrate metabolism in the body.

14. ____ Blood sugar is usually measured a half hour before eating a meal and before bedtime to determine the lowest level of glucose in the blood.

15. ____ A sigmoidoscopy involves inspecting the rectum and a section of the lower intestine with an endoscope.

■ Short Answer Questions

Directions: Read each of the following statements and supply the word(s) necessary in the space provided.

1. List six items of information that should be included in a client's record regarding an examination or special test that has been performed.

   a. _____

   _____

   b. _____

   _____

   c. _____

   _____

   d. _____

   _____

   e. _____

   _____

   f. _____

   _____

2. Identify three factors to be considered when examinations and tests are performed on older adults.

   a. _____

   _____

   b. _____

   _____

   c. _____

   _____

3. Name five client responsibilities that should be included in a teaching plan for clients receiving tests or examinations on an outpatient basis.

   a. _____

   _____

   b. _____

   _____

   c. _____

   _____

   d. _____

   _____

   e. _____

   _____

■ Critical Thinking Exercises

Describe nursing responsibilities for a pregnant woman who is having an amniocentesis (withdrawal of a sample of amniotic fluid for testing). How would the sample be cared for?

Performance Checklist

This section allows you to examine your techniques for assisting with examinations and special tests.

1. Place a check mark in the "S" ("satisfactory") column if you used the recommended technique.
2. Place a check mark in the "NI" ("needs improvement") column if you used some but not all of each recommended technique.
3. Place a check mark in the "U" ("unsatisfactory") column if you forgot to include that particular recommended technique.
4. Note when further practice is indicated, what errors you made, suggestions that will improve your skills, and so on in the section for comments.

RECOMMENDED TECHNIQUE	S	NI	U	Comments
Understand the nature of the procedure, why it is being done, what part of the body is to be entered, and what type of specimen will be collected	☐	☐	☐	_____
Understand the client, diagnosis, and plan of care	☐	☐	☐	_____
Prepare the client psychologically for the procedure	☐	☐	☐	_____
Obtain a permit if one is required	☐	☐	☐	_____
Have the client void prior to the procedure	☐	☐	☐	_____
Gown the client properly	☐	☐	☐	_____
Clean and shave the client's skin at the site of entry, if necessary	☐	☐	☐	_____
Validate that special preparations have been carried out for the procedure	☐	☐	☐	_____
Have the necessary equipment and supplies ready; ensure equipment is in working order	☐	☐	☐	_____
Prepare the working area and position and drape the client appropriately	☐	☐	☐	_____
Clean the skin at the site of entry and handle equipment, as required, to assist the examiner	☐	☐	☐	_____
Care for the client appropriately after the procedure is completed	☐	☐	☐	_____
Assist an examiner appropriately when he or she carries out the following: A lumbar puncture	☐	☐	☐	_____
A thoracentesis	☐	☐	☐	_____
An abdominal paracentesis	☐	☐	☐	_____

CHAPTER 14

Nutrition

■ Summary

Nutrition is a basic human need. If a person is deprived of food for a prolonged period of time, health will be affected and life may be endangered. Most eating habits are learned early in life and usually vary from culture to culture. Research data supports the idea that nutritional status has a great influence on health and well-being. Modifying and regulating food intake are standard techniques used in the treatment of illness.

Nurses should possess certain skills that enable them to assist the client to obtain adequate nutrition within the limits of his or her illness. Several skills and guidelines are included for this purpose.

■ Matching Questions

Directions: For items 1 through 5, match the chief functions in Part B with the common minerals needed by the body in Part A.

PART A

1. ____ Sodium

2. ____ Potassium

3. ____ Calcium

4. ____ Iodine

5. ____ Iron

PART B

a. Buffering action and the formation of bones and teeth

b. Neuromuscular activity, blood coagulation, cell wall permeability, and formation of teeth and bones

c. Activation of enzymes, neuromuscular activity, and formation of teeth and bones

d. Maintenance of water and electrolyte balance

e. Component of hemoglobin and assistance in cellular oxidation

f. Enzyme reactions, neuromuscular activity, and maintenance of fluid and electrolyte balance

g. Regulation of body metabolism and promotion of normal growth

Directions: For items 6 through 8, match the vitamins in Part B with the deficiency diseases in Part A.

PART A

6. ____ Scurvy

7. ____ Rickets

8. ____ Beriberi

PART B

a. Vitamin A

b. Vitamin B

c. Vitamin C

d. Vitamin D

e. Vitamin E

Directions: For items 9 through 13, match the characteristics in Part B with the types of diets in Part A.

PART A

9. ____ Regular/standard

10. ____ Soft

11. ____ Mechanical soft

12. ____ Full liquid

13. ____ Clear liquid

PART B

a. A light diet used for clients with chewing difficulties; provides cooked fruits and vegetables and ground meats

b. A wide variety, such as high-caloric, low-caloric, diabetic, restricted sodium, low-fat, high-protein, and low-roughage diets

c. Unrestricted food selections

d. A diet of fruit and vegetable juices, creamed or blended soups, milk, ices, ice cream, gelatin, junket, custard, and cooked cereal

e. Primarily a regular diet with the omission of fried foods, rich pastries, fat-rich foods, and gas-forming and raw foods

f. A diet of water, clear broth, clear fruit juice, plain gelatin, tea and coffee, and possibly carbonated beverages

g. Foods soft in texture, usually low in residue and easily digestible, few or no spices, and few fruits, vegetables, or meats

■ Multiple-Choice Questions

Directions: For items 1 through 16, circle the letter that corresponds to the best answer for each question.

1. Which of the following best describes nutrition:

   a. The body's need for calories, water, proteins, carbohydrates, fats, vitamins, and minerals

   b. The process whereby the body uses food and fluids to reach and maintain health

   c. The comparison of a certain volume or weight of the energy source with its ability to produce heat

   d. Food is a source of body energy for human beings, and it provides the means by which human beings function

2. A calorie is defined as the amount of heat necessary to raise the temperature of:

   a. 1 pound of water by 1°F

   b. 1 pound of water by 1°C

   c. 1 gram of water by 1°F

   d. 1 gram of water by 1°C

3. The average adult requirement of calories per day is:

   a. 1000–2000

   b. 1500–2500

   c. 1800–3000

   d. 3000–4000

4. Of the following substances, which supplies the body with amino acids:

   a. Proteins

   b. Fats

   c. Carbohydrates

   d. Minerals

5. The caloric yield of fats is:

   a. 4 calories per gram

   b. 5 calories per gram

   c. 7 calories per gram

   d. 9 calories per gram

6. The recommended percentage of dietary fat per day is:

   a. 10%

   b. 20%

   c. 30%

   d. 15%

7. Which of the following provide the body with necessary electrolytes:

   a. Vitamins

   b. Proteins

   c. Minerals

   d. Fats

8. Individuals who eat vegetarian diets maybe lacking:

   a. Amino acids

   b. Vitamins

   c. Electrolytes

   d. Iron

9. Regurgitation commonly occurs in which of the following age groups:

   a. The elderly

   b. The toddler

   c. The infant

   d. The adolescent

10. Which of the following individuals would be at greatest risk for inadequate nutritional intake?

    a. A retired widow

    b. A middle-income family

    c. A person who consumes no meat

    d. A pregnant woman who eats 6 small meals

11. Unsaturated fats that have been hydrogenated and remain solid at room temperature are called:
    a. Lipoproteins
    b. Cholesterol
    c. Lipids
    d. Transfats

12. Foods to which extra amounts of nutritional substances have been added are said to be:
    a. Saturated
    b. Fortified
    c. Supplemented
    d. Enhanced

13. Which of the following represents the normal range of measurement for the triceps skin fold in adult males?
    a. 29.3–17.6 cm
    b. 25.3–15.2 cm
    c. 16.5–9.90 mm
    d. 12.5–7.3 mm

14. Minerals are best described as:
    a. Noncaloric substances that are essential to all cells
    b. Chemical substances that are necessary in minute amounts
    c. Substances that contain as much hydrogen as their molecules can hold
    d. Chemical compounds composed of nitrogen, carbon, hydrogen, and oxygen

15. The term *dysphagia* refers to:
    a. Difficulty swallowing
    b. Impairment of intellectual function
    c. Desire to vomit
    d. Discharge of gas through the mouth

16. Good sources of carbohydrates in food are:
    a. Grains, meat, fish, eggs, tomatoes
    b. Eggs, milk, avocados, nuts, chocolate
    c. Cereals, grains, wheat germ, fruits, vegetables
    d. Seafood, potatoes, soup, peanut butter, corn

■ Alternative Format Questions

1. Among the goals advocated by the government is that an individual's daily caloric intake should be comprised of what percent contributed by fat?

2. The nurse is caring for a client with dysphagia. Which of the following nursing interventions are appropriate? Select all that apply:
    1. Place the client in a sitting position
    2. Have equipment for oral and pharyngeal suctioning at the bedside
    3. Describe the food and indicate its location on the tray
    4. Give short, simple instructions to prompt the client to eat
    5. Be consistent with time and place for eating
    6. Limit distracting stimuli

3. Calculate the body mass index (BMI) of an individual who is 69 inches tall and weighs 160 pounds.

■ True or False Questions

Directions: For items 1 through 10, decide if the statement is true or false and mark T or F in the space provided.

1. ____ An individual's eating habits are determined primarily by hereditary factors.

2. ____ Anorexia is defined as a condition in which there is a general wasting away of body tissue.

3. ____ The synonym for eructation is belching.

4. ____ Flatus refers to intestinal gas released from the rectum.

5. ____ Protein complementation is the combining of animal and plant sources in the same meal.

6. ____ The bulk that helps with elimination comes from the undigestible fiber found in the stems, skins, and leaves of many fruits and vegetables.

7. ____ Many deficiency diseases have been associated with diets in which specific foods, rich in a source of fats, have been lacking.

8. ____ Water-soluble vitamins are stored in the body as reserve for future needs.

9. ____ Consuming megadoses of vitamins can be dangerous.

10. ____ Strict vegetarians should take vitamin B supplements.

■ Short Answer Questions

Directions: Read each of the following statements and supply the word(s) necessary in the space provided.

1. List the six basic food groups and state the number of servings per day for each.

   Food Group   Servings per Day

   a. _____

   _____

   b. _____

   _____

   c. _____

   _____

   d. _____

   _____

   e. _____

   _____

   f. _____

   _____

2. Describe three facts that can be obtained from a current nutritional label.

   a. _____

   _____

   b. _____

   _____

   c. _____

   _____

■ Critical Thinking Exercises

1. Prepare a 3-day menu plan for an economically disadvantaged couple. The wife is 72 and has arthritis. The husband is 74 and has Alzheimer's disease. They are able to consume a regular diet. However, the husband has loose-fitting dentures and often cannot remember where he put them. They have no close family. Consider community resources in your area for transportation, shopping, and meal preparation.

2. Prepare a 1-day menu plan for a child vegetarian. The meals should meet the recommended daily allowance of essential nutrients for this child.

3. Identify daily medications taken by a client in your care. Describe dietary considerations for each of these medications. Discuss how the client would plan to satisfy these conditions.

Performance Checklist

This section allows you to examine your techniques for assisting the client to eat and for assisting to serve meals to hospitalized clients.

1. Place a check mark in the "S" ("satisfactory") column if you used the recommended technique.
2. Place a check mark in the "NI" ("needs improvement") column if you used some but not all of each recommended technique.
3. Place a check mark in the "U" ("unsatisfactory") column if you forgot to include that particular recommended technique.
4. Note when further practice is indicated, what errors you made, suggestions that will improve your skills, and so on in the section for comments.

RECOMMENDED TECHNIQUE	S	NI	U	Comments
Plan ahead so that a period of rest and measures to relieve pain are provided before mealtime	☐	☐	☐	_____
Avoid giving treatments immediately before or after meals	☐	☐	☐	_____
Use available measures to help control noise and odors before mealtimes	☐	☐	☐	_____
See to it that the room is tidy before the meal is served	☐	☐	☐	_____
Offer the client a bedpan or urinal before serving a meal	☐	☐	☐	_____
Offer the client equipment and supplies to wash his or her hands; give oral hygiene as indicated	☐	☐	☐	_____
Provide privacy for seriously ill clients who cannot eat	☐	☐	☐	_____
Assist the client to a comfortable and safe position for eating	☐	☐	☐	_____
Check to see that the correct tray and foods are served to the client	☐	☐	☐	_____
See to it that the tray is complete, tidy, and promptly served	☐	☐	☐	_____
Protect the client and bed linens with a napkin	☐	☐	☐	_____
Sit at the client's bedside while helping him or her to eat	☐	☐	☐	_____
Encourage the client to help himself or herself with eating, as indicated	☐	☐	☐	_____
Serve manageable bits of food in the order of the client's preference; offer fluids intermittently	☐	☐	☐	_____
Allow the client adequate time to chew and swallow	☐	☐	☐	_____

RECOMMENDED TECHNIQUE	S	NI	U	Comments
Note foods the client is not eating, ensure that the client has sufficient food, and report accordingly	☐	☐	☐	_____
Offer support to clients who may not enjoy a special diet	☐	☐	☐	_____
Keep conversation friendly during mealtimes	☐	☐	☐	_____
When a client has limited eyesight, devise a system to indicate when he or she is ready for more food	☐	☐	☐	_____
Remove trays promptly after meals and offer oral hygiene and an opportunity for the client to wash his or her hands	☐	☐	☐	_____
Leave the client clean and comfortable	☐	☐	☐	_____

B. Examine your techniques while caring for a client when anorexia, nausea, and vomiting are present and complete the following form.

RECOMMENDED TECHNIQUE	S	NI	U	Comments
Control odors, noises, and annoying sights as much as possible	☐	☐	☐	_____
Avoid making negative comments about food	☐	☐	☐	_____
Limit the client's activities appropriately	☐	☐	☐	_____
Use deep-breathing exercises to help the client control his or her nausea and vomiting	☐	☐	☐	_____
Limit food and fluid intake appropriately when nausea and vomiting are present	☐	☐	☐	_____
Offer bland foods and avoid spicy and high-fat foods	☐	☐	☐	_____
Use carbonated beverages and ice chips appropriately to relieve nausea and vomiting	☐	☐	☐	_____
Use appropriate measures to prevent vomitus from being aspirated, including using suction, if necessary	☐	☐	☐	_____
After the client vomits, help with oral hygiene	☐	☐	☐	_____
After the client vomits, wash his or her hands and face, change linens, and give a back rub	☐	☐	☐	_____
See to it that the client is in a comfortable position and in a quiet environment after nausea and vomiting	☐	☐	☐	_____

CHAPTER 15

Fluid and Chemical Balance

■ Summary

Water is one of the necessities of life. All of the water in the body contains chemical substances. This chapter presents basic information about how the body maintains fluid and chemical balance. The student will find a summary of the process involved in fluid and chemical balance and a discussion of common imbalances that are likely to occur.

It is part of the nurse's responsibility to assess the client's state of fluid and chemical balance. This chapter describes some of the skills that are useful for gathering data accurately. When alterations occur, the nurse may be required to implement measures described in this chapter to restore chemical balance.

■ Matching Questions

Directions: For items 1 through 6, match the normal adult values in Part B with the serum electrolytes in Part A.

PART A

1. ____ Sodium (Na)

2. ____ Potassium (K)

3. ____ Chloride (Cl)

4. ____ Calcium (Ca)

5. ____ Magnesium (Mg)

6. ____ Bicarbonate (HCO)

PART B

a. 2.1 to 2.6 mEq/liter

b. 22 to 26 mEq/liter

c. 135 to 148 mEq/liter

d. 3.5 to 5.0 mEq/liter

e. 1.3 to 2.1 mEq/liter

f. 90 to 110 mEq/liter

g. 1.7 to 2.6 mEq/liter

Directions: For items 7 through 12, match the signs and symptoms in Part B with the complications in Part A.

PART A

7. ____ Circulatory overload

8. ____ Infiltration

9. ____ Phlebitis

10. ____ Thrombus

11. ____ Pulmonary embolus

12. ____ Air embolism

PART B

a. Shortness of breath, rapid heart rate, drop in blood pressure

b. Redness, warmth, discomfort

c. Elevated blood pressure, shortness of breath, bounding pulse

d. Sudden chest pain, shortness of breath, anxiety

e. Swelling at site, discomfort, decreased skin temperature

f. Swelling, discomfort, slowed infusion rate

Directions: For items 13 through 19, match the causes in Part B with the type of transfusion reactions in Part A.

PART A

13. ____ Incompatibility

14. ____ Febrile

15. ____ Septic

16. ____ Allergic

17. ____ Moderate chilling

18. ____ Overload

19. ____ Hypocalcemia

PART B

a. Sensitivity to foreign substance

b. Multiple transfusions

c. Allergy to foreign protein

d. Rapid rate of infusion

e. Infusion of cold substance

f. Mismatch between donor and recipient

g. Response to microorganisms

■ Multiple-Choice Questions

*Directions: For items 1 through 35, circle the letter
that corresponds to the best answer for each question.*

1. The human body is made up of approximately:

    a. 75% to 95% water

    b. 65% to 75% water

    c. 45% to 75% water

    d. 30% to 45% water

2. Of the following, which individual would have
the most body water:

    a. An elderly person

    b. An adult male

    c. A young child

    d. An infant

3. The total amount of water that most adults consume each day is:

    a. 1200–1500 mL/day

    b. 1500–2500 mL/ day

    c. 1000–2000 mL/day

    d. 2000–3000 mL/day

4. Insensible water loss is fluid lost from the body
via:

    a. The skin and stool

    b. The skin and lungs

    c. The kidneys and skin

    d. The stool and lungs

5. The fluid inside the cells is called:

    a. Extracellular fluid

    b. Intracellular fluid

    c. Interstitial fluid

    d. Intravascular fluid

6. The movement of water from one compartment
within the body to another is regulated by:

    a. Diffusion

    b. Fluid balance

    c. Osmosis

    d. Active transport

7. One of the simplest methods of objectively
assessing fluid balance is:

    a. Asking the client what his or her daily fluid
intake usually averages

    b. Asking the client to describe his or her daily
elimination patterns

    c. Comparing the amount of a client's fluid
intake with fluid output

    d. Summarizing the client's daily diet and
analyzing his or her fluid needs

8. The ratio of fluid intake and output for a
healthy adult is:

    a. Equal amounts of output and intake per day

    b. Twice as much intake as output per day

    c. Twice as much output as intake per day

    d. Two thirds as much output as intake per day

9. When weighing items to determine the client's
output, the criterion is:

    a. One pint (475 mL) of water weighs about 2
pounds (0.94 kg).

    b. One pint (475 mL) of water weighs about 1
pound (0.47 kg).

    c. One pint (475 mL) of water weighs about 1/2
pound (0.71 kg).

    d. One-half pint (237 mL) of water weighs about
1 pound (0.47 kg).

10. When a client is in fluid deficit, a typical sign is:

    a. Light-colored urine

    b. Frequent, moist bowel movements

    c. Warm, flushed, and dry skin

    d. Distended veins in the neck

11. The term for high volume, or amount, of water
present in the blood is:

    a. Hypovolemia

    b. Hypervolemia

    c. Dehydration

    d. Third spacing

12. When fluid becomes trapped in interstitial areas it is known as:
    a. Hypovolemia
    b. Hypervolemia
    c. Dehydration
    d. Third spacing

13. A priority nursing concern related to intravenous therapy is:
    a. That the physician has ordered the correct type of solution
    b. That the correct volume and rate have been ordered
    c. That the correct solution is infused
    d. That the correct equipment is used

14. A crystalloid solution is best described as:
    a. A mixture of water and molecules of protein that remains suspended in the solution
    b. A mixture of water and crystals in a higher concentration than that found in the body
    c. A mixture of water and crystals in a lower concentration than that found in the body
    d. A mixture of water and uniformly dissolved crystals, such as sugar and salt

15. When a hypotonic solution is infused intravenously, it will:
    a. Remain in the intravascular space
    b. Increase the size of the blood cells
    c. Decrease the size of the blood cells
    d. Thin the plasma of the blood

16. When a hypertonic solution is infused intravenously, it will:
    a. Remain in the intravascular space
    b. Increase the size of the blood cells
    c. Decrease the size of the blood cells
    d. Increase the volume of the blood

17. Intravenous solutions will flow into a vein via:
    a. Osmosis
    b. Active transport
    c. Gravity
    d. Diffusion

18. When colloid solutions are given intravenously, the needle size should be:
    a. 21 or 22 gauge
    b. 20 or 21 gauge
    c. 19 or 20 gauge
    d. 18 or 20 gauge

19. Unless there is a specific contraindication, the preferred site for venipuncture is:
    a. A vein on the inner aspect of the elbow
    b. A vein on the lateral aspect of the forearm
    c. A vein on the back of the hand
    d. A vein on the inner aspect of the forearm

20. The commonly accepted time frame for changing the intravenous solution is:
    a. Every 12 hours
    b. Every 18 hours
    c. Every 24 hours
    d. Every 48 hours

21. Unless otherwise ordered, the dressing over a venipuncture site should be changed every:
    a. 24 to 48 hours
    b. 24 to 72 hours
    c. 24 to 36 hours
    d. 12 to 24 hours

22. Swelling and coolness of the skin at the venipuncture site could be indicative of:
    a. Infiltration
    b. Phlebitis
    c. Infection
    d. Air embolism

23. Of the following actions, which should be done first when discontinuing an intravenous infusion:
    a. Apply pressure to the venipuncture site
    b. Remove the needle or catheter without hesitation
    c. Clamp the tubing and remove the tape at the site
    d. Apply antiseptic solution to the venipuncture site

24. Of the following, which is a plasma expander:
    a. Normal saline
    b. Dextran
    c. Dextrose
    d. Ringer's lactate

25. A vein often used for intravenous infusion in infants is:
    a. A vein on the foot
    b. A vein on the forearm
    c. A vein on the back of the hand
    d. A vein on the scalp

26. Of the following, which is a nonelectrolyte:
    a. Sodium
    b. Potassium
    c. Glucose
    d. Magnesium

27. The term for a positively charged ion is:
    a. Cation
    b. Anion
    c. Electrolyte
    d. Milliequivalent

28. The movement of ions from an area of greater concentration to an area of lesser concentration through a semipermeable membrane is called:
    a. Osmosis
    b. Active transport
    c. Diffusion
    d. Dialysis

29. A process of chemical distribution that requires energy to move molecules from an area of lesser concentration to an area of greater concentration through a semipermeable membrane is:
    a. Osmosis
    b. Active transport
    c. Diffusion
    d. Dialysis

30. The major cation in the intracellular fluid is:
    a. Sodium
    b. Chloride
    c. Magnesium
    d. Potassium

31. The chief extracellular anion is:
    a. Sodium
    b. Chloride
    c. Magnesium
    d. Potassium

32. A sealed chamber that provides a means for administering IV medications or solutions periodically is called:
    a. A blood administration unit
    b. A heparin lock
    c. An infusion pump
    d. A volumetric controller

33. The term *parenteral nutrition* refers to:
    a. A technique for providing nutrients through a nasogastric tube
    b. A technique for providing nutrients through the intestinal route
    c. A technique for providing nutrients through the intravenous route
    d. A technique for providing nutrients through an enteral route

34. Peripheral parenteral nutrition may be provided when oral intake is not possible but is expected to resume within:
    a. 7 to 10 days
    b. 10 to 14 days
    c. 14 to 21 days
    d. 21 to 28 days

35. A parenteral lipid emulsion is a mixture of:
    a. Milk, egg yolk, low-density lipids, vitamins, and glycerol
    b. Electrolytes, lipids, milk, egg whites, and glycerin
    c. Water, fat, egg yolk, phospholipids, and glycerin
    d. Water, protein, fat, calcium, and glycerol

■ Alternative Format Questions

1. A physician prescribes normal saline solution by IV to infuse at a rate of 1000 mL every 8 hours. Calculate the number of milliliters of solution the client will receive per hour.

2. A 75-year-old man is admitted to the hospital with GI bleeding. His hemoglobin was 7.0 g/dL. His physician ordered 2 U of packed red blood cells to infuse over a period of 1 hour each. The drip factor on the blood administration set is 10 gtt/mL. Calculate the flow rate in drops per minute.

3. The physician prescribed 25,000 U of heparin in 250 mL of normal saline to infuse at 800 U per hour. The nurse would set the infusion pump to deliver how many milliliters per hour?

■ True or False Questions

Directions: For items 1 through 20, decide if the statement is true or false and mark T or F in the space provided.

1. ____ The term for an electrolyte with a negative charge is cation.

2. ____ Diffusion is the movement of water through a semipermeable membrane from an area of lower concentration of dissolved substances to one of higher concentration.

3. ____ Serum is the synonym for plasma.

4. ____ Intracellular fluid is subdivided into two categories, the interstitial and the intravascular.

5. ____ Glucose is a nonelectrolyte.

6. ____ Most of the water in the body is lost as insensible water loss.

7. ____ Inadequate fluid intake can be the result of a poorly balanced diet.

8. ____ In most situations, it is sufficient to estimate the client's intake and output of fluids.

9. ____ Fluid output is the measurement of the urine excreted by the client.

10. ____ No single sign or symptom in itself necessarily indicates fluid imbalance.

11. ____ The skin is usually warm and flushed when the client is experiencing fluid excess.

12. ____ The consumption of salty foods does not usually affect the intake and retention of fluids.

13. ____ The nurse may independently order and implement measures that replace fluid loss by increasing the client's oral fluid intake.

14. ____ Sodium is the most abundant electrolyte in the intracellular fluid.

15. ____ Intravenous solutions should always be considered a medication.

16. ____ Unvented tubing can be used when administering an IV solution from a glass container.

17. ____ An IV solution must be elevated at least 18 to 24 inches above the venipuncture site because the pressure in the client's vein is higher than the atmospheric pressure.

18. ____ An angiocath is a flexible catheter threaded through a needle into a vein.

19. ____ A colloid solution is a mixture of water and molecules of protein that remain suspended in the solution and do not become dissolved.

20. ____ Cross-matching is the laboratory test that identifies the proteins on red blood cells.

■ Short Answer Questions

Directions: Read each of the following statements and supply the word(s) necessary in the space provided.

1. Identify eight factors that should be considered when selecting a vein for an intravenous infusion, as suggested in this chapter.

   a. _____

   _____

   b. _____

   _____

   c. _____

   _____

   d. _____

   _____

   e. _____

   _____

   f. _____

   _____

   g. _____

   _____

   h. _____

   _____

2. Describe the steps suggested in this chapter for cleansing the venipuncture site.

   a. _____

   _____

   b. _____

   _____

   c. _____

   _____

3. Identify five signs of complications that may occur when a client is receiving intravenous fluids.

   a. _____

   _____

   b. _____

   _____

   c. _____

   _____

   d. _____

   _____

   e. _____

   _____

4. State three techniques for promoting vein distention in order to start an intravenous infusion.

   a. _____

   _____

   b. _____

   _____

   c. _____

   _____

5. List four types of blood products and state the purpose of administration for each.

   Blood Product   Purpose for Administration

   a. _____

   _____

   b. _____

   _____

   c. _____

   _____

   d. _____

   _____

■ Critical Thinking Exercises

The following are practice situations for calculating intravenous infusion rates. Read each statement carefully, state the formula, and compute the rate of flow.

1. A physician orders 1000 mL of solution to be infused over a 4-hour period. Calculate the number of milliliters to be given per hour.

2. The drop factor in the previous situation is 15 drops equal 1 mL. Calculate the number of drops per minute using the amounts in the order given in Question 1.

3. A physician has ordered 2000 mL of solution to be infused over a 24-hour period. Calculate the number of milliliters to be given per hour.

4. Using the information from Question 3, calculate the number of drops per minute when the administration set has a drop factor of 20 drops equal 1 mL.

5. The nurse notes that a client's IV has slowed after 3 hours have passed. He was to receive 3000 mL over a 24-hour period at 42 drops per minute, with a set having a drop factor of 20 drops equal 1 mL. Only 200 mL of the solution has infused, instead of the scheduled 375 mL. A total of 2800 ml remains to be infused. Calculate the new volume per hour.

6. Calculate the new rate of flow for the situation described in Question 5.

Performance Checklist

This section allows you to examine your techniques for controlling oral fluid intake.

1. Place a check mark in the "S" ("satisfactory") column if you used the recommended technique.
2. Place a check mark in the "NI" ("needs improvement") column if you used some but not all of each recommended technique.
3. Place a check mark in the "U" ("unsatisfactory") column if you forgot to include that particular recommended technique.
4. Note when further practice is indicated, what errors you made, suggestions that will improve your skills, and so on in the section for comments.

RECOMMENDED TECHNIQUE	S	NI	U	Comments
Fluid-Intake Increase				
Identify the client	☐	☐	☐	_____
Verify the physician's order	☐	☐	☐	_____
Keep fluids handy at the bedside at all times	☐	☐	☐	_____
Offer a variety of fluids (allow the client to choose what he or she likes, if possible)	☐	☐	☐	_____
Set goals with the client for the amount of fluid to take	☐	☐	☐	_____
Offer foods, as permitted, having high water content	☐	☐	☐	_____
Serve fluids at their proper temperatures	☐	☐	☐	_____
Offer proportionately more fluids early in the day	☐	☐	☐	_____
Fluid-Intake Decrease				
Keep fluids out of sight as much as possible	☐	☐	☐	_____
Use small containers for serving fluids	☐	☐	☐	_____
Avoid serving foods that tend to increase thirst	☐	☐	☐	_____
Set goals with the client for spacing allowable fluids	☐	☐	☐	_____
Use various techniques to maintain good oral hygiene	☐	☐	☐	_____
Offer ice chips, as allowed	☐	☐	☐	_____

B. This section allows you to examine your techniques for initiating an intravenous infusion.

RECOMMENDED TECHNIQUE	S	NI	U	Comments
Identify the client	☐	☐	☐	_____
Verify the physician's order	☐	☐	☐	_____
Explain the procedure	☐	☐	☐	_____

RECOMMENDED TECHNIQUE	S	NI	U	Comments
Assemble appropriate equipment and supplies, including the solution	☐	☐	☐	_____
Wash hands	☐	☐	☐	_____
Select an appropriate and accessible vein for injecting	☐	☐	☐	_____
Use appropriate techniques when a vein can not be felt: Have the client lower his or her arm and make a fist—open and close fist	☐	☐	☐	_____
Gently tap over the vein	☐	☐	☐	_____
Place warm, moist compresses on the vein	☐	☐	☐	_____
Stroke the skin toward the fingers	☐	☐	☐	_____
Place the arm on a supportive surface	☐	☐	☐	_____
Tie the tourniquet 2 to 4 inches above the site of entry, with its ends away from the site, and clean the site correctly	☐	☐	☐	_____
Put on clean gloves	☐	☐	☐	_____
Stabilize the vein and soft tissue with the thumb 2 inches below the site of entry	☐	☐	☐	_____
Hold the needle, bevel side up, at a 45° angle above or to the side of the vein	☐	☐	☐	_____
Pierce the vein and insert the needle about 1/8 to 1/4 inch	☐	☐	☐	_____
When blood comes back through the needle, release the tourniquet and start the flow of solution	☐	☐	☐	_____
Support and secure the catheter in place and adjust the flow of solution to the prescribed rate	☐	☐	☐	_____
Monitor the intravenous infusion regularly and regulate the rate of flow as necessary	☐	☐	☐	_____
Observe the client for complications and report unusual signs or symptoms promptly	☐	☐	☐	_____
Discontinue the infusion properly when the prescribed amount of solution has entered the vein	☐	☐	☐	_____

C. This section allows you to examine your techniques for assisting with a blood transfusion.

RECOMMENDED TECHNIQUE	S	NI	U	Comments
Identify the client	☐	☐	☐	_____
Take the client's vital signs within 30 minutes of obtaining blood	☐	☐	☐	_____
Check and double-check with another person to be sure the proper blood is to be given to the correct client	☐	☐	☐	_____

RECOMMENDED TECHNIQUE	S	NI	U	Comments
Check to see that the blood has not passed its expiration date	☐	☐	☐	_____
Be ready and prepared to give the blood as soon as it arrives from the blood bank	☐	☐	☐	_____
Rotate the blood to mix the red blood cells; do not warm the blood	☐	☐	☐	_____
At the bedside, check the information on the blood bag with client information with another nurse	☐	☐	☐	_____
Start the blood flow and turn off the saline solution	☐	☐	☐	_____
Give the blood slowly; remain with the client for at least 15 minutes. Observe for signs of a reaction (rate 50 mL per hour for the first 15 minutes)	☐	☐	☐	_____
If no signs of a reaction appear, increase the speed of flow to complete the infusion in 2 to 4 hours	☐	☐	☐	_____
Continue to observe the client for a reaction and stop giving blood when any sign of a reaction appears	☐	☐	☐	_____
Assessments are done at 15- to 30-minute intervals during the transfusion	☐	☐	☐	_____
Discontinue the blood transfusion in the same manner as an intravenous infusion when the blood has infused	☐	☐	☐	_____

D. This section allows you to examine your techniques for changing solution containers.

RECOMMENDED TECHNIQUE	S	NI	U	Comments
Determine that the solution to replace the current infusion is available	☐	☐	☐	_____
Identify the client	☐	☐	☐	_____
Wash your hands	☐	☐	☐	_____
Switch the containers when the infusing container is almost empty and the drip chamber still contains fluid	☐	☐	☐	_____
Close the regulator on the tubing	☐	☐	☐	_____
Remove the empty container and tubing from the standard	☐	☐	☐	_____
Pull the spike from the current container without touching the tip	☐	☐	☐	_____
Remove the seal from the replacement solution	☐	☐	☐	_____
Immediately insert the spike into the replacement container	☐	☐	☐	_____
Hang the new solution	☐	☐	☐	_____

RECOMMENDED TECHNIQUE	S	NI	U	Comments
Inspect for the presence of air in the tubing and remove it	☐	☐	☐	_____
Readjust the rate to the ordered or scheduled rate	☐	☐	☐	_____
Record the volume of infused solution	☐	☐	☐	_____
Record the addition of the new solution	☐	☐	☐	_____

E. This section allows you to examine your techniques for changing infusion tubing.

RECOMMENDED TECHNIQUE	S	NI	U	Comments
Obtain sterile infusion tubing like that being currently used	☐	☐	☐	_____
Wash your hands	☐	☐	☐	_____
Tighten the regulator clamp on the replacement tubing	☐	☐	☐	_____
Remove the solution container from the standard	☐	☐	☐	_____
Remove the outdated spike and replace it with the fresh, sterile spike using sterile technique	☐	☐	☐	_____
Replace the solution on the standard	☐	☐	☐	_____
Compress the drip chamber to fill it approximately 1/2 full	☐	☐	☐	_____
Remove the protective cap from the other end and clear the tubing of air by loosening the regulator	☐	☐	☐	_____
Close the regulator and replace the protective cap	☐	☐	☐	_____
Peel back or remove the dressing over the venipuncture site	☐	☐	☐	_____
Put on clean gloves	☐	☐	☐	_____
Disconnect the outdated tubing while holding the venipuncture device firmly	☐	☐	☐	_____
Remove the protective cap and attach the fresh, sterile tubing to the venipuncture device	☐	☐	☐	_____
Loosen the regulator clamp and readjust the rate of flow	☐	☐	☐	_____
Replace the dressing and secure the tubing	☐	☐	☐	_____
Label the tubing with the current date and time	☐	☐	☐	_____
Record the procedure on the correct form	☐	☐	☐	_____

F. This section allows you to examine your techniques for inserting an intermittent venous access device.

RECOMMENDED TECHNIQUE	S	NI	U	Comments
Confirm the medication order to discontinue the continuous intravenous drip and insert a medication lock	☐	☐	☐	_____
Inspect the site to determine if it can be maintained or if a new site is needed	☐	☐	☐	_____
Assemble the necessary equipment	☐	☐	☐	_____
Explain the process to the client	☐	☐	☐	_____
Wash your hands	☐	☐	☐	_____
Prefill the chamber of the medication lock with saline or heparin	☐	☐	☐	_____
Loosen tape and expose the connection between the hub of the catheter and the tubing adapter	☐	☐	☐	_____
Loosen the protective cap from the end of the medication lock	☐	☐	☐	_____
Wear clean gloves	☐	☐	☐	_____
Tighten the roller clamp to close or stop the infusion pump	☐	☐	☐	_____
Apply pressure over the catheter tip. Remove the tip of the tubing from the venipuncture device and insert the medication lock.	☐	☐	☐	_____
Swab the rubber port on the medication lock with alcohol	☐	☐	☐	_____
Gradually instill 2 mL of saline or heparin	☐	☐	☐	_____
Retape and secure the dressing	☐	☐	☐	_____
Flush the lock with 1 or 2 mL of either saline or heparin flush solution after each use or at least every 8 hours	☐	☐	☐	_____
Document assessment data, flush solution, discontinuation of continuous intravenous solution, volume infused, date, time, and insertion of the medication lock	☐	☐	☐	_____

CHAPTER 16

Hygiene

■ Summary

Emphasis in this chapter is placed on nursing measures to promote personal hygiene. Personal cleanliness is an essential part of one's health care practices. When the individual is unable to care for himself or herself, the nurse must possess the skills necessary to provide this aspect of care. The nurse functions in this area as a role model and health care teacher. She must assist the client to differentiate between what is fact and what is fiction while continuing to be supportive of the client's individual method of maintaining personal hygiene.

■ Matching Questions

Directions: For items 1 through 6, match the definitions in Part B with the terms in Part A:

PART A

1. ____ Bridge

2. ____ Caries

3. ____ Gingivitis

4. ____ Plaque

5. ____ Sordes

6. ____ Tartar

PART B

a. Hardened plaque

b. Inflammation of the gums

c. Mucin and grit in saliva

d. Dental appliance

e. Cavities

f. Baby teeth

g. Dried crust on the upper lips

Directions: The following substances may be used for oral care for items 7 through 10. Match the uses in Part B with the substances in Part A.

PART A

7. ____ Antiseptic mouthwash

8. ____ Hydrogen peroxide and water

9. ____ Lemon and glycerin swabs

10. ____ Petroleum jelly

PART B

a. Reduces oral acidity

b. Increases salivation

c. Reduces bacterial growth

d. Removes accumulated secretions

e. Loosens dry, sticky particles

f. Lubricates lips

■ Multiple-Choice Questions

Directions: For items 1 through 14, circle the letter that corresponds to the best answer for each question.

1. The primary concern for nurses when assisting the client with hygiene is:

   a. Personal care does not have to be carried out in an identical fashion for all

   b. Personal care should be carried out in a manner that promotes health for the individual

   c. The exact procedures as prescribed by the health agency must be followed when promoting hygiene

   d. The way in which personal care is promoted is not important, only that it must be done for the client

2. The skin is the main component of which of the following systems:
   a. The immune system
   b. The muscular system
   c. The endocrine system
   d. The integumentary system

3. The oral hygiene practice recommended to break up bacteria lodged between the teeth is:
   a. Using dental floss between the teeth
   b. Directing a jet spray between the teeth
   c. Rinsing the mouth vigorously with a mouthwash
   d. Using an electric toothbrush regularly

4. Of the following procedures, which should be done first when toenails are thick and difficult to cut:
   a. File the rough edges first
   b. Soak the feet in warm water
   c. Massage a cream into the nails
   d. Apply an antiseptic to the nails

5. Which of the following is recommended when grooming hair that is tangled:
   a. Use a fine-tooth comb and start at the ends of the hair
   b. Use a wide-tooth comb and start near the scalp
   c. Use a fine-tooth comb and start near the scalp
   d. Use a wide-tooth comb and start from the ends of the hair

6. Which of the following types of glands found in the skin are responsible for regulating body temperature:
   a. Sudoriferous
   b. Ceruminous
   c. Sebaceous
   d. Ciliary

7. Immersion of the buttocks and perineum in a small basin of continuously circulating water is called a:
   a. Sponge bath
   b. Whirlpool bath
   c. Sitz bath
   d. Medicated bath

8. Of the following substances, which can be used for oral care to reduce oral acidity, dissolve plaque, and soothe oral lesions?
   a. Petroleum jelly
   b. Milk of magnesia
   c. Hydrogen peroxide
   d. Lemon and glycerin

9. An accumulation of cerumen within the ear may cause which of the following sound disturbances for clients with a hearing aid?
   a. Garbled sound
   b. Shrill feedback
   c. Increased noise
   d. Reduced sound

10. The temperature of the water for a tub bath should be:
    a. 105° to 110°F
    b. 110° to 115°F
    c. 90° to 105°F
    d. 100° to 105°F

11. The outermost layer of the skin is called:
    a. The dermis
    b. The keratin layer
    c. The epidermis
    d. The subcutaneous layer

12. In humans, the teeth begin to erupt at which of the following ages?
    a. 6 months of age
    b. 12 months of age
    c. 18 months of age
    d. 24 months of age

13. The term *gingivitis* refers to:
    a. Tooth decay
    b. Hardened plaque
    c. Inflammation of the jaws
    d. Inflammation of the gums

14. The term *partial bath* refers to:
    a. Washing the area around the client's genitals and rectum only
    b. Washing in a manner to remove secretions and excretions from less-soiled to more-soiled areas
    c. Washing areas of the body that are subject to the greatest soiling or odor
    d. Washing all areas of the body at the sink in the client's room

■ Alternative Format Questions

1. All of the following nursing interventions are appropriate when providing the client with a tub bath. Place them in the order in which they would normally be carried out.
   1. Consult the Kardex to verify the type of bath
   2. Clean the tub
   3. Assist the client to the bathing area
   4. Client remains uninjured
   5. Document assessment data
   6. Identify the client

2. A newly admitted client is found to have tinea capitis. Which of the following nursing interventions would be appropriate for this condition? Select all that apply:
   1. Avoid the use of oily cosmetics
   2. Avoid skin-to-skin contact
   3. Keep body areas dry—especially skin folds
   4. Wear clothing that promotes evaporation of perspiration
   5. Wear leather shoes and alternate pairs to reduce damp shoe conditions

3. Which of the following are effects of the use of lemon and glycerin swabs for oral care? Select all that apply:
   1. Lubricates lips
   2. Increases salivation
   3. Reduces oral acidity
   4. Refreshes the mouth
   5. Dissolves plaque

■ True or False Questions

Directions: For items 1 through 12, decide if the statement is true or false and mark T or F in the space provided.

1. ____ It is safe to assume that clients with glasses are not also wearing contact lenses.

2. ____ Many health care agencies require that routine hygienic care be recorded in the nurse's notes.

3. ____ A dental bridge is a prosthesis.

4. ____ The nurse does not have to be tolerant of personal hygiene preferences when the client is in the hospital.

5. ____ Ceruminous glands secrete cerumen, a wax-like substance found in the external ear.

6. ____ Hot water should be used when soaking a client's dentures.

7. ____ A physician's order should be obtained before cutting the toenails of clients with diabetes or vascular disease.

8. ____ The use of preparations made with oil will help loosen tangled hair.

9. ____ The subcutaneous layer separates the skin from skeletal muscle.

10. ____ Goblet cells located within the hair follicles release an oily substance called sebum.

11. ____ The texture, elasticity, and porosity of hair are inherited characteristics.

12. ____ Fingernails and toenails acquire their tough texture from keratin.

■ Short Answer Questions

Directions: Read each of the following statements and supply the word(s) necessary in the space provided.

1. List four of the functions of the skin (as suggested in this chapter).

   a. _____

   _____

b. _____

_____

c. _____

_____

d. _____

_____

2. List four characteristics of healthy nails.

a. _____

_____

b. _____

_____

c. _____

_____

d. _____

3. The usual number of permanent teeth in an adult mouth is _____.

4. List four benefits of bathing.

a. _____

_____

b. _____

_____

c. _____

_____

d. _____

_____

■ Critical Thinking Exercises

1. Complete the form below by writing a teaching plan for a client in each situation. List points to discuss in the teaching plan.

2. Review the nursing care plan included in this chapter. Recall an individual to whom you have recently been assigned. Using the components of the nursing process, develop a plan of care to meet the personal hygiene needs of this individual. Ask your clinical instructor to assist you.

Topic for Teaching	Points to Cover in a Teaching Plan
Measures to promote personal hygiene when the client is a diabetic	
The prevention of tooth and gum diseases	
Promoting personal hygiene when the client is cared for at home	

Performance Checklist

This section allows you to examine your techniques for assisting the client with personal hygiene.

1. Place a check mark in the "S" ("satisfactory") column if you used the recommended technique.
2. Place a check mark in the "NI" ("needs improvement") column if you used some but not all of each recommended technique.
3. Place a check mark in the "U" ("unsatisfactory") column if you forgot to include that particular recommended technique.
4. Note when further practice is indicated, what errors you made, suggestions that will improve your skills, and so on in the section for comments.

RECOMMENDED TECHNIQUE	S	NI	U	Comments
The Bed Bath				
Bring necessary equipment to the bedside and place the client flat in bed with one pillow under his or her head	☐	☐	☐	_____
Remove the top bed linens and cover the client with a bath blanket; care for linens appropriately	☐	☐	☐	_____
Wash your hands	☐	☐	☐	_____
Move the client to the side of the bed near you	☐	☐	☐	_____
Wash, rinse, and dry each body part well and in a logical and convenient order	☐	☐	☐	_____
Fold the washcloth like a mitt or in such a way that there are no loose ends	☐	☐	☐	_____
Make washcloth wet enough to wash, lather, and rinse well but not so wet that it drips water	☐	☐	☐	_____
Do not leave the bar of soap in the water				
Use gentle but firm, long strokes when washing, rinsing, and drying the client	☐	☐	☐	_____
Pay particular attention to areas where skin surfaces touch each other	☐	☐	☐	_____
Change bath water as recommended and also if it becomes too soapy or cool	☐	☐	☐	_____
Soak the client's hands in the bathwater as part of the bathing procedure	☐	☐	☐	_____
Protect bed linens as necessary while bathing various body parts	☐	☐	☐	_____
Use modifications of the bed-bath procedure as indicated	☐	☐	☐	_____

RECOMMENDED TECHNIQUE	S	NI	U	Comments

Oral Hygiene: Self-Help Client

Provide the necessary equipment and supplies so that the client may brush and floss his or her teeth   ☐ ☐ ☐   _____

Oral Hygiene: Helpless Client

Place the client on his or her side with his or her head slightly lowered   ☐ ☐ ☐   _____

Put on gloves   ☐ ☐ ☐   _____

Clean and rinse the mouth, lips, and teeth appropriately and floss the teeth as indicated   ☐ ☐ ☐   _____

Use suction as indicated to prevent the client from aspirating   ☐ ☐ ☐   _____

Lubricate the mouth and lips as indicated   ☐ ☐ ☐   _____

Care of Dentures

Put on gloves   ☐ ☐ ☐   _____

Assist the client to remove and replace dentures as necessary   ☐ ☐ ☐   _____

Care for the dentures over a basin of water or soft surface   ☐ ☐ ☐   _____

Scrub and rinse all surfaces of the dentures thoroughly with appropriate equipment   ☐ ☐ ☐   _____

Store dentures safely and appropriately when they are not being worn   ☐ ☐ ☐   _____

Nail and Hair Care

Groom and clean the fingernails and, if ordered, the toenails with gentleness   ☐ ☐ ☐   _____

Use appropriate equipment to avoid injuries when caring for the nails   ☐ ☐ ☐   _____

Protect the pillow before caring for the hair   ☐ ☐ ☐   _____

Arrange the hair with a proper comb and brush; braid the hair if necessary   ☐ ☐ ☐   _____

See to it that the client's brush and comb are kept clean   ☐ ☐ ☐   _____

Shampoo the client's hair properly, using procedures and equipment recommended by the health agency   ☐ ☐ ☐   _____

Perineal Care: Self-Help Client

Provide the client with proper equipment and supplies for self-care of the perineal area   ☐ ☐ ☐   _____

See to it that the client's privacy is protected while he or she gives himself or herself care   ☐ ☐ ☐   _____

RECOMMENDED TECHNIQUE	S	NI	U	Comments

Perineal Care: Helpless Client

	S	NI	U	
Place the client on a bedpan or protect the bed linens properly when a bedpan is not used	☐	☐	☐	_____
Wear gloves for the procedure or handle supplies with a forceps	☐	☐	☐	_____
Use cotton balls, soap solution, and clear water; thoroughly scrub and rinse the area	☐	☐	☐	_____
Clean the anal area after turning the client to his or her side	☐	☐	☐	_____
Be careful to clean the area well at the foreskin and between the labia	☐	☐	☐	_____
Dry the client; use protective lotion or powder as indicated	☐	☐	☐	_____

CHAPTER 17

Comfort, Rest, and Sleep

■ Summary

Modifying the environment to promote comfort while providing sufficient sensory stimulation and privacy is a major nursing concern. The term environment, as it is used here, refers to the room where the client receives care and the furnishings within it. When the environment is clean, safe, comfortable, and attractive, it can contribute to a sense of well-being and promote rest and recovery. However, no matter how pleasant and comfortable the physical environment or how attractive and homelike the furnishings, recuperation may not occur if the client is unable to rest or sleep.

The need for relief of sleeplessness is among the most common problems clients present. While certain drug therapy may often be indicated, its use does not eliminate the need for high-quality nursing care. Nursing measures for these clients should include actions to promote relaxation and sleep. These measures, accompanied by a description of the characteristics of relaxation and sleep, are presented in this chapter.

■ Matching Questions

Directions: For items 1 through 6, match the descriptions in Part B with the techniques in Part A.

PART A

1. ____ Effleurage

2. ____ Petrissage

3. ____ Frôlement

4. ____ Tapotement

5. ____ Vibration

6. ____ Friction

PART B

a. To brush

b. To set in motion

c. To tap

d. To knead

e. To rub

f. To skim the surface

Directions: For items 7 through 11, match the characteristics in Part B with the stages of sleep in Part A.

PART A

7. ____ Stage 1 NREM

8. ____ Stage 2 NREM

9. ____ Stage 3 NREM

10. ____ Stage 4 NREM

11. ____ REM

PART B

a. Deep sleep; parasomnias occur

b. Vivid, colorful, emotional dreams; very difficult to awaken; pauses in breathing for 15 to 20 seconds

c. Light sleep; easily aroused

d. Early phase of deep sleep; relaxed, no physical movement; difficult to arouse

e. Deep relaxation; can be awakened with effort

■ Multiple-Choice Questions

Directions: For items 1 through 20, circle the letter that corresponds to the best answer for each question.

1. In order for sleep to occur, which of the following is necessary:
   a. The person must be tired
   b. The person must be in a relaxed state
   c. The person must be in a recumbent position
   d. The person must be in comfortable clothing

2. Phenomena that occur every 24 hours are called:
   a. Biorhythms
   b. Ultradian rhythms
   c. Infradian rhythms
   d. Circadian rhythms

3. Sleep is characterized by:
   a. A state of drowsiness and decreased activity
   b. A state of decreased activity and mental stimulation
   c. A state of arousable unconsciousness
   d. A state of emotional rest and excessive sleepiness

4. In which stage of sleep do dreams most often occur:
   a. REM sleep
   b. Stage 2 NREM sleep
   c. Stage 3 NREM sleep
   d. Stage 4 NREM sleep

5. When an individual with insomnia cannot fall asleep within 20 minutes after getting into bed at night, it would be best to:
   a. Stay in bed and concentrate on going to sleep
   b. Stay in bed another 20 minutes and then take a sleeping pill
   c. Not worry about the situation and sleep longer in the morning
   d. Get out of bed and do something else that is quiet, such as reading

6. Of the following colors, which promotes feelings of coolness and relaxation:
   a. Blue and brown
   b. Green and brown
   c. Blue and green
   d. Orange and green

7. Select the room temperature range that is comfortable for most people:
   a. 16° to 21°C (60° to 70°F)
   b. 18° to 24°C (65° to 75°F)
   c. 20° to 23°C (68° to 74°F)
   d. 21° to 25°C (70° to 78°F)

8. All of the following are true about the rapid eye movement phase of sleep except:
   a. It is also called paradoxical sleep because EEG waves are similar to those during wakefulness
   b. It is the lightest stage of sleep
   c. It is a period of active sleep
   d. Eye movements during this phase of sleep are energetic

9. Sleepwalking and bed-wetting usually occur during which stage or phase of sleep:
   a. Stage 4 NREM sleep
   b. Stage 3 NREM sleep
   c. Stage 2 NREM sleep
   d. REM sleep

10. Secretion of the hormone melatonin is triggered by:
    a. Activity
    b. Bright light
    c. Darkness
    d. The environment

11. The term *photoperiod* refers to:
    a. A technique for stimulating light receptors in the eye
    b. A technique for inducing sleep for persons with insomnia
    c. The number of times light therapy can be used effectively
    d. The number of daylight hours to which a person is accustomed

12. Seasonal affective disorder occurs during:
    a. The fall
    b. The winter
    c. The spring
    d. The summer

13. The best sources of L-tryptophan are:
    a. Protein foods and dairy products
    b. Shellfish and vegetables
    c. Dairy products and fruits
    d. Protein foods and legumes

14. Narcolepsy is a condition characterized by:
    a. Excessive anxiety
    b. Excessive sleeping
    c. Excessive fatigue
    d. Excessive sleepiness

15. It is appropriate for a newborn to sleep:
    a. 16 to 20 hours per 24-hour period
    b. 10 to 16 hours in addition to two or three naps
    c. 10 to 12 hours in addition to one or two naps
    d. 8 to 10 hours in addition to one nap or rest period

16. Five- and 6-year-olds spend which of the following percentages in REM sleep:
    a. 50%
    b. 35%
    c. 25%
    d. 20%

17. In severe cases of sleep apnea, which of the following techniques are recommended:
    a. Suggest the individual wear a sleep collar at night
    b. Awaken the individual to restore breathing
    c. Give the individual carbon dioxide before bedtime
    d. Suggest the individual wear a special breathing mask at night

18. Parasomnias are best described as:
    a. Bedtime rituals
    b. Relaxation techniques
    c. Therapeutic use of exercises for sleep
    d. Activities that occur during sleep

19. Nocturnal myoclonus is synonymous with:
    a. Restless leg syndrome
    b. Sleepwalking
    c. Hypopnea syndrome
    d. Bed-wetting

20. All of the following are characteristics of the sundown syndrome except:
    a. Being alert and oriented in the evening
    b. Having disorganized thinking
    c. Feeling restless
    d. Wandering

▪ Alternative Format Questions

1. Alcohol is a depressive drug that promotes sleep. However, its effectiveness is reduced by which of the following? Select all that apply:
   1. Metabolism releases chemicals that block its sedative effects
   2. It causes wakefulness in certain individuals
   3. It reduces normal REM sleep
   4. It causes early awakening
   5. It reduces deep stages of NREM sleep

2. The nurse is caring for a client with a hiatal hernia. The client complains of abdominal pain and sternal pain after eating. The pain makes it difficult for him to sleep. Which of the following instructions should the nurse recommend when teaching this client? Select all that apply:
   1. Avoid constrictive clothing
   2. Lie down for 30 minutes after eating
   3. Decrease intake of caffeine and spicy foods
   4. Eat three meals a day
   5. Sleep in semi-Fowler's position
   6. Maintain a normal body weight

3. A client tells his nurse that he has been taking barbiturate sleeping pills every night for several months. He now wishes to stop taking them. The nurse should advise the client to do the following. Select all that apply:
   1. Continue taking the pills because he will not be able to sleep without them
   2. Take his last pill on a Friday night so he can catch up with sleep on the weekend
   3. Initially skip one pill every third night
   4. Discontinue the pills all at once
   5. Taper his pill intake to every other night before completely stopping the pills

■ True or False Questions

Directions: For items 1 through 10, decide if the statement is true or false and mark T or F in the space provided.

1. ____ During sleep, individuals pass back and forth through the phases and stages of sleep.

2. ____ Snoring occurs during stage 3 NREM sleep.

3. ____ During REM sleep, 15- to 20-second pauses in breathing are normal.

4. ____ Based on current research, REM sleep always precedes NREM sleep.

5. ____ Shift workers have little difficulty adjusting their sleep–wake cycles because indoor lighting is sufficient to suppress melatonin.

6. ____ The term phototherapy refers to a technique for suppressing melatonin by stimulating light receptors in the eye.

7. ____ Symptoms associated with seasonal affective disorder spontaneously disappear as the amount of daylight increases.

8. ____ L-tryptophan is known to facilitate sleep.

9. ____ Tranquilizers are drugs that induce sleep.

10. ____ The incidence of sleep apnea is highest among middle-aged women who snore.

■ Short Answer Questions

Directions: Read each of the following statements and supply the word(s) necessary in the space provided.

1. List four of the components of phototherapy used to relieve the symptoms of seasonal affective disorder as discussed in this chapter.

   a. _____

   _____

   b. _____

   _____

   c. _____

_____

d. _____

_____

2. Identify five tips for client teaching to promote sleep.

   a. _____

   _____

   b. _____

   c. _____

   _____

   d. _____

   _____

   e. _____

   _____

3. State five tips for client teaching related to facilitating the use of progressive relaxation.

   a. _____

   _____

   b. _____

   _____

   c. _____

   _____

   d. _____

   _____

   e. _____

   _____

■ Critical Thinking Exercises

1. Recall an occasion when your sleep was disturbed and you were unable to get as much sleep as you generally need. How did this affect your productivity, ability to concentrate on necessary tasks, relationships, and mood? Draw on this experience to understand how clients with sleep alterations are handicapped.

   Discuss measures nurses can take to promote rest and sleep. Use this experience to project the effect of chronic sleep deprivation on your professional practice.

2. Visit a residential care setting and use observation and interview techniques to identify factors that are compromising the rest and sleep of the residents. Strategize about how the environment and nursing care could be modified to minimize these factors.

3. Describe adjustments you make when promoting rest and sleep in special situations:

a. When the client is an infant or child

b. When the client is elderly

4. Prepare a teaching plan for each of the following topics:

Topic for Teaching	Points to Cover in a Teaching Plan
Sleep and its role in well-being, including the amount required by a variety of age groups	
Drugs used to promote sleep	

Performance Checklist

This section allows you to examine your techniques for maintaining the client's environment.

1. Place a check mark in the "S" ("satisfactory") column if you used the recommended technique.
2. Place a check mark in the "NI" ("needs improvement") column if you used some but not all of each recommended technique.
3. Place a check mark in the "U" ("unsatisfactory") column if you forgot to include that particular recommended technique.
4. Note when further practice is indicated, what errors you made, suggestions that will improve your skills, and so on in the section for comments.

RECOMMENDED TECHNIQUE	S	NI	U	Comments
The Room				
Has attractive and practical floor and wall coverings and wall accessories	☐	☐	☐	_____
Provides good lighting for the client and for health workers	☐	☐	☐	_____
Has provisions for regulating temperature, humidity, and ventilation				
Has features so that privacy is ensured	☐	☐	☐	_____
Has an adjustable bed with an over-the-bed table	☐	☐	☐	_____
Has several pillows and a mattress that is sufficiently firm to provide good body alignment	☐	☐	☐	_____
Has chairs that are comfortable and convenient for the client and visitors				
Has personal care items and a bedside stand available	☐	☐	☐	_____
Has diversionary items, such as a television, radio, and telephone	☐	☐	☐	_____
To Provide Privacy				
Use cubicle drapes and screens appropriately	☐	☐	☐	_____
Close room door when giving care	☐	☐	☐	_____
Drape client appropriately when giving care	☐	☐	☐	_____
Provide privacy when the client uses a bedpan or urinal	☐	☐	☐	_____
Knock before entering a room	☐	☐	☐	_____
Help visitors find the client they wish to visit	☐	☐	☐	_____

RECOMMENDED TECHNIQUE	S	NI	U	Comments

To Control Noise

RECOMMENDED TECHNIQUE	S	NI	U	Comments
Handle equipment as quietly as possible; handle dinnerware and trays quietly	☐	☐	☐	_____
Answer telephone promptly and speak in a normal tone of voice	☐	☐	☐	_____
Avoid calling down corridors	☐	☐	☐	_____
Avoid laughing and chatting in corridors and lounges	☐	☐	☐	_____
Limit reporting to the nurses' station and conference rooms	☐	☐	☐	_____
Help keep television sets and radios at a low volume	☐	☐	☐	_____

To Control Odors

RECOMMENDED TECHNIQUE	S	NI	U	Comments
Discard waste and refuse promptly	☐	☐	☐	_____
Empty bedpans, urinals, and emesis basins promptly	☐	☐	☐	_____
Remove leftover food from rooms promptly	☐	☐	☐	_____
Use personal grooming measures for yourself and for clients to prevent unpleasant odors	☐	☐	☐	_____

B. Examine your techniques when stripping and making an unoccupied bed and complete the following form.

RECOMMENDED TECHNIQUE	S	NI	U	Comments
Bring hamper to the bedside	☐	☐	☐	_____
Avoid touching uniform with soiled linens and avoid shaking linens during the procedure	☐	☐	☐	_____
Bring necessary linens to the bedside and arrange them in order of their use on clean furniture	☐	☐	☐	_____
Assist the client from the bed	☐	☐	☐	_____
Place the bed in the high position and drop bed side rails	☐	☐	☐	_____
Put on gloves as necessary	☐	☐	☐	_____
Loosen linens while moving around the bed	☐	☐	☐	_____
Roll all soiled linens snugly in the bottom sheet and place them directly into the hamper	☐	☐	☐	_____
Remove gloves and wash your hands	☐	☐	☐	_____
Place bottom linens on the bed, one piece at a time, and unfold them in place after centering them	☐	☐	☐	_____
Secure bottom linens in place	☐	☐	☐	_____
Center and unfold top linens on the bed; secure them well but allow for toe room	☐	☐	☐	_____

RECOMMENDED TECHNIQUE	S	NI	U	Comments
Cover pillows and position them properly on the bed	☐	☐	☐	_____
Place the signal device so that it is conveniently located for use	☐	☐	☐	_____
Examine your technique when assisting the client with a sleep disturbance	☐	☐	☐	_____
Know the client's diagnosis and usual patterns of sleep	☐	☐	☐	_____
Provide for an environment that promotes sleep	☐	☐	☐	_____
Allow the client to observe usual bedtime habits to the extent possible	☐	☐	☐	_____
Remove causes of restlessness and sleeplessness, such as pain, and use techniques to help with relaxation	☐	☐	☐	_____
Take steps to avoid waking a sleeping client	☐	☐	☐	_____
Use prescribed medications for restlessness and sleeplessness judiciously	☐	☐	☐	_____
Consult others for assistance with the care of the restless and sleepless client, as necessary	☐	☐	☐	_____
Record techniques you have found helpful when assisting the restless and sleepless client	☐	☐	☐	_____
Document date, time, assessment data, and care according to agency requirements	☐	☐	☐	_____

CHAPTER **18**

Safety

■ Summary

No age group is immune to accidental injury. However, there are distinct differences among various age groups that contribute to their risks and to the type of accident or injury that may occur. These differences are highlighted in this chapter. The appropriate steps to be taken when fires, accidents, or injuries occur are suggested so that students may familiarize themselves with nursing responsibilities surrounding these incidents.

■ Matching Questions

Directions: For items 1 through 10, match the definitions in Part B with the terms in Part A.

PART A

1. _____ Hazards

2. _____ Burns

3. _____ Asphyxiation

4. _____ Drowning

5. _____ Macroshock

6. _____ Poisoning

7. _____ Restraint

8. _____ Microshock

9. _____ Ground

10. _____ Safety

PART B

a. Measures that prevent unintentional injuries

b. Distribution of low-amperage electricity over a large body area

c. A device that restricts movement

d. A device that diverts electrical energy to earth

e. A type of skin injury from chemicals

f. Ingestion or inhalation of a toxic substance

g. Distribution of low-voltage, high-amperage electricity over a large body area

h. Inability to breathe

i. Fluid that interferes with ventilation

j. Potentially dangerous conditions in the physical surroundings

■ Multiple Choice Questions

Directions: For items 1 through 12, circle the letter that corresponds to the best answer for each question.

1. A Class B fire extinguisher contains:
   a. Water under pressure
   b. Carbon dioxide
   c. Dry chemicals
   d. Graphite

2. The first measure the nurse must carry out when a fire occurs is:
   a. Notifying the switchboard using the proper code
   b. Turning off the oxygen supply near the fire
   c. Using the appropriate fire extinguisher
   d. Evacuating the people from the room with the fire

3. When an accident occurs, which of the following steps should be taken first:
   a. Report the accident to the proper person promptly
   b. Comfort and reassure the client who was involved
   c. Check the condition of the involved client
   d. Call for the assistance of other health personnel

4. When an accident occurs, which of the following steps should be taken last:
   a. Reporting the accident to the proper authorities
   b. Entering all of the information on an accident report
   c. Notifying the physician that the client has had an accident
   d. Comforting and reassuring the client involved

5. A thermal burn is a skin injury caused by:
   a. Heat
   b. Lightning
   c. Steam
   d. Electricity

6. The term *asphyxiation* means:
   a. The inability to breathe
   b. Fluid in the airway
   c. Discharge of electricity through the body
   d. Inhalation of a toxic substance

7. The body is susceptible to electrical shock because:
   a. It is well insulated
   b. It is grounded
   c. It acts as a resistor
   d. It is a good conductor

8. The most prevalent type of accident experienced by older adults is:
   a. Poisoning
   b. Falls
   c. Burns
   d. Asphyxiation

9. Which of the following acronyms incorporates the steps found in most fire plans:
   a. ABC
   b. OBRA
   c. NFPA
   d. RACE

10. Macroshock is best described as:
    a. The distribution of low-amperage electricity over a large body area
    b. The distribution of high-amperage electricity over a large body area

c. A fatal electrical current delivered directly to the heart
d. Resistance to the movement of electric current offered by intact skin

11. Class A fire extinguishers are used for fires involving:
    a. Flammable liquid
    b. Electricity
    c. Paper or wood
    d. Any type of fire

12. Risks associated with the use of physical restraints include:
    a. Constipation, incontinence, infection
    b. Falls, confusion, asphyxiation
    c. Dementia, disorientation, disability
    d. Visual impairment, hypotension, urinary urgency

■ Alternative Format Questions

1. The nurse is preparing a teaching plan about preventing poisoning for the parents of a toddler. Which of the following points should the nurse include in the plan? Select all that apply:
   1. Install child-resistant latches on cupboard doors
   2. Store toxic substances in empty food containers
   3. Never keep medications in your purse
   4. Ask for tamper-proof lids on prescriptions
   5. Keep plants out of reach or outside

2. All of the following interventions are appropriate when treating a victim of suspected poisoning with a corrosive substance. Place them in order of priority.
   1. Treat symptoms
   2. Prevent vomiting
   3. Maintain breathing and cardiac function
   4. Dilute with water or milk
   5. Identify the substance, quantity ingested, and time and date of occurrence
   6. Hydrate the client

3. The nurse is conducting an infant nutrition class for parents. Which of the following foods should the nurse tell parents is safe to introduce during the first year of life? Select all that apply:

   1. Sliced roast beef
   2. Pureed fruits
   3. Whole milk
   4. Rice cereal
   5. Strained vegetables
   6. Fruit juice

■ True or False Questions

Directions: For items 1 through 10, decide if the statement is true or false and mark T or F in the space provided.

1. _____ One of the general reasons to use restraints is to provide for as much movement as possible within the restraint.

2. _____ In the event of a fire, it is best to place bath blankets at the threshold of doors where smoke is leaking.

3. _____ Smoke is sometimes more deadly than the fire with which it is associated.

4. _____ Carbon monoxide can be present in the absence of smoke.

5. _____ Victims of warm-water drownings are more likely to be resuscitated than those who drown in cold water.

6. _____ Poisonings never occur in health care institutions.

7. _____ Educating children is the only way to prevent childhood poisoning in the home.

8. _____ Falls may be prevented by determining which clients are at risk.

9. _____ Restrained clients are more likely to die during hospitalization than clients who are not restrained.

10. _____ Among older adults who fall, 90% are eventually transferred to a nursing home.

■ Short Answer Questions

Directions: Read each of the following statements and supply the word(s) necessary in the space provided.

1. State (briefly) why it is necessary to obtain a physician's written order before restraints are applied.

2. List three methods to help prevent falls as suggested in this chapter.

   a. _____

   _____

   b. _____

   _____

   c. _____

   _____

3. List the risk factors suggested in this chapter for accidental falls. _____

   _____

   _____

4. List the seven steps the nurse should follow when a fire occurs.

   a. _____

   _____

   b. _____

   _____

   c. _____

   _____

   d. _____

   _____

   e. _____

   _____

   f. _____

   _____

   g. _____

   _____

5. List the six steps the nurse should follow when using a fire extinguisher.

a. _____

_____

b. _____

_____

c. _____

_____

d. _____

_____

e. _____

_____

f. _____

_____

■ Critical Thinking Exercises

1 Describe adjustments necessary to provide a safe and comfortable environment:

a. When the client is an infant or child

b. When the client is helpless

c. When the client is elderly

2. Identify nursing strategies that would be likely to secure client cooperation in making these changes.

Performance Checklist

A. This section allows you to examine your techniques for maintaining safety in the client's environment.

1. Place a check mark in the "S" ("satisfactory") column if you used the recommended technique.
2. Place a check mark in the "NI" ("needs improvement") column if you used some but not all of each recommended technique.
3. Place a check mark in the "U" ("unsatisfactory") column if you forgot to include that particular recommended technique.
4. Note whether further practice is indicated, what errors you made, suggestions that will improve your skills, and so on in the section for comments.

RECOMMENDED TECHNIQUE	S	NI	U	Comments
To Use Restraints				
Obtain a physician's order as soon as possible	☐	☐	☐	_____
Explain to the client and family why restraints are to be used	☐	☐	☐	_____
Allow some mobility and do not apply restraints too tightly	☐	☐	☐	_____
Protect skin and bony prominences	☐	☐	☐	_____
Position the client comfortably before applying restraints	☐	☐	☐	_____
Keep the client in sight whenever restraints are used	☐	☐	☐	_____
Apply restraints to parts of the body correctly and safely	☐	☐	☐	_____
Fasten restraints to the bed's frame, not the side rails	☐	☐	☐	_____
Give appropriate nursing care to the restrained client	☐	☐	☐	_____
To Prevent Falls				
Place bed in a low position for the ambulatory client	☐	☐	☐	_____
Use nonskid mats or strips in tubs and showers	☐	☐	☐	_____
Use tub and shower stools and handrails appropriately	☐	☐	☐	_____
Use equipment and supplies only for their intended purposes	☐	☐	☐	_____
Have clients use good walking shoes when ambulating	☐	☐	☐	_____
Do not allow litter to gather on floors and in corridors	☐	☐	☐	_____
Have clients in wheelchairs use wide doorways, ramps, and elevators	☐	☐	☐	_____

RECOMMENDED TECHNIQUE	S	NI	U	Comments
See to it that spilled liquids are wiped up promptly	☐	☐	☐	_____

To Prevent Electrical Injuries

	S	NI	U	Comments
Use plugs and outlets with grounds whenever possible	☐	☐	☐	_____
Remove plugs from wall sockets by grasping the plugs	☐	☐	☐	_____
Use electrical equipment for its intended purpose only	☐	☐	☐	_____
See to it that electrical equipment is in good working order	☐	☐	☐	_____
Keep electrical equipment away from bathtubs, sinks, and showers	☐	☐	☐	_____
Avoid wearing wet shoes or standing in water when using equipment	☐	☐	☐	_____
Do not kink electrical cords or use frayed cords	☐	☐	☐	_____

To Prevent Fires

	S	NI	U	Comments
Know where emergency exits and fire extinguishers are	☐	☐	☐	_____
Use appropriate precautions when oxygen is in use	☐	☐	☐	_____
Help enforce smoking regulations	☐	☐	☐	_____
Observe clients for safety when they smoke	☐	☐	☐	_____
Avoid storing materials that may lead to spontaneous combustion	☐	☐	☐	_____

To Prevent Poisoning

	S	NI	U	Comments
Know where emergency instructions are posted	☐	☐	☐	_____
Help see to it that poisonous substances are conspicuously labeled	☐	☐	☐	_____
Store poisonous substances properly	☐	☐	☐	_____
Do not place poisonous substances in another container	☐	☐	☐	_____
See to it that medications are stored securely and properly	☐	☐	☐	_____

To Prevent Scalds and Burns

	S	NI	U	Comments
Check the temperature of bath and shower water	☐	☐	☐	_____
Agitate water when adding hot water to a tub	☐	☐	☐	_____
Use heating pads according to agency policy	☐	☐	☐	_____

RECOMMENDED TECHNIQUE	S	NI	U	Comments
To Prevent Drowning and Asphyxiation				
Offer small bits of food to clients while helping them to eat	☐	☐	☐	_____
Offer liquids to helpless clients with care	☐	☐	☐	_____
Do not leave a client alone in a tub or shower if they are weak or cognitively impaired	☐	☐	☐	_____
Never leave a child alone in a tub, shower, or bathroom	☐	☐	☐	_____
Miscellaneous				
Observe practices of medical and surgical asepsis	☐	☐	☐	_____
See to it that the call device is always handy for use	☐	☐	☐	_____

B. Examine your techniques, or those of another nurse, when an accident occurs and complete the following form.

RECOMMENDED TECHNIQUE	S	NI	U	Comments
Check the client's condition immediately	☐	☐	☐	_____
Call for assistance	☐	☐	☐	_____
Begin resuscitation measures if needed.	☐	☐	☐	_____
Do not move the client until it is safe to do so	☐	☐	☐	_____
Comfort and reassure the client appropriately	☐	☐	☐	_____
Report accident and assessment data to the physician	☐	☐	☐	_____
Document the accident properly, including preparing an incident report	☐	☐	☐	_____

CHAPTER 19

Pain Management

■ Summary

Pain is an unpleasant sensation usually associated with disease or injury. It also has an emotional aspect referred to as suffering. Research shows that the pain experience is highly subjective and individualized. Pain exists when and to what extent the client says it does.

Pain is probably the major cause of physical distress among clients. This chapter provides information about pain and techniques for pain relief.

■ Matching Questions

Directions: For items 1 through 5, match the descriptions in Part B with the standards in Part A.

PART A

1. _____ Standard I

2. _____ Standard II

3. _____ Standard III

4. _____ Standard IV

5. _____ Standard V

PART B

a. Adherence to standards is monitored by an interdisciplinary committee

b. Clients are informed verbally and in writing that pain relief is important

c. Acute pain and cancer pain are recognized and effectively treated

d. Information about analgesics is readily available

e. Explicit policies for use of advanced analgesic technologies are defined

Directions: For items 6 through 10, match the descriptions in Part B with the types of pain in Part A.

PART A

6. _____ Cutaneous

7. _____ Visceral

8. _____ Neuropathic

9. _____ Referred

10. _____ Phantom

PART B

a. Pain with atypical characteristics

b. Discomfort perceived away from the site of stimulation

c. Discomfort arising from internal organs

d. Deep pain in tissues that have been surgically removed

e. Discomfort that originates at the skin level

■ Multiple-Choice Questions

Directions: For items 1 through 10, circle the letter that corresponds to the best answer for each question.

1. Which of the following statements most accurately describes a characteristic of pain:

   a. Pain is objective in nature

   b. Responses to pain vary widely

   c. Pain is always associated with bodily damage

   d. Pain is not a demanding situation

2. Acute pain is best described as:

   a. Physical discomfort that exists less than 6 months

   b. Physical discomfort that usually lasts longer than 6 months

   c. Physical discomfort that usually lasts longer than 2 months

   d. Physical discomfort that usually lasts less than 2 months

3. Of the following statements, which best defines referred pain:
   a. Physical discomfort that exists less than 6 months
   b. Physical discomfort that exists in the part of the body that is injured
   c. Pain in an area of the body that results from some mental or emotional origin
   d. Pain in an area of the body that is some distance from the part that is injured

4. Acupuncture and acupressure may stimulate the production of which of the following chemicals to relieve pain:
   a. Morphine
   b. Endorphins
   c. Insulin
   d. Adrenaline

5. Biofeedback is best described as:
   a. A training program that helps the individual by substituting for his or her drug therapy
   b. A training program that produces a subconscious condition that is used to control pain
   c. A training program that helps the individual become aware of certain body changes
   d. A program used to produce simple pressure on various body parts to help reduce pain

6. The client's discomfort is most likely relieved by a placebo in which of the following situations:
   a. When the discomfort is only mild
   b. When the discomfort is imagined or anticipated
   c. When the client is almost recovered
   d. When the client has confidence in his or her caregivers

7. One of the advantages for using transcutaneous electrical nerve stimulation (TENS) is:
   a. It can be used for pregnant women
   b. It can only be used intermittently
   c. It is nonnarcotic without toxic effects
   d. It requires no training in its use

8. A parenteral dose of 10 mg of morphine sulfate given every 3 to 4 hours is equal to which of the following dosages of the same drug given orally?
   a. 7.5 mg by mouth every 3 to 4 hours
   b. 30 mg by mouth every 3 to 4 hours
   c. 150 mg by mouth every 3 to 4 hours
   d. 300 mg by mouth every 2 to 3 hours

9. An equianalgesic dose of a medication refers to:
   a. The amount required to provide a favorable response over time
   b. The amount associated with sympathetic nervous system responses
   c. An unpleasant sensation associated with the adjusted oral dose over time
   d. The adjusted oral dose that provides the same relief as a parenteral dose

10. Nondrug interventions for pain relief are most likely to be used for which of the following types of pain?
    a. Acute pain
    b. Chronic pain
    c. Visceral pain
    d. Cutaneous pain

■ Alternative Format Questions

1. A physician ordered ¼ gr of morphine sulfate for pain relief for a client. The nurse knows that the medication is available labeled only in milligrams. Convert the ordered dose to milligrams.

2. The physician ordered 50 mg of meperidine HCl (Demerol) pain relief for a client. The nurse knows that on her unit, meperidine HCl is available only in single-dose units containing 100 mg per milliliter. Calculate the dose in milliliters to be given to this client.

3. From the following descriptors, select those that are characteristic of chronic pain. Select all that apply:

1. Recent onset of pain
2. Nonspecific, generalized pain
3. Poor response to drug therapy
4. Increasing amount of drug required for acceptable pain control
5. Decreased suffering with time
6. Pain relief as healing takes place

■ True or False Questions

Directions: For items 1 through 12, decide if the statement is true or false and mark T or F in the space provided.

1. ____ Pain threshold is the ability of an individual to endure pain.

2. ____ Discomfort in a location distant from the diseased or injured part of the body is known as phantom limb pain.

3. ____ The point at which the sensation of pain becomes noticeable appears to be about the same among healthy persons.

4. ____ Individuals from different cultures tolerate pain in the same manner.

5. ____ Anxiety and fear are common emotions accompanying pain.

6. ____ The human body is able to adapt to the sensation of pain.

7. ____ When the client is allowed to help select methods to relieve his or her pain, he or she usually has better results.

8. ____ Patient-controlled analgesia (PCA) is used primarily in hospitals for clients with chronic pain.

9. ____ The initial dose administered through a PCA system is the same as the amount released each time the client activates the system.

10. ____ The TENS unit is contraindicated in pregnancy because its effect is unknown.

11. ____ Addiction is a pattern of compulsive drug use accompanied by a continued craving for the drug and a need to use the drug for effects other than pain relief.

12. ____ Hypnosis is a trancelike state during which perception and memory are altered.

■ Short Answer Questions

1. List eight of the advantages of using PCA suggested in this chapter.

a. _____
   _____
b. _____
   _____
c. _____
   _____
d. _____
   _____
e. _____
   _____
f. _____
   _____
g. _____
   _____
h. _____
   _____

2. Identify five components of pain assessment as suggested in this chapter.

a. _____
   _____
b. _____
   _____
c. _____
   _____
d. _____
   _____
e. _____
   _____

■ Critical Thinking Exercises

1. Plan a teaching program for a woman in labor and complete the following form.

2. Read the following case study and use your nursing process skills to prepare a nursing care plan related to pain management for this client.

A 24-month-old infant with AIDS is hospitalized with infectious diarrhea. She is well known to the pediatric staff, and there is real concern that she might not pull through this admission. She has suffered many of the complications of AIDS and is no stranger to pain. At the present time, the skin on her buttocks is raw and excoriated, and tears stream down her face whenever she is moved. Her blood pressure also shoots up when she is touched. The severity of her illness has left her extremely weak and listless, and her foster mother reports that she no longer recognizes her child. When alone in her crib, she seldom moves and moans softly. Several nurses have expressed great frustration caring for her because they find it hard to perform even simple nursing measures, such as turning, diapering, and weighing her when they see how much pain these procedures cause.

Topic for Teaching	Points to Cover in a Teaching Plan
Pain and its role in the labor process	
Measures to control pain	

Performance Checklist

A. This section allows you to examine your techniques for assisting the client with pain control.

1. Place a check mark in the "S" ("satisfactory") column if you used the recommended technique.
2. Place a check mark in the "NI" ("needs improvement") column if you used some but not all of each recommended technique.
3. Place a check mark in the "U" ("unsatisfactory") column if you forgot to include that particular recommended technique.
4. Note whether further practice is indicated, what errors you made, suggestions that will improve your skills, and so on in the section for comments.

RECOMMENDED TECHNIQUE	S	NI	U	Comments
Know the client's diagnosis, his or her plan of therapy, and his or her usual responses to pain	☐	☐	☐	_____
Determine the nature of the client's pain accurately	☐	☐	☐	_____
Observe the client in pain at least every 2 hours while awake and note any signs or symptoms that accompany his or her pain	☐	☐	☐	_____
Take appropriate steps to decrease or remove factors that contribute to the client's pain	☐	☐	☐	_____
Use various techniques to help a client relax and obtain relief from pain	☐	☐	☐	_____
Remain with the client in pain and listen if the client wishes to talk about his or her pain	☐	☐	☐	_____
Use prescribed medications for pain as ordered	☐	☐	☐	_____
Consult others for assistance with the care of the client in pain as necessary	☐	☐	☐	_____
Record techniques you have found helpful when assisting the client in pain	☐	☐	☐	_____

CHAPTER 20

Oxygenation

■ Summary

Oxygen is essential for almost every form of animal and plant life. It is used by each cell of the human body to metabolize nutrients and produce energy. This chapter presents information on the bedside procedure for measuring oxygen content of the blood, the type of oxygen equipment used in oxygen therapy, and the skills needed to maintain respiratory function. Tips for physical assessment of the client receiving oxygen therapy are also presented.

■ Matching Questions

Directions: For items 1 through 10, match the definition in Part B with the term in Part A.

PART A

1. _____ External respiration

2. _____ Ventilation

3. _____ Respiration

4. _A_ Internal respiration

5. _J_ Hypoxemia

6. _G_ Oxygen saturation

7. _C_ Deep breathing

8. _I_ Incentive spirometry

9. _F_ Pursed-lip breathing

10. _B_ Hypoxia

PART B

a. Transfer of oxygen across cellular membranes

b. Inadequate oxygen at the cellular level

c. A technique for maximizing ventilation

d. Transfer of oxygen from alveoli to blood

e. Movement of air in and out of the lungs

f. Controlled ventilation in which expiration is prolonged

g. The percent of oxygen bound to hemoglobin

h. Mechanism by which oxygen is delivered to the cells

i. A technique for measuring volume of air inhaled

j. Insufficient oxygen within arterial blood

Directions: For items 11 through 14, match the characteristics in Part B with the types of masks in Part A.

PART A

11. _d_ Simple mask

12. _c_ Partial rebreather mask

13. _b_ Nonrebreather mask

14. _a_ Venti mask

PART B

a. Is designed so all exhaled air leaves mask

b. Has large, ringed tube and dial system for specific amount of oxygen

c. Is attached to reservoir bag; one third of exhaled air enters bag

d. Fits over nose and mouth

■ Multiple Choice Questions

Directions: For items 1 through 10, circle the letter that corresponds to the best answer for each question.

1. The client's response to oxygen therapy is most accurately determined by:
   a. Examinations of the arterial blood gases
   b. Changes in the color of his or her skin and nail beds
   c. Changes in his or her vital signs
   d. Changes in his or her level of consciousness

2. One of the earliest signs of oxygen toxicity is:
   a. A productive cough
   b. A dry cough
   c. Loss of consciousness
   d. Flushing of the skin

3. To crack an oxygen tank means to:
   a. Stabilize the tank on a stand
   b. Attach a humidifier to the tank
   c. Regulate the flowmeter of the tank
   d. Clean the tank's outlet of debris

4. For clients with chronic lung conditions, oxygen via nasal cannula is usually prescribed at:
   a. 2 to 3 liters per minute
   b. 2 to 4 liters per minute
   c. 3 to 6 liters per minute
   d. 4 to 7 liters per minute

5. For a client with a chronic lung condition, high levels of oxygen may decrease or even stop respirations because:
   a. His body is not accustomed to breathing correctly
   b. The oxygen level in the body will go too high
   c. His body is accustomed to higher-than-normal carbon dioxide levels
   d. His body is accustomed to lower-than-normal carbon dioxide levels

6. The Venturi mask delivers a supply of up to:
   a. 10% oxygen
   b. 20% oxygen
   c. 30% oxygen
   d. 40% oxygen

7. Lung collapse is primarily caused by:
   a. The loss of negative pressure within the pleural space
   b. The loss of negative pressure within the lungs
   c. The loss of positive pressure within the pleural space
   d. The loss of fluid pressure within the pleural cavity

8. The water-seal chest drainage system is designed to prevent:
   a. Negative pressure from reentering the lungs
   b. Negative pressure from reentering the pleural cavity
   c. Atmospheric air from reentering the lungs
   d. Atmospheric air from reentering the pleural space

9. Clients receiving oxygen via the transtracheal method usually achieve adequate oxygenation with:
   a. More oxygen flow than other methods
   b. Less oxygen flow than other methods
   c. The same amount of oxygen flow as other methods
   d. A method that does not affect the amount of oxygen used

10. Oxygen delivered at 4 L per minute for a period of time is humidified because:
    a. It is a means of decreasing the amount of oxygen used
    b. The addition of water can deliver the exact amount of oxygen required
    c. Oxygen is very drying to mucous membranes
    d. Oxygen has a bad taste if it is not humidified

■ Alternative Format Questions

1. A client is admitted from the emergency department with a diagnosis of pneumothorax. Which of the following signs and symptoms support this diagnosis? Select all that apply:
   1. Presence of shoulder, neck, or chest pain
   2. Normal chest x-ray
   3. Hypotension
   4. Normal breath sounds
   5. Dyspnea and cyanosis
   6. Palpitations

2. A 33-year-old woman with primary pulmonary hypertension is being evaluated. The nurse asks the client what treatments she is currently receiving for her disease. The client is most likely to be receiving which of the following treatments? Select all that apply:
   1. Oxygen therapy
   2. Aminoglycosides
   3. Diuretics
   4. Vasodilators
   5. Antihistamines
   6. Sulfonamides

3. The nurse is performing an admission evaluation of a client with chronic obstructive pulmonary disease (COPD). As the nurse completes his initial physical assessment, which of the following signs and symptoms would be expected? Select all that apply:
   1. Decreased respiratory rate
   2. Dyspnea on exertion
   3. Barrel chest
   4. Short expiratory phase
   5. Clubbed fingers and toes
   6. Fever

■ True or False Questions

Directions: For items 1 through 10, decide if the statement is true or false and mark T or F in the space provided.

1. ____ Hypoxemia is defined as a deficiency in the amount of oxygen in inspired air.

2. ____ Oxygen is a flammable gas.

3. ____ Oxygen is usually administered via cannula for clients suffering with smoke inhalation or carbon monoxide poisoning.

4. ____ Lung collapse is caused by the loss of positive pressure within the pleural space.

5. ____ No lung sounds are heard over the areas in which the lung has deflated.

6. ____ A water-seal drainage system should be emptied routinely.

7. ____ Failure of the water to fluctuate within the water-seal drainage system may mean that the client's lung has expanded.

8. ____ A major advantage of the nasal cannula is that it allows 10 or more liters of oxygen to be administered without causing drying of the mucous membranes.

9. ____ High percentages of oxygen via nasal cannula are needed by clients with chronic lung diseases.

10. ____ Because transtracheal catheters are made of plastic, they can be cleaned and reused.

■ Short Answer Questions

Directions: Read each of the following statements and supply the word(s) necessary in the space provided.

1. Identify the nursing guidelines for the safe use of oxygen as suggested in this chapter.

   a. _____

   _____

   b. _____

   _____

   c. _____

   _____

   d. _____

   _____

   e. _____

   _____

   f. _____

   _____

   g. _____

   _____

2. Identify five common signs of inadequate oxygenation.

   a. _____

   _____

   b. _____

   _____

   c. _____

   _____

   d. _____

   _____

   e. _____

   _____

3. List seven components that are part of the evaluation of the effectiveness of oxygen administration.

   a. _____

   b. _____

   _____

c. _____

_____

d. _____

_____

e. _____

_____

f. _____

_____

g. _____

_____

4. List four suggested actions that should be taken when using oxygen dispensed from a tank.

a. _____

_____

b. _____

_____

c. _____

_____

d. _____

_____

5. List five methods of administering oxygen.

a. _____

_____

b. _____

_____

c. _____

_____

d. _____

_____

e. _____

_____

■ Critical Thinking Exercises

Arrange with your clinical instructor to spend some time observing the respiratory therapist administer various types of respiratory treatments. Describe each, including the purpose or goal, kinds of clients treated, and results. Identify nursing activities appropriate for effective client care and coordination of these activities. Determine when and how you might need to be the client's advocate when he or she is receiving respiratory therapy.

Performance Checklist

A. This section allows you to examine your techniques for assisting a client receiving oxygen therapy.

1. Place a check mark in the "S" ("satisfactory") column if you used the recommended technique.

2. Place a check mark in the "NI" ("needs improvement") column if you used some but not all of each recommended technique.

3. Place a check mark in the "U" ("unsatisfactory") column if you forgot to include that particular recommended technique.

4. Note whether further practice is indicated, what errors you made, suggestions that will improve your skills, and so on in the section for comments.

RECOMMENDED TECHNIQUE	S	NI	U	Comments
Wash your hands	☐	☐	☐	_____
Fill a humidifier bottle with distilled water to the appropriate level if administering 4 or more L/minute	☐	☐	☐	_____
Place a cannula into the client's nostrils so that skin irritation is avoided	☐	☐	☐	_____
Place a lubricated catheter properly into a nostril a distance about equal to the distance from nostril to earlobe	☐	☐	☐	_____
Check the placement of a catheter in the oropharynx and secure it to the nose	☐	☐	☐	_____
Place a mask over the face and secure it in place	☐	☐	☐	_____
Change a disposable cannula, catheter, or mask, or clean a reusable one, at least every 8 hours and more often if indicated	☐	☐	☐	_____
Check at regular intervals that the client is receiving humidified oxygen at the prescribed rate	☐	☐	☐	_____
Observe the client for oxygen toxicity	☐	☐	☐	_____
Check the supply of oxygen at regular intervals and know the agency policy for obtaining additional oxygen	☐	☐	☐	_____
Check at regular intervals that the cannula, catheter, or mask is not irritating the skin	☐	☐	☐	_____
Reassess the client's oxygen status every 2 to 4 hours	☐	☐	☐	_____
Offer skin, nasal, and oral hygiene at least every 4 to 8 hours	☐	☐	☐	_____
Observe precautions at all times for the safe delivery of oxygen	☐	☐	☐	_____
Post "no smoking" signs	☐	☐	☐	_____
Note that electrical equipment is in good working order	☐	☐	☐	_____

RECOMMENDED TECHNIQUE	S	NI	U	Comments
Avoid petroleum and acetone products	☐	☐	☐	_____
Check to see that oil and grease are not used near oxygen equipment	☐	☐	☐	_____
See to it that there are no open flames in the presence of oxygen	☐	☐	☐	_____
See to it that fire extinguishers are handy and know how to use them	☐	☐	☐	_____
If oxygen is in a tank, ensure that the tank is secured properly on its stand	☐	☐	☐	_____
Avoid wearing clothing that produces static electricity when around oxygen	☐	☐	☐	_____

B. Examine your techniques for maintaining water-seal drainage and complete the following form.

RECOMMENDED TECHNIQUE	S	NI	U	Comments
Review client's medical record to determine the condition that necessitated the chest-tube insertion	☐	☐	☐	_____
Determine if there are one or two chest tubes and note the date of insertion	☐	☐	☐	_____
Check medical orders to determine if drainage is being collected by gravity or with suction	☐	☐	☐	_____
Perform physical assessment as soon after report as possible	☐	☐	☐	_____
Take a roll of tape and a container of distilled water with you	☐	☐	☐	_____
Introduce yourself and explain purpose of interaction	☐	☐	☐	_____
Wash your hands	☐	☐	☐	_____
Check to see that hemostats are at bedside	☐	☐	☐	_____
Turn off suction regulator; assess client's lung sounds	☐	☐	☐	_____
Inspect the dressing for signs of soiling or looseness	☐	☐	☐	_____
Palpate the skin around the insertion site to feel for and listen for air crackling in the tissue	☐	☐	☐	_____
Inspect all connections; reinforce loose ones with tape	☐	☐	☐	_____
Make sure tubing is unkinked and hangs freely into the drainage system	☐	☐	☐	_____
Observe that the fluid level in the water-seal chamber is at the 2-cm level	☐	☐	☐	_____

RECOMMENDED TECHNIQUE	S	NI	U	Comments
Add distilled water to mark if the fluid level is below the 2-cm mark	☐	☐	☐	_____
Note if water is rising and falling with each respiration	☐	☐	☐	_____
Observe for continuous bubbling in the water-seal chamber	☐	☐	☐	_____
Correct for continuous bubbling as appropriate	☐	☐	☐	_____
Maintain water level in suction chamber at 20 cm	☐	☐	☐	_____
Regulate suction to produce gentle bubbling				
Observe nature and amount of drainage	☐	☐	☐	_____
Keep drainage system below the chest	☐	☐	☐	_____
Curl and secure tubing as appropriate	☐	☐	☐	_____
Encourage coughing and deep breathing at least every 2 hours while awake	☐	☐	☐	_____
Instruct client to move about in bed, ambulate, and exercise shoulder on the side with the tubing	☐	☐	☐	_____
Never clamp tubing for long periods of time	☐	☐	☐	_____
Mark drainage level on the collection chamber at the end of your shift	☐	☐	☐	_____
Document assessment findings, care provided, and amount of drainage during the period of care	☐	☐	☐	_____

CHAPTER 21

Asepsis

■ Summary

Microorganisms are naturally present in the environment. Some are beneficial; some are not. Some are harmless to most individuals, others are harmful to a great many people, and many others are harmless except in certain circumstances.

Preventing infections is one of the priorities in nursing. This chapter discusses how microorganisms survive and how to use aseptic techniques (measures that reduce or eliminate microorganisms).

■ Matching Questions

Directions: For items 1 through 5, match the examples in Part B with the routes of transmission in Part A.

PART A

1. _____ Direct contact

2. _____ Droplet

3. _____ Airborne

4. _____ Vehicle

5. _____ Vector

PART B

a. Drinking contaminated water

b. Inhalation

c. Sexual intercourse

d. Mosquitoes

e. Sneezing

Directions: For questions 6 through 10, match the descriptions in Part B with the organisms in Part A.

PART A

6. _____ Aerobic bacteria

7. _____ Fungi

8. _____ Helminths

9. _____ Protozoans

10. _____ Viruses

PART B

a. Single-celled animals

b. Yeasts and molds

c. Smallest microorganisms known to cause infections

d. Microorganisms that require oxygen to live

e. Infectious worms

■ Multiple-Choice Questions

Directions: For items 1 through 16, circle the letter that corresponds to the best answer for each question.

1. The term used for harmless microorganisms is:
   a. Nonpathogens
   b. Aerobic
   c. Anaerobic
   d. Pathogens

2. One example of an adaptive change in a microorganism is:
   a. They become anaerobic
   b. They become aerobic
   c. They become spore forming
   d. They become alkaline

3. The best examples of a portal of entry are:
   a. Nose, throat, mouth, ear, eye
   b. Hands, equipment, instruments
   c. Humans and animals
   d. Any break in the skin

4. The best examples of the vehicle of transmission are:
   a. Nose, throat, mouth, ear, eye
   b. Hands, equipment, instruments
   c. Humans and animals
   d. Any break in the skin

5. Soaps and detergents are examples of:
   a. Disinfectants
   b. Antimicrobial agents
   c. Antiseptics
   d. Bacteriostatic agents

6. The best definition of an antiseptic is:
   a. A chemical agent used to reduce the growth of microorganisms on living tissue
   b. A chemical that kills or suppresses the growth or reproduction of microorganisms
   c. A substance that is capable of destroying or killing microorganisms, but not necessarily spores
   d. A substance that is capable of killing or destroying all microorganisms

7. Of the following, which is the best definition of a disinfectant:
   a. A chemical agent used to reduce the growth of microorganisms on living tissue
   b. A chemical that kills or suppresses the growth or reproduction of microorganisms
   c. A substance that is capable of destroying or killing microorganisms, but not necessarily spores
   d. A substance that is capable of killing or destroying all microorganisms

8. An infection that the client acquires in the hospital is called:
   a. A local infection
   b. A secondary infection
   c. An endogenous infection
   d. A nosocomial infection

9. The single most effective way to prevent nosocomial infections is to:
   a. Isolate clients with infections
   b. Wash all equipment with detergents
   c. Cover the mouth and nose when coughing
   d. Practice conscientious hand washing

10. In the health care agency, the care given to cleaning contaminated supplies and equipment is called:
   a. Medical asepsis
   b. Concurrent disinfection
   c. Terminal disinfection
   d. Surgical asepsis

11. Which of the following methods of heat sterilization should be used for sharp instruments:
   a. Boiling water
   b. Free-flowing steam
   c. Dry heat
   d. Steam under pressure

12. Surgical asepsis is based on which of the following principles:
   a. Health practitioners are continuously striving to eliminate pathogens
   b. It is the practice that reduces the number of pathogens on surfaces
   c. Areas that are free of microorganisms must be protected from contamination
   d. Areas that are contaminated must be washed with antiseptics and sterilized

13. When creating a sterile field, the nurse should open the sterile package in such a way that:
   a. The outermost triangle edge is moved away from the nurse
   b. The outermost triangle edge is moved to the left of the nurse
   c. The outermost triangle edge is moved to the right of the nurse
   d. The outermost triangle edge is moved toward the nurse

14. When opening a sterile package, the nurse should unfold:
   a. The left side first
   b. The nearest side first
   c. The far side first
   d. The right side first

15. Opened wrappers are considered sterile:
   a. Within 2 inches of the edge
   b. Within 1 inch of the edge
   c. Out to the hem on the edge
   d. Out to and including the edge

16. Why is it important to avoid talking over a sterile area?

    a. Microbes are everywhere, not just on physical objects

    b. Microorganisms are present in the moisture from respiratory secretions

    c. Air currents can carry organisms, which can then be deposited onto sterile areas

    d. Moisture on sterile cloth or a paper can act as a wick, pulling in microbes

■ Alternative Format Questions

1. Hand washing is the single most effective way to prevent infections. Place the following steps in the order in which they should be carried out:

    1. Wet hands with warm water

    2. Lather hands with soap

    3. Rinse hands

    4. Turn faucet off

    5. Rinse soap

    6. Dispense paper towel

2. The nurse is interviewing a mother who anxiously states, "The school nurse sent a note home saying there's been a case of hepatitis A in my daughter's sixth-grade class. Isn't that what drug users get? Should I keep my daughter home from school? How can I keep her from catching it?" Which of the following points would be important to share with this mother? Select all that apply:

    1. The incubation period for hepatitis A

    2. An explanation that hepatitis A is transmitted by contact with blood and body fluids

    3. The signs and symptoms, which are the same as that of the flu

    4. A demonstration of proper hand washing

    5. A discussion of the availability of immunizations

3. Health care personnel caring for a client with tuberculosis would require a particulate filter respirator. Which of the following are important points to remember when using this type of mask? Select all that apply:

    1. The minimum specification is N95

    2. Particulate filter respirators must carry a seal of approval

    3. They can be shared by all personnel caring for the client

    4. Certain changes can cause leakage

    5. They must be discarded in a waterproof container after use

■ True or False Questions

Directions: For items 1 through 10, decide if the statement is true or false and mark T or F in the space provided.

1. _____ A microorganism that requires free oxygen in order to exist is called an anaerobic microorganism.

2. _____ The terms *antiseptic* and *bacteriostatic* are synonymous.

3. _____ Medical asepsis and clean technique are the same.

4. _____ A person or animal on which or in which microorganisms live is called a reservoir.

5. _____ Sterilization is the practice that helps confine or reduce the number of microorganisms.

6. _____ Wearing gloves is the single most effective way to prevent nosocomial infections.

7. _____ All bacteria are affected by antibiotics.

8. _____ When cleaning supplies and equipment that have been contaminated with bodily secretions, it is best to rinse with hot water first.

9. _____ As a general rule, it is best to consider that the greater the number of microorganisms, the longer it will take to destroy them.

10. _____ A reliable method of sterilization is to soak objects in a solution of 70% ethyl alcohol for 10 to 20 minutes.

■ Short Answer Questions

Directions: Read each of the following statements and supply the word(s) necessary in the space provided.

1. Identify the five conditions most microorganisms need to grow and survive.

   a. _____

   _____

   b. _____

   _____

   c. _____

   _____

   d. _____

   _____

   e. _____

   _____

2. List five factors that can result in reduced resistance to the entry of disease-causing organisms.

   a. _____

   _____

   b. _____

   _____

   c. _____

   _____

   d. _____

   _____

   e. _____

   _____

3. Identify 10 of the guidelines suggested in this chapter for safe and effective practices of medical asepsis when soap or detergent and water are used to clean supplies and equipment.

   a. _____   f. _____

   b. _____   g. _____

   c. _____   h. _____

   d. _____   i. _____

   e. _____   j. _____

4. Describe the effect of the body's biological defense mechanisms on microorganisms. _____

   _____

   _____

5. List the 10 guidelines for hand washing suggested in this chapter.

   a. _____   f. _____

   b. _____   g. _____

   c. _____   h. _____

   d. _____   i. _____

   e. _____   j. _____

■ Critical Thinking Exercises

1. Describe the role of the infection control nurse in the hospital.

2. Describe how the nurse would practice asepsis in the client's home while doing a dressing change.

Performance Checklist

This section allows you to examine your techniques for controlling the spread of microorganisms in the client's environment.

1. Place a check mark in the "S" ("satisfactory") column if you used the recommended technique.
2. Place a check mark in the "NI" ("needs improvement") column if you used some but not all of each recommended technique.
3. Place a check mark in the "U" ("unsatisfactory") column if you forgot to include that particular recommended technique.
4. Note whether further practice is indicated, what errors you made, suggestions that will improve your skills, and so on in the section for comments.

RECOMMENDED TECHNIQUE	S	NI	U	Comments
Medical Asepsis When Giving Care				
Wash hands before and after giving care	☐	☐	☐	_____
Handle all discharges correctly	☐	☐	☐	_____
Place damp or wet items in a waterproof bag	☐	☐	☐	_____
Discard disposable equipment according to agency policy	☐	☐	☐	_____
Flush away contents of bedpans and urinals promptly	☐	☐	☐	_____
Use equipment for one client only	☐	☐	☐	_____
Cover breaks in the skin with sterile dressings	☐	☐	☐	_____
Prevent soiled equipment and supplies from touching your uniform	☐	☐	☐	_____
Consider the floor heavily contaminated	☐	☐	☐	_____
Avoid raising dust and lint	☐	☐	☐	_____
Clean the least soiled areas first and the heavily soiled areas last	☐	☐	☐	_____
Pour liquids to be discarded directly into a drain or toilet	☐	☐	☐	_____
Avoid spilling and splashing liquids	☐	☐	☐	_____
Help keep the client's room as clean, bright, dry, and airy as possible	☐	☐	☐	_____
Do not use equipment when there is any doubt about its cleanliness or sterility	☐	☐	☐	_____
Personal Grooming				
Keep hair cut short or secured well if long	☐	☐	☐	_____
Wear only plain-band rings	☐	☐	☐	_____
Wear a wristwatch high enough so that it does not become contaminated	☐	☐	☐	_____
Do not wear loose-fitting bracelets	☐	☐	☐	_____

RECOMMENDED TECHNIQUE	S	NI	U	Comments
Keep fingernails short and well groomed	☐	☐	☐	_____
Follow agency policy about the use of nail polish	☐	☐	☐	_____

Practices of Everyday Living

	S	NI	U	Comments
Cover the nose and mouth when coughing or sneezing and wash your hands	☐	☐	☐	_____
Wash hands before handling food	☐	☐	☐	_____
Use individual personal care items	☐	☐	☐	_____
Wash hands after using the bathroom	☐	☐	☐	_____

Hand Washing

	S	NI	U	Comments
Stand near the sink but without touching it with your uniform	☐	☐	☐	_____
Observe agency policy about opening and closing faucets or use foot and knee controls properly	☐	☐	☐	_____
Keep hands and forearms lower than elbows and avoid touching the sink during the entire procedure	☐	☐	☐	_____
Use warm water and enough soap to produce a good lather on the hands and wrists	☐	☐	☐	_____
If bar soap is used, keep the bar in your hands until the end of washing, and drop it into the dish without touching it	☐	☐	☐	_____
Use firm, rubbing, and circular motions while cleaning the palms, backs of hands, fingers, and wrists	☐	☐	☐	_____
Wash for recommended periods for light and heavy soilage	☐	☐	☐	_____
Rinse and soap two to three times when soilage is especially heavy	☐	☐	☐	_____
Finish by rinsing washed areas well under running water	☐	☐	☐	_____
Clean surfaces under nails at least once a day and whenever hands are heavily soiled	☐	☐	☐	_____
Pat hands and wrists dry	☐	☐	☐	_____
Apply lotion to hands and wrists as necessary	☐	☐	☐	_____

Surgical Asepsis

	S	NI	U	Comments
Open sterile trays by folding top layer away from you and bottom layer toward you	☐	☐	☐	_____
Touch only the out side of the wrapper when opening a tray	☐	☐	☐	_____
Do not walk away from a sterile field or reach across it	☐	☐	☐	_____

RECOMMENDED TECHNIQUE	S	NI	U	Comments
Avoid talking, coughing, or sneezing over a sterile field	☐	☐	☐	_____
Hold sterile objects above the level of the waist	☐	☐	☐	_____
See to it that a sterile field remains dry	☐	☐	☐	_____
Handle sterile equipment with sterile forceps or with hands after putting on sterile gloves	☐	☐	☐	_____
Don sterile gloves in such a way that the hands do not touch the outside surface of the gloves	☐	☐	☐	_____
Avoid drafts in the work area	☐	☐	☐	_____
Use only sterile equipment and supplies	☐	☐	☐	_____
Replace items if there is doubt about their sterility	☐	☐	☐	_____

CHAPTER 22

Infection Control

■ Summary

Infectious diseases (diseases spread from one person to another) are also called contagious or communicable diseases and community-acquired infections. They were once the leading cause of death, but because of vaccines, aggressive public health measures, and advances in drug therapy, that is no longer true. Nevertheless, infectious diseases have not disappeared. In fact, the microorganisms that cause tuberculosis, gonorrhea, and some forms of wound and respiratory infections have developed drug-resistant strains. The current epidemic of AIDS, an infectious disease spread by human immunodeficiency virus (HIV) in blood and some body fluids, makes it clear that the war against pathogens has not been won.

This chapter discusses precautions that confine the reservoir of infectious agents and block their transmission from one host to another. To understand the concepts of infection control, it is important to understand the chain of infection (see Chapter 21) and the course of an infection.

■ Matching Questions

Directions: For items 1 through 5, match the characteristics in Part B with the stages in Part A.

PART A

1. ____ Incubation period

2. ____ Prodromal stage

3. ____ Acute stage

4. ____ Convalescent stage

5. ____ Resolution

PART B

a. Symptoms severe and specific

b. Pathogen destroyed

c. Host overcomes infectious agent

d. No recognizable symptoms

e. Initial symptoms appear

■ Multiple-Choice Questions

Directions, For items 1 through 10, circle the letter that corresponds to the best answer for each question.

1. The term *infection* refers to:
   a. A condition in which microorganisms are present and the host is injured
   b. A condition in which microorganisms develop resistance to drugs
   c. A condition in which microorganisms are present but the host is not damaged
   d. A condition in which microorganisms become more contagious

2. The primary goal of infection control is:
   a. To contain infectious microorganisms in one place
   b. To prevent infectious microorganisms from reproducing
   c. To prevent the spread of infectious microorganisms
   d. To control the effect of infectious microorganisms

3. The single most important means of preventing the spread of microorganisms is:
   a. Wearing barrier gowns when caring for clients with a contagious disease
   b. Wearing a mask when caring for clients with a contagious disease
   c. Washing your hands between clients even though they do not have a contagious disease
   d. Wearing gloves when you care for a client who may have a contagious disease

4. Gloves are required as barriers in which of the following situations:

   a. When direct contact with the source of microorganisms will occur

   b. To replace the need for hand washing when client care is finished

   c. When microorganisms present on the hands grow and multiply rapidly

   d. When the nurse does not want to have contact with the client

5. Standard precautions are best described as:

   a. Infection-control measures used when caring for clients with AIDS

   b. Infection-control measures used when caring for older adults

   c. Infection-control measures used when caring for clients with infections

   d. Infection-control measures used when caring for all clients

6. Why should a client with a contagious disease be placed in a private room:

   a. To control the number of visitors

   b. To keep the client away from others

   c. To control the spread of the disease

   d. To remind the hospital staff to use isolation techniques

7. For which of the following communicable diseases would you place the client in droplet isolation:

   a. Diarrhea

   b. Rubella

   c. Tuberculosis

   d. Chickenpox

8. For which of the following communicable diseases would you place the client on contact precautions:

   a. Diarrhea

   b. Tuberculosis

   c. Chickenpox

   d. Rabies

9. For which of the following communicable diseases would you place the client in airborne isolation?

   a. Hepatitis

   b. Tuberculosis

   c. Rubeola

   d. Conjunctivitis

10. From the following, which would be most likely to contain HIV or the hepatitis B virus?

    a. Tears

    b. Semen

    c. Perspiration

    d. Stool

■ Alternative Format Questions

1. The nurse is caring for a client with HIV. She is being assisted by a licensed practical nurse (LPN). Which statements by the LPN indicate her understanding of HIV transmission? Select all that apply:

   1. "I'll wear a gown, mask, and gloves for all client contact."

   2. "I don't need to wear any personal protective equipment because nurses have a low risk of occupational exposure."

   3. "I'll wear a mask if the client has a cough caused by an upper respiratory infection."

   4. "I'll wear a mask, gown, and gloves when splashing of body fluids is likely."

   5. "I will wash my hands after client care."

2. All of the following apply to removal of soiled personal protective equipment. Place each piece in the order in which it would be carried out.

   1. Remove the mask, touching only the ties

   2. Remove soiled gloves

   3. Untie the waist ties of the gown if tied at the waist in front

   4. Remove eyewear

   5. Remove soiled gown by rolling it up with soiled part inside

   6. Wash hands

3. A parent is planning to enroll her 9-month-old infant in a day care facility. The parent asks the nurse what to look for as indicators that the day care facility is adhering to good infection-control measures. How should the nurse reply? Select all that apply:

1. The facility keeps boxes of gloves in the director's office
2. Diapers are discarded into covered receptacles
3. Toys are kept on the floor for the children to share
4. Disposable papers are used on the diaper-changing tables
5. Facilities for hand washing are located in every classroom
6. Soiled clothing and cloth diapers are sent home in labeled paper bags

■ True or False Questions

Directions: For items 1 through 10, decide if the statement is true or false and mark T or F in the space provided.

1. _F_ The most recent guidelines from the Centers for Disease Control (CDC) state that there are three types of suggested infection-control techniques: protective, category, and disease specific.

2. ____ During the incubation period, the infectious agent may leave the host and infect others.

3. _F_ The nursing diagnosis Risk for Infection Transmission is not a diagnostic category currently approved by the North American Nursing Diagnosis Association.

4. _F_ The humidity in the environment is the cause of droplet-spread microorganisms.

5. _F_ When removing a mask, you should handle it only by the strings.

6. _F_ When removing an isolation gown, you should untie the waist strings before washing your hands or removing your gloves.

7. _T_ Children with the same contagious disease may be placed in a room together.

8. _F_ Gloves are considered to be a total and complete barrier to microorganisms.

9. _T_ All hospital personnel should follow the recommended standard precautions.

10. _F_ If an individual has received the hepatitis B vaccination, it is not necessary to be as careful when in contact with blood or body fluids.

■ Short Answer Questions

Directions: Read each of the following statements and supply the word(s) necessary in the space provided.

1. Write the standard precautions recommended in this chapter.

a. _____
b. _____
c. _____
d. _____
e. _____
f. _____
g. _____
h. _____

2. Identify three methods of contracting AIDS.

a. _____
b. _____
c. _____

■ Critical Thinking Exercises

Describe one technique for infection control for a client with the nursing diagnosis Risk for Infection Transmission.

a. Describe its purpose

b. Describe its basic requirements

c. List two examples of illnesses for which this technique may be used

d. Write a plan of care to meet the psychological needs of this client

Performance Checklist

This section allows you to examine your techniques for preventing the spread of communicable diseases.

1. Place a check mark in the "S" ("satisfactory") column if you used the recommended technique.
2. Place a check mark in the "NI" ("needs improvement") column if you used some but not all of each recommended technique.
3. Place a check mark in the "U" ("unsatisfactory") column if you forgot to include that particular recommended technique.
4. Note whether further practice is indicated, what errors you made, suggestions that will improve your skills, and so on in the section for comments.

RECOMMENDED TECHNIQUE	S	NI	U	Comments
Removal of Isolation Garments				
Untie or unfasten waist ties	☐	☐	☐	_____
Remove gloves and dispose of them in the proper container	☐	☐	☐	_____
Wash hands	☐	☐	☐	_____
Turn off the faucet with a paper towel	☐	☐	☐	_____
Remove the mask and discard it in the disposable trash or laundry container	☐	☐	☐	_____
Untie or unfasten the neck closure	☐	☐	☐	_____
Remove the gown	☐	☐	☐	_____
Discard the gown in the trash container if it is a disposable type or in the soiled linen container if it is made of fabric	☐	☐	☐	_____
Wash hands	☐	☐	☐	_____
Open the isolation door with a clean paper towel, touching the doorknob only	☐	☐	☐	_____
Discard the paper towel into the wastebasket inside the client's room	☐	☐	☐	_____
Leave the room taking care not to touch anything	☐	☐	☐	_____
Go directly to the utility room and wash your hands one final time	☐	☐	☐	_____

Performance Checklist

CHAPTER 23

Body Mechanics, Positioning, and Moving

■ Summary

Though many people are not active enough to improve their level of health, some are so inactive that their health actually deteriorates. Multiple complications can occur among individuals whose activity and movement are limited.

This chapter describes how to turn, move, position, exercise, and promote mobility in the inactive client in order to prevent complications. The use of several types of pressure-relieving mattresses and specialty beds that help prevent complications for immobile clients is discussed.

■ Matching Questions

Directions: For items 1 through 5, match the indications for its use given in Part B with the pressure-relieving device given in Part A.

PART A

1. ____ Foam mattress

2. ____ Static or alternating air

3. ____ Oscillating support bed

4. ____ Low-air-loss bed

5. ____ Air-fluidized bed

PART B

a. Burns that require frequent dressing changes or topical applications

b. Changes in position occur spontaneously or require minimal assistance

c. Seldom transferred from bed

d. At high risk for systemic effects of immobility, such as pneumonia and skin breakdown

e. Alteration of position is limited, less than adequate, or impossible

f. Presence of a superficial or single deep break in the skin, but pressure is easily relieved

Directions: For items 6 through 11, match the definitions in Part B with the terms in Part A.

PART A

6. ____ Gravity

7. ____ Balance

8. ____ Center of gravity

9. ____ Line of gravity

10. ____ Base of support

11. ____ Alignment

PART B

a. The area on which an object rests

b. The point at which the mass of an object is centered

c. The capacity to do work

d. Having parts of an object in proper relationship to one another

e. A force that pulls objects toward the center of the earth

f. An imaginary, vertical line that passes through the center of gravity

g. Having a steady position with weight distributed equally on the base of support

■ Multiple-Choice Questions

Directions: For items 1 through 14, circle the letter that corresponds to the best answer for each question.

1. Which of the following are associated with disuse syndrome:
   a. Contractures, diarrhea, and vomiting
   b. Atelectasis, increased appetite, and muscle weakness
   c. Muscle weakness, atelectasis, and contractures
   d. Atelectasis, contractures, and diarrhea

2. Which of the following is the best definition of *footdrop*:
   a. The result of allowing the joint to be bent and unmoved for long periods of time
   b. The result of prolonged plantar flexion, lack of movement of the ankle joint, and shortening of muscles at the back of the calf
   c. The result of prolonged dorsiflexion, lack of movement of the ankle joint, and shortening of muscles at the back of the calf
   d. The result of allowing the joint to be stabilized and unmoved for short periods of time

3. The term that refers to the position of the body or the way in which it is held is:
   a. Balance
   b. Posture
   c. Body mechanics
   d. Flexibility

4. It is recommended that the feet be separated in the standing position in order to:
   a. Distribute the body weight evenly
   b. Provide a wide base of support
   c. Prevent the strain of locked knees
   d. Relieve stress on the arches of the feet

5. Which of the following best defines *body mechanics*:
   a. The efficient use of the body as a machine
   b. The ratio of lean mass to fat mass
   c. The structures of the body used for support and movement
   d. The potential to respond when stimulated to work

6. The primary reason for recommending the "use of the longest and strongest muscles to provide the energy needed for a task" is:
   a. This technique overcomes slouching and uses muscles properly to prevent strain and injury to the abdominal wall
   b. This technique uses gravity and reduces the strain placed on a group of muscles
   c. This technique will provide the greatest strength and potential for performing work
   d. This technique will provide a base of support and enhance the balance of the body

7. One should push, pull, or roll objects whenever possible because:
   a. This technique will reduce strain and injury on the muscles of the lower back
   b. This technique reduces the strain on a group of muscles by using the body weight as a lever
   c. This technique uses gravity and reduces the strain placed on a group of muscles
   d. This technique improves balance by keeping the weight of the object close to the center of gravity

8. The reason for keeping the work area as close to the body as possible is:
   a. Stretching will cause poor balance as the line of gravity falls outside the body's base of support
   b. Stretching will cause strain and injury to the muscles of the legs and arms
   c. Stretching will cause the client to feel uncomfortable because the nurse's movements are "jerky"
   d. Stretching will make the nurse uncomfortable and therefore possibly harm the client

9. How often should an inactive client's position be changed:
   a. At least every 2 hours
   b. At least every 3 hours
   c. At least every 4 hours
   d. At least once a shift

10. The best placement for a turning sheet under the client would be:
    a. Between the upper back and the thighs
    b. Between the head and the buttocks
    c. Between the waist and the knees
    d. Between the buttocks and the ankles

11. Evaporation of moisture and the escape of heat is best provided by which of the following mattresses:
    a. Static air mattress
    b. Alternating air mattress
    c. Water mattress
    d. Foam mattress

12. One of the primary concerns when using the supine position is that the client may develop footdrop. The second concern is:

    a. The formation of contractures of the legs

    b. The interference with proper breathing

    c. The development of decubitus ulcers on the back

    d. The interference with chest expansion

13. Which of the following is a primary concern when using the lateral position:

    a. The formation of contractures of the legs

    b. The interference with proper breathing

    c. The development of decubitus ulcers on the back

    d. The formation of footdrop

14. Of the following, which position is especially helpful for clients with dyspnea:

    a. Semi-Fowler's position

    b. High Fowler's position

    c. Supine position

    d. Prone position

■ Alternative Format Questions

1. When the client is placed in a semi-Fowler's position, the head and torso are elevated _____ degrees.

2. A mechanical lift maybe used to transfer some clients from the bed to a chair, stretcher, tub, or toilet and back again. Which of the following are nursing concerns when using a mechanical lift? Select all that apply:

    1. Agency policy for operation of the lift

    2. The weight of the person to be moved

    3. The client's ability to move

    4. The condition of the equipment

    5. Indications for using the lift

    6. The size of the seat on the lift

3. As an alternative to the supine position, clients maybe placed in the prone position. Which of the following are benefits of this position? Select all that apply:

    1. It provides drainage from the bronchioles

    2. It makes it easier to talk with and assess the client

    3. It improves oxygenation in certain critically ill clients

    4. It stretches the trunk and extremities

    5. It creates a potential for footdrop

    6. It produces less pressure on the hip

■ True or False Questions

Directions: For items 1 through 10, decide if the statement is true or false and mark T or F in the space provided.

1. _____ Good posture includes holding the head erect with the face forward and with the chin elevated.

2. _____ It is not necessary to worry about good posture when lying down.

3. _____ The helpless client's position should be changed every 1 to 2 hours.

4. _____ Egg-crate mattresses provide greater pressure reduction than the waffle-shaped mattresses.

5. _____ Trochanter rolls are placed between the client's legs to prevent external rotation.

6. _____ When transferring a client, the joints should be supported to prevent injury and strain of the muscles.

7. _____ When transferring a client from the bed to a chair, the nurse should place the chair alongside the bed on the client's weaker side.

8. _____ Persons with short-term memory loss may be unable to follow directions regarding positioning and transferring.

9. ____ Impaired physical mobility is an appropriate nursing diagnosis for clients requiring assistance with body mechanics, positioning, and movement.

10. ____ The term *transfer* refers to moving clients from a bed to a chair.

■ Short Answer Questions

Directions: Read each of the following statements and supply the word(s) necessary in the space provided.

1. Identify the characteristics of good posture in a standing, sitting, and lying position.

   a. Standing:

      1. _____

      2. _____

   b. Sitting:

      1. _____

      2. _____

   c. Lying:

      1. _____

      2. _____

2. Describe three principles of correct body mechanics.

   a. _____
   _____

   b. _____
   _____

   c. _____
   _____

3. List five positioning devices and the purpose of each.

   a. _____
   _____

   b. _____
   _____

   c. _____
   _____

   d. _____
   _____

   e. _____
   _____

4. Name three pressure-relieving devices and an advantage of each.

   a. _____
   _____

   b. _____
   _____

   c. _____
   _____

5. List five measures to prevent inactivity in older adults.

   a. _____
   _____

   b. _____
   _____

   c. _____
   _____

   d. _____
   _____

   e. _____
   _____

■ Critical Thinking Exercises

1. Assess a bedridden client for whom you are caring who is at risk for or suffers from disuse syndrome and complete the following form.

Body System	Signs or Symptoms of Disuse Syndrome Are Present	Techniques That Are or Should Be Used to Overcome or Prevent Disuse Syndrome
Muscular system	Yes _____ No _____	
Skeletal system	Yes _____ No _____	
Cardiovascular system	Yes _____ No _____	
Respiratory system	Yes _____ No _____	
Urinary system	Yes _____ No _____	
Gastrointestinal system	Yes _____ No _____	
Integumentary system	Yes _____ No _____	
Metabolic functions	Yes _____ No _____	
Psychosocial functions	Yes _____ No _____	

2. Plan a teaching program for a client for whom you are caring and complete the following form.

Topic for Teaching	Points to Cover in a Teaching Plan
The importance of changing positions of the bedridden client	
Dangers of inactivity	

Performance Checklist

A. This section allows you to examine your technique for assisting the client with improving posture and body mechanics.

1. Place a check mark in the "S" ("satisfactory") column if you used the recommended technique.

2. Place a check mark in the "NI" ("needs improvement") column if you used some but not all of each recommended technique.

3. Place a check mark in the "U" ("unsatisfactory") column if you forgot to include the particular recommended technique.

4. Note whether further practice is indicated, what errors you made, suggestions that will improve your skills, and so on in the section for comments.

RECOMMENDED TECHNIQUE	S	NI	U	Comments
Posture When Standing				
Place feet parallel to each other, at right angles to the lower legs	☐	☐	☐	_____
Place feet about 10 to 20 centimeters (4 to 8 inches) apart	☐	☐	☐	_____
Distribute weight equally on both feet	☐	☐	☐	_____
Slightly bend knees	☐	☐	☐	_____
Use an internal girdle and a long midriff	☐	☐	☐	_____
Hold the head erect with the chin slightly tucked	☐	☐	☐	_____
Posture When Sitting				
Place both feet on the floor, legs uncrossed	☐	☐	☐	_____
Keep knees bent and popliteal area free from the edge of the chair	☐	☐	☐	_____
Hold the head erect with the chin slightly tucked	☐	☐	☐	_____

B. Examine how well you are using your body mechanics when at work by completing the following form.

RECOMMENDED TECHNIQUE	S	NI	U	Comments
Keep the work area as close to the body as possible	☐	☐	☐	_____
Face the work area	☐	☐	☐	_____
Keep the work area at a comfortable height	☐	☐	☐	_____
Lower the body to reach a low work area; return to standing by lifting the body with the thigh and hip muscles	☐	☐	☐	_____
Stand on a sturdy stool or stepladder when obtaining articles out of easy reach	☐	☐	☐	_____
Pivot to turn the body	☐	☐	☐	_____

RECOMMENDED TECHNIQUE	S	NI	U	Comments
Carry objects as close to the body as possible without contaminating the uniform	☐	☐	☐	_____
Lean toward objects being pushed and away from objects being pulled	☐	☐	☐	_____
Roll and slide objects rather than lift them whenever possible	☐	☐	☐	_____
Use the longest and strongest muscles of the body	☐	☐	☐	_____
Use an internal girdle and a long midriff	☐	☐	☐	_____
Move muscles smoothly and evenly	☐	☐	☐	_____
Maintain a good posture when working	☐	☐	☐	_____
Rest after strenuous work or exercise	☐	☐	☐	_____

Turning the Client From Her Back Onto Her Side

	S	NI	U	
Have the client flex her knees and place her arms across her chest	☐	☐	☐	_____
Place your hands on the client's far shoulder and hip and gently roll the client toward you	☐	☐	☐	_____
Put up the bedside rails and move to the opposite side of the bed	☐	☐	☐	_____
Move the client's shoulders, then his or her hips, or both together if the client is not heavy, to the center of the bed	☐	☐	☐	_____

or

	S	NI	U	
Use techniques just described but roll the client away from you, rather than toward you	☐	☐	☐	_____

Turning the Client Toward You: Back Onto His Abdomen

	S	NI	U	
Place the client's arm near you under his buttock, palm up, and bring his far leg over the leg near you	☐	☐	☐	_____
Turn the client's face away from you	☐	☐	☐	_____
Grasp the client's far hand and hip with your hands and gently roll the client toward you onto his or her abdomen	☐	☐	☐	_____
Move the client into the center of the bed properly	☐	☐	☐	_____

Turning the Client Away From You: Back Onto Her Abdomen

	S	NI	U	
Put up the bedside rails on the far side of the bed and move the client toward you	☐	☐	☐	_____
Place the client's arm away from you, under her buttock, palm up, and bring her near leg over her far leg	☐	☐	☐	_____
Turn the client's face toward you	☐	☐	☐	_____

RECOMMENDED TECHNIQUE	S	NI	U	Comments
Place your arm under the client's near leg and your other arm under the client's far shoulder	☐	☐	☐	_____
Gently roll the client away from you onto his or her abdomen	☐	☐	☐	_____

Turning the Client From His Abdomen Onto His Back

	S	NI	U	Comments
Place the client's far hand under his far thigh and cross his near leg over his far leg	☐	☐	☐	_____
Turn the client's face toward you	☐	☐	☐	_____
Reach under the client to grasp his far hand; place your other hand on his near hip	☐	☐	☐	_____
Pull the client's hand while pushing on his hip and gently roll him away from you onto his back	☐	☐	☐	_____

or

	S	NI	U	Comments
Place the client's far hand under his far thigh and cross his near leg over his far leg	☐	☐	☐	_____
Turn the client's face toward you	☐	☐	☐	_____
Put your arm between the client's legs and thighs and place your hand on his far thigh	☐	☐	☐	_____
Put your other arm under the client's shoulders and place your hand on his far shoulder	☐	☐	☐	_____
Straighten both of your arms as you gently roll the client onto his back	☐	☐	☐	_____

Moving the Client Up in Bed

	S	NI	U	Comments
Remove pillows from under the client's head and place one against the bed's headboard	☐	☐	☐	_____
Have the client flex her knees; place one of your arms under the client's shoulders and the other under her hip	☐	☐	☐	_____
Using a wide base of support, rock toward the head of the bed as the client pushes with her feet	☐	☐	☐	_____
Obtain an assistant if the client is too heavy for one person to move	☐	☐	☐	_____

The Three-Carrier Lift

	S	NI	U	Comments
Place the stretcher at a right angle to the foot of the bed and lock its wheels	☐	☐	☐	_____
Place the tallest carrier at the client's head and shoulders and the other two at his legs and waist	☐	☐	☐	_____
Have the three carriers place their hands well under the client and have them move him or her to the near side of the bed	☐	☐	☐	_____

RECOMMENDED TECHNIQUE	S	NI	U	Comments
Have the three carriers logroll the client onto their chests and then pivot toward the stretcher	☐	☐	☐	_____
Carry the client to the stretcher and gently place him or her on it	☐	☐	☐	_____

C. This section allows you to examine your techniques for assisting the client with positioning.

RECOMMENDED TECHNIQUE	S	NI	U	Comments

The Back-Lying Position

	S	NI	U	Comments
Place a small pillow under the client's upper shoulders, neck, and head; the cervical spine is extended	☐	☐	☐	_____
Bring the arms out to the side, flex the elbows, and place the forearms on pillows in pronation	☐	☐	☐	_____
Extend the wrists and place a hand roll in the client's elbows; the elbows are above shoulder level	☐	☐	☐	_____
Place a small roll at the proximal area under the knees so that they are only slightly flexed, at right angles to the lower legs	☐	☐	☐	_____
Place sandbags or trochanter rolls alongside the client's hips and thighs	☐	☐	☐	_____
Arrange top bed linens over the footboard so they do not rest on the feet	☐	☐	☐	_____

The Side-Lying Position

	S	NI	U	Comments
Place a small pillow under the client's neck so that the neck is in a position of extension	☐	☐	☐	_____
Place the client's arm on the side on which he or she is lying so that the elbow is flexed about 90°	☐	☐	☐	_____
Place the flexed arm alongside a pillow at the client's head	☐	☐	☐	_____
Place a pillow under the arm on the opposite side on which the client is lying	☐	☐	☐	_____
Slightly flex the knee on the side on which the client is lying	☐	☐	☐	_____
Place pillow(s) under the thigh, leg, and foot of the leg opposite the side on which the client is lying; flex the knee slightly	☐	☐	☐	_____
Pull the hip on which the client is lying backward slightly	☐	☐	☐	_____

RECOMMENDED TECHNIQUE	S	NI	U	Comments

The Face-Lying Position

Move the client down in bed after she is on her abdomen so that her feet are over the edge of the mattress ☐ ☐ ☐ _____

or

Instead of the above technique, support the legs on pillows so that the toes do not touch the bed ☐ ☐ ☐ _____

Place the client's arms alongside his or her head or body, depending on the client's comfort ☐ ☐ ☐ _____

Place a very small pillow under the client's head if this is comfortable ☐ ☐ ☐ _____

Slip a small pillow under the client between the bottom ribs and the upper abdomen if this is comfortable ☐ ☐ ☐ _____

Fowler's Position

Raise the head of the bed to the desired height ☐ ☐ ☐ _____

Allow the client's head to rest against the mattress or on a small pillow, depending on comfort ☐ ☐ ☐ _____

Position the client so that the angle of elevation begins at the hips ☐ ☐ ☐ _____

Support the forearms on pillows so that they are elevated enough to prevent a pull on the client's shoulders ☐ ☐ ☐ _____

Support the hands on pillows so that they are in natural alignment, with the forearms higher than the elbows ☐ ☐ ☐ _____

Elevate the knees a bit for short periods of time only, if this adds to the client's comfort ☐ ☐ ☐ _____

Support the feet at right angles to the lower legs and keep the top bed linens off the toes ☐ ☐ ☐ _____

CHAPTER 24

Therapeutic Exercise

■ Summary

Human beings need activity and exercise for optimal well-being. The need to move about is directly related to quality of life. There is currently renewed and continuous interest in and awareness of the importance of exercise, which has led many Americans to participate in some form of physical activity.

This chapter is intended to assist nursing students to assess the individual's level of fitness, identify risk factors, and provide suggestions to prevent complications associated with inactivity.

■ Matching Questions

Directions: For items 1 through 11, match the descriptions in Part B with the terms in Part A.

PART A

1. _____ Abduction

2. _____ Adduction

3. _____ Extension

4. _____ Flexion

5. _____ Hyperextension

6. _____ External rotation

7. _____ Internal rotation

8. _____ Pronation

9. _____ Supination

10. _____ Distal

11. _____ Proximal

PART B

a. The act of positioning the forearm so that the palm of the hand faces upward

b. The act of turning inward

c. The act of moving so that the angle between adjoining parts is reduced; bending

d. Nearest to the center of the body

e. The act of positioning the forearm so that the palm of the hand faces downward

f. The act of moving a body part away from the center of the body

g. Farthest from the center of the body

h. The act of straightening or increasing an angle that brings parts into or toward a straight line

i. The act of turning outward

j. The act of moving so that the angle between adjoining parts is made larger than its normal or average range, or more than 180 degrees

k. The act of moving a body part toward the center of the body

■ Multiple-Choice Questions

Directions: For items 1 through 10, circle the letter that corresponds to the best answer for each question.

1. Exercise is best described as:

   a. The movement that accompanies the activities of daily living

   b. The increased capacity to perform work with greater ease

   c. The movement intended to increase strength, stamina, and overall body tone

   d. The amount of movement that is possible in the normal joints of the body

2. Of the following types of exercise, which is performed with the assistance of another person:

   a. Passive exercise

   b. Active exercise

   c. Aerobic exercise

   d. Isometric exercise

3. Which of the following best defines *isometric exercise*:

   a. The contracting and relaxing of muscles during exercise to increase the capacity of the heart and lungs

   b. The contracting and relaxing of muscles with no movement to increase the capacity of the heart and lungs

   c. The contracting and relaxing of muscles with little or no movement and no increased heart and lung capacity

   d. A type of exercise that involves movement and work that challenges the heart and lungs

4. Which of the following is the formula for computing the target heart rate:

   a. 120 − age × 70% = target heart rate

   b. 220 − age × 50% = target heart rate

   c. 220 − age × 60% = target heart rate

   d. 120 − age × 50% = target heart rate

5. Aerobic exercise is an example of which of the following:

   a. Isotonic exercise

   b. Isometric exercise

   c. Therapeutic exercise

   d. Range-of-motion exercise

6. Isometric exercises are best described as:

   a. Exercises involving movement and work

   b. Exercises performed with assistance

   c. Exercises performed against resistance

   d. Exercises performed independently

7. "A state in which an individual is perceptually unaware of and inattentive to one side of the body" is the definition of which of the following nursing diagnoses:

   a. Impaired Physical Mobility

   b. Risk for Disuse Syndrome

   c. Unilateral Neglect

   d. Activity Intolerance

8. An exercise test that does not stress a person to exhaustion is called a (an):

   a. Ambulatory electrocardiogram

   b. Submaximal fitness test

   c. Walk-a-mile test

   d. Recovery index

9. The term *body composition* refers to:

   a. A guide for determining a person's fitness level

   b. A measure of energy and oxygen consumption during exercise

   c. The amount of body tissue that is lean versus that which is fat

   d. A therapeutic activity performed with assistance

10. Which of the following *best* describes range-of-motion exercises?

    a. Therapeutic activity performed independently

    b. Therapeutic activity performed against resistance

    c. Permanent loss of ability to perform therapeutic activities

    d. Therapeutic activity in which joints are moved

■ Alternative Format Questions

1. Calculate the target heart rate for a 55-year-old who is beginning an exercise program.

2. A 50-year-old female completed a 3-minute step test. Her pulse rate, taken for 30 seconds, was 45 at 1 minute, 40 at 2 minutes, and 30 at 3 minutes.

   Calculate the client's recovery index.

3. A female client who completes the walk-a-mile test in 10 minutes would have used an MET (metabolic energy equivalent) of ____.

■ True or False Questions

Directions: For items 1 through 15, decide if the statement is true or false and mark T or F in the space provided.

1. ____ Aerobic exercise is a form of active exercise that involves movement and work.

2. ____ Stamina is the ability to sustain effort.

3. ____ A preliminary step to fitness is preventing strain and injury through the development of good posture and body mechanics.

4. ____ Fatigue is accentuated by the buildup of chemicals when muscles are overused or misused.

5. ____ Athletes generally have increased pulse rates because of continuous activity and exercise.

6. ____ Flexibility is the amount of movement that is possible for a joint.

7. ____ One of the chief minerals that allows bones to be strong and compact is sodium.

8. ____ Softening of the bones is called osteoporosis.

9. ____ Caution should be used when planning any type of exercise program.

10. ____ A stress electrocardiogram is done while the client alternates going up and down two steps.

11. ____ Fitness refers to a person's capacity to perform physical activity.

12. ____ Rocking chairs are a good method for promoting exercise for the elderly.

13. ____ According to the Healthy People 2010 National Strategies for Improving Physical Activity and Fitness, children should be involved in activities that require flexibility and effort.

14. ____ The object of exercise should be to promote health while avoiding injury or complications from overexertion.

15. ____ Metabolic energy equivalent (MET) is the measure of energy and oxygen consumption that one's body can support.

■ Short Answer Questions

Directions: Read each of the following statements and supply the word(s) necessary in the space provided.

1. Describe six of the basic guidelines for assisting with range of motion as suggested in this chapter.

   a. _____
   _____

   b. _____
   _____

   c. _____
   _____

   d. _____
   _____

   e. _____
   _____

   f. _____
   _____

2. Identify five benefits of physical exercise.

   a. _____
   _____

   b. _____
   _____

   c. _____
   _____

   d. _____
   _____

   e. _____
   _____

3. Identify eight items necessary for client teaching in order to develop a safe exercise program.

a. _____

_____

b. _____

_____

c. _____

_____

d. _____

_____

e. _____

_____

f. _____

_____

g. _____

_____

h. _____

_____

■ Critical Thinking Exercises

List the members found on a comprehensive rehabilitation team. Describe the role of each member. Explain how the group would develop a collaborative plan of care for a client. How would the client's progress be evaluated?

Performance Checklist

A. This section allows you to examine your techniques for assisting with range-of-motion exercises.

1. Place a check mark in the "S" ("satisfactory") column if you used the recommended technique.

2. Place a check mark in the "NI" ("needs improvement") column if you used some but not all of each recommended technique.

3. Place a check mark in the "U" ("unsatisfactory") column if you forgot to include that particular recommended technique.

4. Note whether further practice is indicated, what errors you made, suggestions that will improve your skills, and so on in the section for comments.

RECOMMENDED TECHNIQUE	S	NI	U	Comments
Know the client's diagnosis and why the exercises are used	☐	☐	☐	_____
Explain to the client what exercise will be used, why it is used, and how it will be done	☐	☐	☐	_____
Avoid overexertion and fatigue	☐	☐	☐	_____
Start exercising gradually and work slowly with smooth, rhythmic, and regular motions	☐	☐	☐	_____
Use a firm but comfortable grip on the client when moving body parts	☐	☐	☐	_____
Move the joint until there is resistance but no pain	☐	☐	☐	_____
Support the part being exercised well at the proximal parts of the joints; do not grasp muscle groups	☐	☐	☐	_____
Return the joint to a neutral position when finishing each exercise	☐	☐	☐	_____
Stop the exercises if spasticity of muscles occurs	☐	☐	☐	_____
Keep friction at a minimum when moving the extremities	☐	☐	☐	_____
Use the exercises as prescribed, usually two times a day	☐	☐	☐	_____
Do each exercise two to five times, depending on the client's needs	☐	☐	☐	_____
Check the client's respiratory and pulse rates and evaluate when exercising may be too strenuous	☐	☐	☐	_____
Use passive exercises as necessary but encourage the use of active exercises when possible	☐	☐	☐	_____
Extend, hyperextend, flex, and rotate the neck, back, shoulder, and hip joints appropriately	☐	☐	☐	_____

RECOMMENDED TECHNIQUE	S	NI	U	Comments
Abduct and adduct the arms	☐	☐	☐	_____
Extend, hyperextend, flex, and rotate the elbow, wrist, finger, and thumb joints appropriately	☐	☐	☐	_____
Abduct and adduct the legs	☐	☐	☐	_____
Extend, hyperextend, flex, and rotate the knee, ankle, and toe joints appropriately	☐	☐	☐	_____
Observe any special orders when conducting range-of-motion exercises	☐	☐	☐	_____

B. This section allows you to examine your techniques for using a continuous passive motion machine.

RECOMMENDED TECHNIQUE	S	NI	U	Comments
Review the exercise prescription for the client	☐	☐	☐	_____
Determine the client's need for pain-relieving medication before you start	☐	☐	☐	_____
Develop a schedule with the client for using the machine	☐	☐	☐	_____
Obtain the continuous-passive-motion machine and a piece of sheepskin for making a cradle for the calf	☐	☐	☐	_____
Wear gloves to empty any wound-drainage containers and change dressings	☐	☐	☐	_____
Wash your hands	☐	☐	☐	_____
Explain the procedure to the client	☐	☐	☐	_____
Position the client appropriately for comfort during the exercise period	☐	☐	☐	_____
Place the machine on the bed and position the client appropriately	☐	☐	☐	_____
Position the knee correctly	☐	☐	☐	_____
Support and stabilize the leg	☐	☐	☐	_____
Adjust machine to a lower prescribed rate and turn it on	☐	☐	☐	_____
Observe the client's response	☐	☐	☐	_____
Readjust the alignment of the leg or the position of the machine as needed	☐	☐	☐	_____
Increase the degree of flexion and number of cycles gradually to prescribed levels	☐	☐	☐	_____
Turn machine off at end of the exercise period with the leg extended	☐	☐	☐	_____
Release straps; support joints at the knee and ankle while lifting the leg	☐	☐	☐	_____
Remove the machine; encourage active range-of-motion and isometric exercises	☐	☐	☐	_____
Document assessment data, use of machine, level of exercise, and client's response	☐	☐	☐	_____

CHAPTER 25

Mechanical Immobilization

■ Summary

Mechanical immobilization is used for clients who have sustained trauma to the musculoskeletal system. These injuries are painful and do not heal as rapidly as the skin or soft tissue does. They require a period of inactivity during the time that the body requires to repair the damaged structures.

Treatment requires mechanical immobilization devices that cover, attach to, and confine areas of the body for varying and extended periods of time. The purpose of these devices is to inactivate the injured area and prevent further trauma while avoiding injury to other body structures as they are used. This chapter describes the specialized skills and techniques needed to care for clients who require mechanical immobilization.

■ Matching Questions

Directions: For items 1 through 6, match the descriptions in Part B with the devices in Part A.

PART A

1. _____ Braces

2. _____ Cast

3. _____ Immobilizer

4. _____ Sling

5. _____ Splint

6. _____ Petal

PART B

a. Device that immobilizes an injured body part

b. Cloth device used to elevate, cradle, and support

c. Custom-made devices designed to support weak structures

d. Adhesive tape reinforcement to protect the skin

e. A rigid mold placed around a body part

f. A commercial splint made from cloth or foam

■ Multiple-Choice Questions

Directions: For items 1 through 10, circle the letter that corresponds to the best answer for each question.

1. A device that is used to support or align a body part and prevent or correct deformities is called a(n):
   a. Window
   b. Functional brace
   c. External fixator
   d. Orthosis

2. A foam or rigid splint used to treat athletic neck injuries is called a(n):
   a. Molded splint
   b. Internal fixator
   c. Cervical collar
   d. Brace

3. When applying a splinting device to an injured lower leg, the device should extend:
   a. From mid-thigh to the ankle
   b. From below the knee to the ankle
   c. From mid-thigh to below the ankle
   d. From below the knee to the toes

4. Which of the following is the first action when applying a triangular sling to support an injured arm?
   a. Place the upper end of the base of the triangle around the back of the neck on the unaffected side
   b. Place the upper end of the base of the triangle around the back of the neck on the affected side
   c. Place the base of the open triangle along the length of the client's chest on the unaffected side
   d. Place the base of the open triangle along the length of the client's chest on the affected side

5. Newly applied plaster casts may remain wet for:
   a. 24 to 48 hours
   b. 24 to 36 hours
   c. 20 to 30 hours
   d. 12 to 24 hours

6. The most appropriate way to dry a plaster cast is to:
   a. Expose the surface to a heat cradle
   b. Use an electric fan to circulate air on it
   c. Apply electric heating pads to the surface
   d. Expose the surface to room air circulation

7. Following surgery and the application of a cast, the nurse's primary concern should be:
   a. Assessing for pain and discomfort
   b. Assessing for swelling and bleeding
   c. Assessing the cast for hot spots
   d. Assessing the cast for wetness

8. An assessment technique recommended for determining the extent and effects of swelling and circulation of a casted area is:
   a. Assessing the pulse
   b. Assessing the blood pressure
   c. Assessing capillary refill
   d. Assessing the level of pain

9. To avoid compromised circulation to an area protected by a pneumatic splint, examination and treatment should take place within:
   a. 5–15 minutes
   b. 15–30 minutes
   c. 30–45 minutes
   d. 45–60 minutes

10. Custom-made devices that are designed to support weakened structures during periods of activity are called:
    a. Braces
    b. Splints
    c. Slings
    d. Casts

■ Alternative Format Questions

1. The nurse is planning the care for a client with a cast on his right leg. Which of the following statements should the nurse include in the client's nursing care plan? Select all that apply:
   1. Swab the cast with alcohol to clean it
   2. Cover the cast until it is dry to avoid chilling the client
   3. Assess circulation and sensation in exposed toes often
   4. Pad the edges of the cast
   5. Elevate the cast on pillows
   6. Apply ice packs to the cast at the level of the injury

2. The nurse is planning the care of a client who has been placed in traction. Which of the following statements should be included on the nursing care plan. Select all that apply:
   1. Provide a trapeze or over-bed frame
   2. Position the client so that his or her body is in a line opposite the pull of traction
   3. Apply traction as ordered
   4. Allow weights to rest on the floor
   5. Apply clean linens from the bottom toward the top of the bed
   6. Tuck the top sheet securely beneath the mattress

3. The nurse is caring for a client who is wearing a cervical collar after sustaining an athletic neck injury. Which of the following would indicate that the client's neurological function is intact? Select all that apply:
   1. He can elevate both arms
   2. He can rotate both wrists
   3. He can make a fist
   4. He can touch his thumbs to his little fingers
   5. He can spread his fingers
   6. He can hold a ball

■ True or False Questions

Directions: For items 1 through 12, decide if the statement is true or false and mark T or F in the space provided.

1. _____ A splint is a device designed to support weakened body structures during weight bearing.

2. _____ Pneumatic and traction splints are intended for brief periods of use immediately after an injury.

3. _____ A pneumatic splint should be fully inflated to produce sufficient pressure on the injured area.

4. _____ Casts made of the newer synthetic materials take 24 to 48 hours to dry.

5. _____ The nurse should use only the palms of the hands to move and reposition the cast while it is wet.

6. _____ A wet cast should be covered to protect the client from chills.

7. _____ The blanching test is used to assess the warmth of tissues.

8. _____ Bleeding under a cast is characterized by dark red areas on the cast.

9. _____ Rough edges of a cast may be repaired by applying petals made from adhesive tape.

10. _____ The electric cast saw must be used by a physician because it will cut the client's skin.

11. _____ Following cast removal, the skin should be scrubbed to forcibly remove the loose skin.

12. _____ Clients in skeletal traction must avoid active range of motion.

■ Short Answer Questions

Directions: Read each of the following statements and supply the word(s) necessary in the space provided.

1. Identify the five general purposes of mechanical immobilization.

   a. _____

   _____

   b. _____

   _____

   c. _____

   _____

   d. _____

   _____

   e. _____

   _____

2. Identify 10 of the important techniques that should be followed when applying an emergency splint.

   a. _____

   _____

   b. _____

   _____

   c. _____

   _____

   d. _____

   _____

   e. _____

   _____

   f. _____

   _____

   g. _____

   _____

   h. _____

   _____

   i. _____

   _____

   j. _____

   _____

3. List the three types of casts.

a. _____

_____

b. _____

_____

c. _____

_____

4. Identify four principles for maintaining effective traction.

a. _____

_____

b. _____

_____

c. _____

_____

d. _____

_____

■ Critical Thinking Exercise

Prepare a teaching plan for a client who is right-handed with a broken right wrist that has been placed in a cast. Complete the following form.

Topic for Teaching	Points to Cover in a Teaching Program
Accommodations necessary for:	
a. Eating	
b. Dressing	
c. Hygiene	
d. Toileting	
e. Working	

Performance Checklist

A. This section allows you to examine your techniques for caring for the client who has a cast.

1. Place a check mark in the "S" ("satisfactory") column if you used the recommended technique.
2. Place a check mark in the "NI" ("needs improvement") column if you used some but not all of each recommended technique.
3. Place a check mark in the "U" ("unsatisfactory") column if you forgot to include that particular recommended technique.
4. Note whether further practice is indicated, what errors you made, suggestions that will improve your skills, and so on in the section for comments.

RECOMMENDED TECHNIQUE	S	NI	U	Comments
Know the type of fracture the client has and why a particular type of cast was applied	☐	☐	☐	_____
Elevate the cast and allow nothing to rest on it	☐	☐	☐	_____
Expose the cast to air or use appropriate devices to promote drying of a new fiberglass cast	☐	☐	☐	_____
Look for signs or symptoms that indicate the cast is too tight	☐	☐	☐	_____
Look for signs or symptoms that indicate there is bleeding under the cast	☐	☐	☐	_____
Look for signs or symptoms that indicate there is an infection in tissues under the cast	☐	☐	☐	_____
Make the previous three observations at frequent intervals, the first two at least every hour during the first 24 hours	☐	☐	☐	_____
Report any unusual signs or symptoms promptly	☐	☐	☐	_____
Petal a cast properly	☐	☐	☐	_____
Keep the cast clean and do not introduce various devices under the cast	☐	☐	☐	_____
Protect a cast placed near the perineal area appropriately	☐	☐	☐	_____
Use range-of-motion and isometric exercises	☐	☐	☐	_____
Teach the client and family about proper cast care	☐	☐	☐	_____

B. This section allows you to examine your technique while caring for the client in traction.

RECOMMENDED TECHNIQUE	S	NI	U	Comments
Inspect the mechanical equipment for the application of traction	☐	☐	☐	_____
Provide a trapeze if the type of traction allows the client to raise his or her body weight	☐	☐	☐	_____
Position or reposition the client so that his or her body is centered in the bed and in the opposite line of pull	☐	☐	☐	_____
Avoid tucking top linens beneath the mattress	☐	☐	☐	_____
Instruct the client and nursing personnel as to the length of time the client is to be attached to the traction	☐	☐	☐	_____
Identify the positions that the client may assume	☐	☐	☐	_____
Depress the mattress to wash and rub posterior parts of the body	☐	☐	☐	_____
Make the bed by removing bottom linens from the head toward the toes	☐	☐	☐	_____
Provide pressure-relieving devices under bony prominences	☐	☐	☐	_____
Apply elbow and heel protectors as needed	☐	☐	☐	_____
Omit the use of pillows unless specified	☐	☐	☐	_____
Provide fracture bedpan for bowel elimination if lifting the hips alters the line of pull	☐	☐	☐	_____
Encourage active range of motion and isometric and isotonic exercises as much as possible	☐	☐	☐	_____
Encourage frequent dorsiflexion of unrestricted lower extremities	☐	☐	☐	_____
Inspect the skin for potential and possible areas of irritation and breakdown frequently	☐	☐	☐	_____
Cleanse the skin around skeletal pin-insertion sites	☐	☐	☐	_____
Apply or change dressings around skeletal pin-insertion sites using sterile technique	☐	☐	☐	_____
Cover any sharp points on traction devices	☐	☐	☐	_____
Assess the color, temperature, and mobility of all areas where traction is applied	☐	☐	☐	_____
Record the frequency of bowel movements	☐	☐	☐	_____
Provide diversionary activities as necessary	☐	☐	☐	_____

CHAPTER 26

Ambulatory Aids

■ Summary

This chapter provides information on the nursing activities and mechanical devices used to promote mobility in debilitated clients. Activities to prepare the client for ambulation and exercises to strengthen and tone muscles are described.

■ Matching Questions

Directions: For items 1 through 4, match the methods of use in Part B with the crutch-walking gaits in Part A.

PART A

1. _____ Two-point gait

2. _____ Three-point gait

3. _____ Four-point gait

4. _____ Swing-through gait

PART B

a. Only one point is moved forward at a time (e.g., left crutch, right foot, right crutch, left foot)

b. The crutches are advanced together. The body weight is shifted from the legs to the hand grips. The legs are swung either slightly beyond or parallel with the crutches.

c. The client bears weight on both feet. The right crutch and the left foot are moved forward. Then, the left foot and right crutch move forward.

d. Both crutches and the leg that cannot bear weight move forward, and then the foot permitted to bear weight comes through

■ Multiple-Choice Questions

Directions: For items 1 through 10, circle the letter that corresponds to the best answer for each question.

1. Muscle tone refers to:
   a. The muscle's ability to respond
   b. The muscle's power to perform
   c. The muscle's ability to contract
   d. The muscle's strength at rest

2. Quadriceps setting is an example of:
   a. Isotonic exercise
   b. Aerobic exercise
   c. Isometric exercise
   d. Passive exercise

3. For optimum use, a cane must be adjusted to an appropriate height for the client as follows:
   a. The handle should be parallel with the client's hip, allowing the elbow to extend
   b. The handle should be parallel with the client's hip, allowing 30° of elbow flexion
   c. The handle should allow the client to lean forward 15° with the elbow flexed 10°
   d. The handle should allow the client to stand straight with the elbow flexed 15°

4. Clients who require the use of crutches for ambulation but who are unable to bear weight on their hands and wrists would most likely use:
   a. Lofstrand crutches
   b. Axillary crutches
   c. Canadian crutches
   d. Platform crutches

5. The most stable form of ambulatory aid is:
   a. A cane
   b. Crutches
   c. A walking belt
   d. A walker

6. Quadriceps setting is done in which of the following ways:
   a. The client pinches the buttocks together and then relaxes
   b. The client sits in bed and raises the buttocks up by pushing down with his or her hands
   c. The client lies on his or her abdomen and lifts the head and shoulders off the bed with his or her arms
   d. The client pulls the kneecaps toward the hips by pushing down on his or her knees

7. When a client is using a cane, he should:
   a. Place the cane about 10 centimeters (4 inches) to the side of the foot and hold it on the involved side
   b. Place the cane about 10 centimeters (4 inches) to the side of the foot and hold it on the uninvolved side
   c. Place the cane about 5 centimeters (2.5 inches) to the side of the foot and hold it on the involved side
   d. Place the cane about 5 centimeters (2.5 inches) to the side of the foot and hold it on the uninvolved side

8. In which of the following situations would the individual use the three-point gait for crutch walking?
   a. The client must be able to bear some weight on each leg
   b. Weight bearing is allowed on one leg and no weight or only limited weight on the other leg
   c. Weight bearing must be permitted on both feet, but they may have weak or limited ability
   d. One or both legs are involved, and the client usually has leg braces or a cast

9. Which of the following are appropriate for walking on stairs with a cane?
   a. Use the cane rather than the stair rail
   b. Keep your back straight
   c. Take each step going up with the stronger leg first
   d. Move the cane forward with the stronger extremity

10. When using a walker, clients are instructed to:
    a. Stand within the walker
    b. Advance the walker 10 to 12 inches
    c. Always step with the stronger extremity
    d. Flex their hips and knees when walking

■ Alternative Format Questions

1. The nurse is preparing a client with an above-the-knee amputation for discharge. Which of the following statements should be part of the discharge teaching? Select all that apply:
   1. Weigh yourself once a week
   2. Cleanse the stump each morning
   3. Lie supine two or three times a day
   4. Start slowly and increase wearing time of the prosthesis each day
   5. Cover the prosthetic foot with a sock and shoe
   6. Wash, rinse, and twist the nylon sheath to remove excess water

2. When a client is being raised from a supine to a standing position on a tilt table, the maximum degree of tilt at each increment is _____ degrees.

3. When the client is standing erect, the shoulder rest of the crutch should be positioned _____ finger widths below the axilla?

■ True or False Questions

Directions: For items 1 through 10, decide if the statement is true or false and mark T or F in the space provided.

1. ____ Most clients are capable of performing quadriceps and gluteal setting exercises independently.

2. ____ The nurse should place a rolled towel under the knees before the client attempts the quadriceps setting exercise.

3. ____ Crutches should fit snugly into the axilla to prevent falls.

4. ____ A cane is a handheld device that is used by clients who have weakness on one side of their bodies.

5. ____ When assisting a client to ambulate using a walking belt, the nurse should hold onto the handles of the belt and walk behind the client.

6. ____ It is possible to obtain an approximate measurement for crutch length by subtracting 40 centimeters from the client's height.

7. ____ In older adults, postural changes may result in a swaying or shuffling gait.

8. ____ When walking downstairs while using a cane, take each step with the stronger leg first.

9. ____ A walker is the most stable form of ambulatory aid.

10. ____ Antiembolism stockings are not necessary for clients being placed on a tilt table for preambulation therapy.

■ Short Answer Questions

Directions: Read each of the following statements and supply the word(s) necessary in the space provided.

1. List four devices and techniques that provide support and assistance with walking.

   a. _____

   _____

   b. _____

   _____

   c. _____

   _____

   d. _____

   _____

2. List three common aids for ambulation.

   a. _____

   _____

   b. _____

   _____

   c. _____

   _____

3. Describe three characteristics of appropriately fitted crutches.

   a. _____

   _____

   b. _____

   _____

   c. _____

   _____

4. Explain the reason for using a tilt table as part of preambulation therapy. _____

   _____

   _____

■ Critical Thinking Exercise

Describe how the nurse could demonstrate respect for individual decision making when the clients requiring the use of ambulatory aids are a preschooler, adolescent, and older adult.

a. Preschooler

b. Adolescent

c. Older adult

Performance Checklist

A. This section allows you to examine your techniques for caring for the client who has an ambulatory aid or needs assistance with ambulation.

1. Place a check mark in the "S" ("satisfactory") column if you used the recommended technique.
2. Place a check mark in the "NI" ("needs improvement") column if you used some but not all of each recommended technique.
3. Place a check mark in the "U" ("unsatisfactory") column if you forgot to include that particular recommended technique.
4. Note whether further practice is indicated, what errors you made, suggestions that will improve your skills, and so on in the section for comments.

RECOMMENDED TECHNIQUE	S	NI	U	Comments
Have the client use quadriceps drills by having him or her contract and relax muscles on the front of the thigh	☐	☐	☐	_____
Have the client fix his or her buttocks by pinching them together and then relaxing them	☐	☐	☐	_____
Use push-ups properly, as indicated, if this exercise is recommended	☐	☐	☐	_____
Prepare the client for dangling by placing him in the Fowler's position for a few minutes	☐	☐	☐	_____
Pivot the client so that his or her legs dangle over the edge of the bed, feet resting on a footstool or on the floor	☐	☐	☐	_____
Properly assist the client to a chair. Walk alongside the client, using a walking belt when he or she is ready to ambulate.	☐	☐	☐	_____
Demonstrate the proper use of a walking belt, a cane, and crutches when the client requires these devices	☐	☐	☐	_____

B. This section allows you to examine your techniques for assisting with crutch walking.

RECOMMENDED TECHNIQUE	S	NI	U	Comments
Review the medical orders for the type of activity and crutch-walking gait	☐	☐	☐	_____
Observe the condition of the client's axilla and palms	☐	☐	☐	_____
Inspect the condition of the axillary pads and rubber crutch tips	☐	☐	☐	_____
Ask if there are any symptoms such as pain, numbness, or tingling in the fingers or joints	☐	☐	☐	_____
Assist the client to put on a robe, clothing, and appropriate walking shoes	☐	☐	☐	_____

RECOMMENDED TECHNIQUE	S	NI	U	Comments
Apply a walking belt as necessary	☐	☐	☐	_____
Clear the pathway where the client will walk	☐	☐	☐	_____
Wash your hands	☐	☐	☐	_____
Assist the client to a standing position	☐	☐	☐	_____
Offer the crutches and observe that they are placed correctly	☐	☐	☐	_____
Remind the client to stand straight with the shoulders relaxed	☐	☐	☐	_____
Position yourself to the side and slightly behind the client	☐	☐	☐	_____
Position yourself on the client's weaker side	☐	☐	☐	_____
Instruct the client to move forward	☐	☐	☐	_____
Observe that the client uses the prescribed gait	☐	☐	☐	_____
Stop if there is evidence of fatigue or intolerance for the activity	☐	☐	☐	_____
Evaluate the client's tolerance of the activity	☐	☐	☐	_____
Document the activity	☐	☐	☐	_____

CHAPTER 27

Perioperative Care

■ Summary

Certain illnesses must be treated through surgery. Surgery involves the entering of tissues and removal or reconstructing of structures that are diseased, injured, or malformed. This chapter discusses basic care of the surgical client. It includes care that applies, in general, to all surgical clients, regardless of diagnosis or type of surgery. The discussion also includes laser surgery and blood donors from autologous and directed donor sources.

■ Matching Questions

Directions: For items 1 through 5, match the examples in Part B with the types of surgery in Part A.

PART A

1. ____ Optional

2. ____ Elective

3. ____ Required

4. ____ Urgent

5. ____ Emergency

PART B

a. Surgery for the removal of a cataract

b. Surgery to relieve an intestinal obstruction

c. Surgery for the removal of a superficial cyst

d. Surgery for cosmetic purposes

e. Surgery for the removal of a malignant tumor

Directions: For items 6 through 12, match the descriptions in Part B with the complications in Part A.

PART A

6. ____ Airway occlusion

7. ____ Evisceration

8. ____ Adynamic ileus

9. ____ Hypoxemia

10. ____ Urinary retention

11. ____ Dehiscence

12. ____ Shock

PART B

a. Inadequate oxygenation of blood

b. Severe, rapid blood loss

c. Obstruction of the trachea from swelling

d. Inability to void

e. Separation of incision

f. Lack of bowel motility

g. Protrusion of abdominal organs through incision

h. Inadequate blood flow

■ Multiple-Choice Questions

Directions: For items 1 through 10, circle the letter that corresponds to the best answer for each question.

1. Which of the following is the primary disadvantage of outpatient surgery:

    a. It requires that care of the client following discharge be carried out by unskilled individuals

    b. It allows for fewer delays in assessing and preparing a client once he or she arrives for surgery

    c. It requires intensive preoperative teaching in a short amount of time

    d. It reduces the time for establishing a nurse–client relationship

2. With which type of anesthesia does the client experience loss of feeling in the lower half of the body only?

    a. General anesthesia

    b. Regional anesthesia

    c. Local anesthesia

    d. Topical anesthesia

3. Which of the following is true of directed donors?

    a. They must be at least 21 years old

    b. They must meet volunteer donor medical history criteria

    c. They must weigh at least 95 pounds

    d. They may donate 1 unit every 56 days

4. A postoperative client's question, "How am I doing?" may really mean:

    a. "I'm doing fine, don't you think?"

    b. "I'm worried about my family."

    c. "Is the surgery all over?"

    d. "Do you think I'll make it?"

5. The postoperative complication that deep-breathing exercises help most to prevent is:

    a. Hiccups

    b. Phlebitis

    c. Atelectasis

    d. Nausea

6. Which type of cough should the client be taught to use postoperatively?

    a. Hard

    b. Hacking

    c. Whooping

    d. Forced

7. To prevent the formation of thrombi and emboli in the postoperative client, the nurse should:

    a. Have the client lie still

    b. Place pillows under the knees

    c. Raise the knee gatch

    d. Teach foot and leg exercises

8. Mr. J. states that he is worried about his planned operation. Of the following comments the nurse can make, which would be the most appropriate response?

    a. "Don't worry, Mr. J. Your surgeon has done this many times."

    b. "There is really no need to worry; it will be okay"

    c. "Tell me what worries you about the surgery"

    d. "Mrs. S. had the same surgery yesterday, and she is fine"

9. Plume produced during laser surgery can be hazardous because the:

    a. Smell is damaging to the nasal tissues

    b. Smoke may cause burning and watering of the eyes

    c. Airborne cells and viruses may be inhaled

    d. Water may produce routes for contamination

10. When a 7-year-old male client states that he doesn't want to cry after his operation, the nurse's best response would be:

    a. "It is all right if you cry."

    b. "Big boys don't cry."

    c. "It will not help if you cry."

    d. "Crying will only make things worse."

■ Alternative Format Questions

1. When applying a pneumatic compression device, the air pressure should be set at_____.

2. What information should be included when teaching postcircumcision care to parents of a newborn who is being discharged from the hospital? Select all that apply:

    1. The infant must void before discharge

    2. Petroleum jelly should be applied to the penis with each diaper change

    3. Tub baths can be given while the circumcision heals

4. Blood on the front of the diaper should be reported

5. Circumcision care will be required for 2 to 4 days after discharge

6. The plastic ring will come off by itself in about 7 to 10 days

3. Which of the following statements by the client indicate that preoperative teaching for gallbladder surgery has been effective? Select all that apply:

   1. "I can have tea or water up to 2 hours before my surgery"

   2. "I will not be allowed to cough after surgery because it might open my incision"

   3. "I must stop taking my anticoagulant 3 days before my surgery"

   4. "I will have to do some leg exercises in bed after my surgery"

   5. "I will not be able to eat after surgery"

■ True or False Questions

Directions: For items 1 through 15, decide if the statement is true or false and mark T or F in the space provided.

1. ____ The separation of a wound with exposure of body organs is known as dehiscence.

2. ____ Clients scheduled for outpatient surgery must check into the hospital the night before.

3. ____ The nurse shares the responsibility for assessing factors that pose a hazard for the client undergoing surgery.

4. ____ An autologous transfusion is made from one's own blood.

5. ____ Shaving the surgical area the night before surgery is the safest method for preventing the growth of microorganisms.

6. ____ The individual who is donating blood as a directed donor must weigh at least 95 pounds.

7. ____ An individual designated as a directed donor may give blood once every week.

8. ____ It is generally agreed that forced coughing should be routinely performed postoperatively.

9. ____ It is a nursing responsibility to check that a surgical consent has been obtained before proceeding with the preparation of a client for surgery.

10. ____ The special skin preparation prior to surgery is done to sterilize the skin.

11. ____ The nurse who is caring for the preoperative client is responsible for checking to make sure all the items on the preoperative checklist have been completed.

12. ____ It is important to give the operative client's family the exact time their family member will return from the recovery room.

13. ____ When teaching clients deep breathing, the nurse should emphasize that the breathing should be done rapidly.

14. ____ It is best to apply antiembolism stockings after the client has been out of bed and has exercised his or her legs.

15. ____ Hypovolemic shock is caused by blood loss resulting from hemorrhage.

■ Short Answer Questions

Directions: Read each of the following statements and supply the word(s) necessary in the space provided.

1. List the equipment and supplies that are likely to be needed in readiness for the postoperative client's room, as suggested in this chapter.

   a. _____

   _____

   b. _____

   _____

   c. _____

   _____

   d. _____

   _____

2. List the advantages of laser surgery suggested in this chapter.

   a. _____

   _____

   b. _____

   _____

   c. _____

   _____

   d. _____

   _____

   e. _____

   _____

   f. _____

   _____

   g. _____

   _____

   h. _____

   _____

   i. _____

   _____

3. List six areas commonly addressed in discharge instructions.

   a. _____

   _____

   b. _____

   _____

   c. _____

   _____

   d. _____

   _____

   e. _____

   _____

   f. _____

   _____

4. Identify eight general types of measures included in postoperative care, as suggested in this chapter.

   a. _____

   _____

   b. _____

   _____

   c. _____

   _____

   d. _____

   _____

   e. _____

   _____

   f. _____

   _____

   g. _____

   _____

   h. _____

   _____

■ Critical Thinking Exercises

1. Describe adjustments you make when caring for preoperative and postoperative clients:

   a. When the client is an infant or child

   b. When the client has diabetes mellitus

   c. When the client is obese

   d. When the client is elderly

Performance Checklist

A. This section allows you to examine your techniques for caring for the client who is having surgery.

1. Place a check mark in the "S" ("satisfactory") column if you used the recommended technique.
2. Place a check mark in the "NI" ("needs improvement") column if you used some but not all of each recommended technique.
3. Place a check mark in the "U" ("unsatisfactory") column if you forgot to include that particular recommended technique.
4. Note whether further practice is indicated, what errors you made, suggestions that will improve your skills, and so on in the section for comments.

RECOMMENDED TECHNIQUE	S	NI	U	Comments
Changing position of the client	☐	☐	☐	_____
Increasing activity for the client	☐	☐	☐	_____
Preparing the client for ambulation	☐	☐	☐	_____
Helping the client to walk	☐	☐	☐	_____
Having the client perform self-care	☐	☐	☐	_____
Anticipating other topics, depending on the client's needs	☐	☐	☐	_____

Teaching Deep Breathing

	S	NI	U	Comments
Position the client for comfort	☐	☐	☐	_____
Help the client relax to allow for total lung expansion	☐	☐	☐	_____
Have the client take a deep breath to the count of five to seven, with 1 second per count	☐	☐	☐	_____
Teach the client to make his or her abdomen larger while inhaling	☐	☐	☐	_____
Have the client hold his or her breath to the count of three after inhaling deeply	☐	☐	☐	_____
Have the client exhale against pursed lips for about twice as long as it took him or her to inhale	☐	☐	☐	_____
Teach the client to contract her abdomen toward her spine while exhaling	☐	☐	☐	_____
Repeat inhaling and exhaling several times with a few seconds rest between respirations	☐	☐	☐	_____
Watch for signs that the client may be breathing too rapidly and instruct him or her to rest between breaths	☐	☐	☐	_____
Have the client practice deep breathing until he or she is able to do so correctly	☐	☐	☐	_____
Teach the client how to use incentive spirometry with equipment of the agency's choice	☐	☐	☐	_____

RECOMMENDED TECHNIQUE	S	NI	U	Comments
Teaching Leg and Foot Exercises				
Have the client sit with his or her head raised	☐	☐	☐	_____
Teach the client to bend one knee, raise the leg, hold the position, and then extend the leg	☐	☐	☐	_____
Have the client do the same exercise with the other leg	☐	☐	☐	_____
Have the client draw imaginary circles with the great toes	☐	☐	☐	_____
Have the client repeat the exercise five times every 2 hours	☐	☐	☐	_____
Teaching Coughing				
Determine what the client will be able to do postoperatively in relation to coughing	☐	☐	☐	_____
Position the client in Fowler's position, unless contraindicated	☐	☐	☐	_____
Splint the area well where the operative site will be	☐	☐	☐	_____
Inhale deeply through the nose	☐	☐	☐	_____
Do forced coughing three times in a row while exhaling	☐	☐	☐	_____
Repeat the exercise if secretions remain	☐	☐	☐	_____
Miscellaneous Preoperative Teaching				
Instruct client on the use of a bedpan and urinal	☐	☐	☐	_____
Describe commonly used tubes	☐	☐	☐	_____
Inform client of the frequency of vital signs	☐	☐	☐	_____
Discuss measures to control discomfort and sleeplessness	☐	☐	☐	_____
Review diet and fluid restrictions with client	☐	☐	☐	_____
Teach client immediate preoperative and postoperative care	☐	☐	☐	_____
Make client aware of visiting privileges	☐	☐	☐	_____

B. This section allows you to examine your techniques for preparing a client for a surgical procedure.

RECOMMENDED TECHNIQUE	S	NI	U	Comments
Determine that the client has had a complete examination and is familiar with his or her condition	☐	☐	☐	_____
Assist with measures to help the client so that he or she is well rested and in a good nutritional state	☐	☐	☐	_____

RECOMMENDED TECHNIQUE	S	NI	U	Comments
Note that the proper consent for surgery has been completed	☐	☐	☐	_____
Check vital signs preoperatively, including immediately before surgery, and report abnormalities promptly	☐	☐	☐	_____
See to it that the incision area is properly prepared, including shaving the area as necessary	☐	☐	☐	_____
Administer a cleansing enema preoperatively if ordered	☐	☐	☐	_____
Attend to the client's hygienic needs the night before and immediately before surgery	☐	☐	☐	_____
Administer prescribed medications the day or night before and immediately before surgery	☐	☐	☐	_____
See to it that the client has had nothing by mouth as ordered	☐	☐	☐	_____
Care for valuables according to agency policy	☐	☐	☐	_____
Remove cosmetics, hairpins, and hair clips; secure long hair in place	☐	☐	☐	_____
Gown and cap the client for surgery; use antiembolic stockings if agency policy requires	☐	☐	☐	_____
See to it that the client voids immediately before surgery and report promptly if he or she does not	☐	☐	☐	_____
Assist with transferring the client to surgery and check the client's identity with operating-room personnel	☐	☐	☐	_____

C. This section allows you to examine your techniques for receiving a client from the recovery room.

RECOMMENDED TECHNIQUE	S	NI	U	Comments
Have the room and bed ready to receive the client	☐	☐	☐	_____
Verify the identity of the client with recovery-room personnel	☐	☐	☐	_____
Assist recovery-room personnel to transfer the client to his or her bed	☐	☐	☐	_____
Position the client properly in bed	☐	☐	☐	_____
Obtain a report on the client's condition from recovery-room personnel	☐	☐	☐	_____
Check vital signs, including skin color, and report anything unusual	☐	☐	☐	_____
Check the dressings for evidence of excessive bleeding and report unusual findings	☐	☐	☐	_____

RECOMMENDED TECHNIQUE	S	NI	U	Comments
Check the client's postoperative orders and carry out those that need to be taken care of immediately	☐	☐	☐	_____
Check the client for level of consciousness and help him or her to become oriented	☐	☐	☐	_____
Put bedside rails in place and leave the signal device handy when it is safe to leave the client	☐	☐	☐	_____
Notify relatives that the client has returned from surgery and tell them when they may visit	☐	☐	☐	_____
Continue to check vital signs, level of consciousness, and dressings according to agency policy	☐	☐	☐	_____

D. This section allows you to examine your techniques for applying antiembolism stockings.

RECOMMENDED TECHNIQUE	S	NI	U	Comments
Wash your hands	☐	☐	☐	_____
Measure client for appropriate size, if indicated	☐	☐	☐	_____
Plan to apply the stockings before the client is out of bed in the morning	☐	☐	☐	_____
Check to see that the client's legs are dry and clean before applying the stockings	☐	☐	☐	_____
Use powder or cornstarch on the skin, as indicated; avoid massaging the legs	☐	☐	☐	_____
Turn stocking inside out, insert toes, and pull stocking over foot	☐	☐	☐	_____
Gather and pull remaining stocking over the leg	☐	☐	☐	_____
Remove the stockings twice a day for 20 minutes and then reapply them	☐	☐	☐	_____
Avoid turning down the tops of the stockings and ensure that they are free of wrinkles	☐	☐	☐	_____
See to it that the stockings are laundered as necessary	☐	☐	☐	_____

CHAPTER **28**

Wound Care

[handwritten notes:] resolution – recovery of injured cells
regeneration – replacement c̄ new cells
scar formation –
non-functioning substitute

■ Summary

Everyone acquires a wound at one time or another in his or her life. The body's responses to injury and the healing process are normal, protective mechanisms. Even though the body has a remarkable ability to recover when tissue is injured, there are certain actions that can be taken to support or assist these mechanisms. This chapter discusses general principles related to wound healing, the body's responses to tissue injury, and the body's responses to heat and cold. Clients who have problems with tissue healing are likely to have nursing diagnoses similar to the ones listed in this chapter. The nursing care plan was developed for a client with Impaired Tissue Integrity.

■ Matching Questions

Directions: For items 1 through 6, match the descriptions in Part B with the types of wounds in Part A.

PART A

1. __G__ Incision
2. __C__ Laceration
3. __F__ Abrasion
4. __A__ Avulsion
5. __E__ Ulceration
6. __D__ Puncture

PART B

a. Stripping away of large areas of skin and underlying tissue, leaving cartilage and bone exposed
b. An opening of skin, underlying tissue, or mucous membrane caused by a narrow, sharp, pointed object
c. A separation of skin and tissue in which the edges are torn and irregular
d. Injury of soft tissue underlying the skin from the force caused by contact with a hard object

e. A shallow area in which skin or mucous membrane is missing
f. A wound in which the surface layers of skin are scraped away
g. A clean separation of skin and tissue with smooth, even edges

Directions: For items 7 through 9, match the descriptions in Part B with the pressure classifications in Part A.

PART A

7. __d__ Stage I
8. __c__ Stage II
9. __a__ Stage III

PART B

a. The break in the skin extends to the subcutaneous tissue
b. The ulcer involves loss of all layers, exposing muscle and bone
c. Redness of the area is usually accompanied by blistering or a shallow break in the skin
d. The skin does not return to normal color, even when the pressure is relieved

■ Multiple-Choice Questions

Directions: For items 1 through 15, circle the letter that corresponds to the best answer for each question.

1. During the inflammation process, which of the following characteristics occurs first:
   a. Decreased functioning
   b. Pain
   c. Redness
   d. Swelling

2. The components of a scar are:
   a. Fibroblasts and collagen
   b. Fibroblasts and neutrophils

    c. Neutrophils and monocytes

    d. Monocytes and collagens

3. The replacement of damaged cells with identical new cells during wound healing is known as:

    a. Scar formation

    b. Resolution

    c. Regeneration

    d. Granulation

4. Granulation tissue is best described as:

    a. The production of nonfunctioning substitute cells

    b. The recovery of injured cells during wound healing

    c. Pinkish-red tissue containing capillary projections

    d. The temporary building blocks of fibroblasts and collagen

5. The single most effective method of preventing wound infections is:

    a. Careful cleansing of the wound

    b. The application of sterile dressings

    c. Practicing surgical asepsis

    d. Using careful hand-washing practices

6. The primary cause of a pressure sore is:

    a. Unrelieved compression of the skin cells and muscle tissue

    b. Unrelieved compression of muscle cells and subcutaneous tissue

    c. Unrelieved compression of capillaries supplying bone and muscle tissue

    d. Unrelieved compression of capillaries supplying the skin and underlying tissue

7. Of the following, which is the earliest sign of excessive pressure:

    a. Pale appearance of the skin

    b. Ulcer formation on the skin

    c. Dark or cyanotic color to the skin

    d. Reddened appearance of the skin

8. Of the following individuals, who would be most prone to pressure sores:

    a. Mr. J., age 45, weight 172 pounds, height 6 feet, 1 inch

    b. Ms. K., age 16, weight 105 pounds, height 5 feet, 4 inches

    c. Mrs. R., age 73, weight 98 pounds, height 5 feet, 6 inches

    d. Mr. L., age 59, weight 165 pounds, height 5 feet, 7 inches

9. One of the common reasons for dressing a wound is:

    a. To absorb drainage

    b. To restrict microorganisms

    c. To control edema

    d. To prevent friction

10. If changing a dressing is likely to be a painful experience, the nurse should:

    a. Give prescribed medication about 45 to 60 minutes before to reduce discomfort

    b. Give prescribed medication about 30 to 45 minutes before to reduce discomfort

    c. Give prescribed medication about 15 to 30 minutes before to reduce discomfort

    d. Give prescribed medication about 5 to 10 minutes before to reduce discomfort

11. The wound-closure materials least likely to compress tissues if swelling occurs are:

    a. Silk sutures

    b. Metal staples

    c. Nylon sutures

    d. Wire sutures

12. It is important to ease a dressing from all the edges toward the center of a wound because:

    a. This will prevent contamination of the wound and enhance the healing process

    b. Wounds heal toward the center, and pulling toward the edge could cause further tissue damage

    c. Wounds heal away from the center, and pulling toward the edge could cause further tissue damage

    d. This approach helps to avoid tearing fragile skin that could be pulled away with the dressing

13. The approximate temperature of an irrigating solution for an eye irrigation should be:
    a. Body temperature
    b. Warm to touch
    c. Cool to touch
    d. Room temperature

14. Which of the following age groups would be most likely to experience a thermal injury from application of heat or cold:
    a. Preschool children
    b. School-age children
    c. Adults
    d. Older adults

15. The purpose of the spiral-reverse turn method of bandaging is:
    a. To anchor and secure a bandage when it is started and ended
    b. To wrap a part that is cylindrical in shape, such as an arm or leg
    c. To bandage a cone-shaped body part, such as the thigh or leg
    d. To bandage the thumb, breast, shoulder, groin, or hip

■ Alternative Format Questions

1. A hydrocolloid dressing (Duoderm), if intact, can remain in place for _____ week(s).

   duoderm X 1 wk

2. The nurse is assessing the skin of a newly admitted client. When she inspects the client's back, she finds a wound at the sacrum that has a shallow crater, extends to the subcutaneous tissue, and has purulent drainage. The client states that it is not painful. These observations are characteristic of a pressure ulcer at stage ___III___?

3. The nurse is caring for a postpartum client who has an episiotomy. She is preparing the sitz bath for the client's use. The temperature of the water for the sitz bath container should be no hotter than _____° Fahrenheit.

■ True or False Questions

Directions: For items 1 through 12, decide if the statement is true or false and mark T or F in the space provided.

1. ____ Second intention is a type of wound healing in which the edges are directly next to one another.

2. ____ Third intention is a type of wound healing in which widely separated edges must heal inward toward the center.

3. ____ A spica turn is an adaptation of the figure-of-8 turning technique in which all turns overlap and cross each other, forming a sharp angle.

4. ____ Shearing force is the friction of sheets against the skin.

5. ____ Pressure sores frequently occur over the ears.

6. ____ When the surface of the skin is broken over a pressure sore, the nurse must maintain a dry environment.

7. ____ Two of the principal goals of wound care are comfort and good dressing applications.

8. ____ The best feature of transparent dressings is that they are not permeable.

9. ____ Hydrocolloid dressings promote healing and comfort because they do not cause trauma when removed or reapplied.

10. ____ It is necessary to follow sterile technique when performing any type of irrigation.

11. ____ The drainage basin used to receive the solution during irrigations must be sterile.

12. ____ Irrigation is contraindicated with situations in which a live insect has become lodged in the auditory canal.

■ Short Answer Questions

Directions: Read each of the following statements and supply the word(s) necessary in the space provided.

1. List the sequence of events that are associated with the inflammatory response.

   a. _____

   _____

   b. _____

   _____

   c. _____

   _____

   d. _____

   _____

2. List six common purposes of a dressing.

   a. _____

   _____

   b. _____

   _____

   c. _____

   _____

   d. _____

   _____

   e. _____

   _____

   f. _____

   _____

3. List items of equipment and supplies for changing a dressing on a clean, open wound as suggested in this chapter.

   a. _____

   _____

   b. _____

   _____

   c. _____

   _____

   d. _____

   _____

e. _____

_____

f. _____

_____

g. _____

_____

h. _____

_____

4. Discuss four nursing measures when caring for a wound with a drain as suggested in this chapter.

   a. _____

   _____

   b. _____

   _____

   c. _____

   _____

   d. _____

   _____

5. Describe ten basic techniques for securing a dressing as recommended in this chapter.

   a. _____

   _____

   b. _____

   _____

   c. _____

   _____

   d. _____

   _____

   e. _____

   _____

   f. _____

   _____

   g. _____

   _____

   h. _____

   _____

   i. _____

   _____

j. _____

_____

6. List the purposes of bandages and binders as suggested in this chapter.

a. _____

_____

b. _____

_____

c. _____

_____

■ Critical Thinking Exercise

1. Describe adjustments you make when promoting tissue healing:

a. When the client is an infant or child

b. When the client is unconscious

c. When the client is elderly

Performance Checklist

A. This section allows you to examine your techniques for caring for the client who requires a dressing change.

1. Place a check mark in the "S" ("satisfactory") column if you used the recommended technique.

2. Place a check mark in the "NI " ("needs improvement") column if you used some but not all of each recommended technique.

3. Place a check mark in the "U" ("unsatisfactory") column if you forgot to include that particular recommended technique.

4. Note whether further practice is indicated, what errors you made, suggestions that will improve your skills, and so on in the section for comments.

RECOMMENDED TECHNIQUE	S	NI	U	Comments
Wash your hands	☐	☐	☐	
Set up a sterile field with all necessary supplies and equipment	☐	☐	☐	
Remove adhesive securing the dressing while pulling it toward the wound	☐	☐	☐	
Remove and discard the soiled dressings in a waterproof container	☐	☐	☐	
If the dressing sticks to the wound, moisten it with sterile water or normal saline	☐	☐	☐	
Wash your hands again	☐	☐	☐	
Cleanse the wound with the antimicrobial agent	☐	☐	☐	
Allow the antimicrobial agent to dry before applying fresh dressings	☐	☐	☐	
Inspect the wound carefully and note any abnormalities	☐	☐	☐	
Cover the wound with sterile dressings	☐	☐	☐	
Secure the dressing in place with tape	☐	☐	☐	
Use gloves according to agency policy; observe aseptic technique throughout the procedure	☐	☐	☐	

B. This section allows you to examine your techniques for irrigating a wound, shortening a drain, packing a wound, and dressing a draining wound.

RECOMMENDED TECHNIQUE	S	NI	U	Comments
Assemble necessary equipment, including solution for the irrigation and supplies for the dressing change	☐	☐	☐	
Position and drape the client appropriately	☐	☐	☐	
Remove adhesive securing the dressing while pulling it toward the wound	☐	☐	☐	

RECOMMENDED TECHNIQUE	S	NI	U	Comments
Remove and discard the soiled dressings in a waterproof container	☐	☐	☐	_____
Prepare the prescribed solution for the wound irrigation correctly	☐	☐	☐	_____
Wash your hands	☐	☐	☐	_____
Apply personal protective equipment as needed	☐	☐	☐	_____
Inspect the wound carefully and estimate the amount of drainage	☐	☐	☐	_____
Position the client so that solution will flow from the wound into a collecting basin	☐	☐	☐	_____
Irrigate the wound generously but carefully, being sure to irrigate pockets in the wound	☐	☐	☐	_____
If a drain is present, shorten it correctly as prescribed	☐	☐	☐	_____
If the wound needs packing, pack as prescribed	☐	☐	☐	_____
Clean the wound and the skin immediately around it	☐	☐	☐	_____
Allow the wound to dry and apply skin protectant of the agency's choice, as indicated	☐	☐	☐	_____
Apply a wet-to-dry dressing as prescribed	☐	☐	☐	_____
If wet-to-dry dressings are not used, cover the wound with sterile dressings	☐	☐	☐	_____
Loosely pack dressing, depending on the amount of drainage	☐	☐	☐	_____
Secure the dressing				
Use gloves according to agency policy; observe aseptic technique throughout the procedure	☐	☐	☐	_____
See that the dressing is changed often enough to prevent it from becoming soaked	☐	☐	☐	_____

C. This section allows you to examine your techniques for using roller bandages.

RECOMMENDED TECHNIQUE	S	NI	U	Comments
Elevate and support the limb	☐	☐	☐	_____
Wrap in a distal-to-proximal direction	☐	☐	☐	_____
Avoid gaps between each turn of the bandage	☐	☐	☐	_____
Exert equal, but not excessive, tension with each turn	☐	☐	☐	_____
Keep the bandage free of wrinkles	☐	☐	☐	_____
Secure the end of the roller bandage with metal clips	☐	☐	☐	_____
Assess the color and sensation of exposed fingers and toes	☐	☐	☐	_____

RECOMMENDED TECHNIQUE	S	NI	U	Comments
Remove the bandage for hygiene and replace it twice daily	☐	☐	☐	_____
Demonstrate the ability to apply roller bandages using the following turns correctly	☐	☐	☐	_____
Circular turn	☐	☐	☐	_____
Spiral turn	☐	☐	☐	_____
Spiral-reverse turn	☐	☐	☐	_____
Figure-of-8 turn	☐	☐	☐	_____
Spica	☐	☐	☐	_____
Recurrent turn	☐	☐	☐	_____
Demonstrate the ability to apply a T binder correctly	☐	☐	☐	_____

CHAPTER 29

Gastrointestinal Intubation

■ Summary

Intubation is the term used for placing a tube into a structure of the body. When the tube is inserted into the stomach by passing it through the nose or mouth, it is called gastric intubation. If the tube passes through the intestinal tract and stops after it exits the stomach, it is called intestinal intubation. Tubes may also be inserted through a surgically created opening called an ostomy. Certain clients, especially those experiencing abdominal or gastrointestinal surgery, may require the placement of such a tube. This chapter discusses the uses for gastrointestinal tubes and the nursing guidelines and skills required for managing client care in these situations.

■ Matching Questions

Directions: For items 1 through 6, match the purposes in Part B with the types of gastrointestinal tubes in Part A.

PART A

1. _A_ Ewald
2. _d_ Levin
3. _C_ Salem sump
4. _E_ Sengstaken-Blakemore
5. _b_ Keofeed
6. _F_ Maxter

PART B

a. Intestinal decompression
b. Decompression
c. Lavage
d. Compression
e. Diagnostics
f. Gavage

Directions: For items 7 through 10, match the disadvantages in Part B with the feeding tubes in Part A.

PART A

7. _b_ Nasogastric
8. _d_ Nasointestinal
9. _A_ Gastrostomy
10. _C_ Jejunostomy

PART B

a. Must wait 24 hours after initial placement to use
b. Potentiates gastric reflux
c. Increases incidence for infection
d. Requires x-ray to verify placement

Directions: For items 11 through 20, match the solutions in Part B with the problem in Part A.

PART A

11. _h_ Diarrhea
12. _b_ Nausea and vomiting
13. _A_ Aspiration
14. _C_ Constipation
15. _f_ Elevated blood glucose
16. ____ Middle ear inflammation
17. _J_ Sore throat
18. _E_ Plugged feeding tube
19. _d_ Dumping syndrome
20. ____ Elevated electrolytes

dumping Syndrome

PART B

a. Check placement before instilling liquids
b. Administer small, continuous volume
c. Increase supplemental water
d. Hang only 4 hours' worth of formula
e. Dilute crushed drugs
f. Change formula
g. Change position every 2 hours
h. Increase concentration
i. Allow feeding to instill by gravity
j. Use smaller tube

■ Multiple-Choice Questions

Directions: For items 1 through 15, circle the letter that corresponds to the best answer for each question.

1. Highly concentrated tube feedings can result in:
   a. Constipation
   b. Nausea and vomiting
   c. Aspiration
   d. Diarrhea

2. Lack of fiber in a tube feeding can cause:
   a. Constipation
   b. Nausea and vomiting
   c. Aspiration
   d. Diarrhea

3. The nursing activity most likely to prevent the clogging of a nasogastric feeding tube is:
   a. Attaching the tubing to suction after each feeding
   b. Flushing the tubing with water and clamping it after each feeding
   c. Clamping the tubing before all of the nourishment has drained
   d. Aspirating as much as possible from the tubing using a 50-mL syringe

4. When a client is unable to eat or drink normally over a long period of time, which of the following would be the best alternative:
   a. Giving liquid nutrients through a tube leading from the nose to the stomach or intestine
   b. Giving solutions through tubing inserted into a peripheral vein
   c. Giving continuous tube feedings regulated via an electric feeding pump
   d. Giving feedings through a tube inserted through the skin and tissue of the abdomen

5. The process of removing poisonous substances through gastric intubation is called:
   a. Gavage
   b. Decompression
   c. Lavage
   d. Tamponade

6. Feeding-tube obstruction may occur if the formula is administered at a rate that is less than:
   a. 30 mL per hour
   b. 50 mL per hour
   c. 70 mL per hour
   d. 90 mL per hour

7. Which of the following feeding tubes is least likely to become obstructed:
   a. Nasogastric
   b. Nasointestinal
   c. Jejunostomy
   d. Gastrostomy

8. An advantage of the gastrostomy over other feeding tubes is:
   a. It has reduced potential for reflux and aspiration
   b. It is easy to insert
   c. It accommodates crushed medications
   d. It accommodates long-term use

9. Which of the following gastrointestinal tubes has the largest diameter:
   a. Sengstaken-Blakemore
   b. Levin
   c. Ewald
   d. Keofeed

10. Instillation of a large volume of liquid nourishment into the stomach in a fairly short time describes:
    a. A bolus feeding
    b. A cyclic feeding
    c. An intermittent feeding
    d. A continuous feeding

11. Most formulas used for tube feedings have a caloric value of:
    a. 1.5 to 2.0 kcal/mL
    b. 0.5 to 1.5 kcal/mL
    c. 0.5 to 2.0 kcal/mL
    d. 1.5 to 2.5 kcal/mL

12. Bolus formula feedings are the least desirable because they:

    a. Mimic the natural filling and emptying of the stomach

    b. Are given by gravity drip over an hour's time

    c. Are given during the late evening hours and during sleep

    d. Cause gastric reflux and increase the risk of aspiration

13. Gastric residual is best described as:

    a. A volume equal to 20% of the total volume of the previous hour's tube feeding

    b. The volume of liquid left in the stomach after allowing sufficient time for emptying to occur

    c. The volume of liquid from the stomach that empties into the small intestine

    d. The extra volume of formula from a feeding that will cause reflux and aspiration

14. Which of the following amounts represents an accurate estimate of the daily water requirement for adults receiving tube feedings:

    a. 30 mL/kg of weight

    b. 50 mL/kg of weight

    c. 70 mL/kg of weight

    d. 90 mL/kg of weight

15. Instilling a tube feeding rapidly can result in:

    a. Nausea and vomiting

    b. Constipation

    c. Weight loss

    d. Sore throat

■ Alternative Format Questions

1. The nurse is assisting with insertion of an intestinal decompression tube. Which of the following activities would be appropriate? Select all that apply:

    1. Ambulate the client

    2. Place the client on his or her right side for 2 hours

    3. Advance the tube several inches each hour

    4. Request x-ray confirmation of placement

    5. Cut off any excess tubing

    6. Clamp the tubing

2. To estimate the length of the tube required for placement of a nasointestinal tube, the nurse determines the NEX measurement and adds _____ inches.

3. Regardless of the feeding schedule, tube feeding administration sets are generally replaced every _____ hours.

■ True or False Questions

Directions: For items 1 through 10, decide if the statement is true or false and mark T or F in the space provided.

1. _____ When preparing to give nourishment by gastric gavage, the nurse should warm the solution before administering it.

2. _____ A surgical opening into the stomach through the abdominal wall is called a gastrostomy.

3. _____ Nasogastric tube feedings are the method of choice when the client requires an alternative to oral feeding for longer than a month.

4. _____ Incorrect nasogastric tube placement may cause aspiration.

5. _____ The distance from the earlobe to the xiphoid process approximates the length of tubing required for a nasogastric tube to reach the stomach.

6. _____ The least accurate test for determining the correct placement of a nasogastric tube is placing the end of the tube into a glass of water.

7. _____ The stylet for a small-diameter feeding tube should be reinserted while the tube is in the client.

8. _____ The purpose for measuring gastric residual is to determine if the rate or volume is more than the physiological capacity of the client.

9. _____ Intestinal decompression refers to the enteral feeding of clients who cannot tolerate oral nourishment.

10. _____ If the gastrostomy is accidentally extubated, the nurse may insert a mercury-weighted tube into the opening to maintain patency until reintubation can be accomplished.

■ Short Answer Questions

Directions: Read each of the following statements and supply the word(s) necessary in the space provided.

1. Describe the approved methods for determining if a nasogastric tube is in the client's stomach.

   a. _____

   b. _____

   c. _____

2. List the steps utilized for administering an intermittent feeding.

   a. _____

   b. _____

   c. _____

   d. _____

   e. _____

   f. _____

   g. _____

   h. _____

   i. _____

   j. _____

   k. _____

   l. _____

3. Describe four schedules for administering tube feedings.

   a. _____

   b. _____

   c. _____

   d. _____

4. Identify four purposes for gastrointestinal intubation.

   a. _____

   b. _____

   c. _____

   d. _____

■ Critical Thinking Exercise

You are the nurse caring for a client who has just had a nasogastric feeding tube removed. The client tells you he is hungry and would like something to eat and drink. Identify appropriate nursing activities to supply nourishment and fluid for this client. State the rationale for your choices.

Performance Checklist

A. This section allows you to examine your techniques for caring for the client who has gastrointestinal intubation.

1. Place a check mark in the "S" ("satisfactory") column if you used the recommended technique.
2. Place a check mark in the "NI" ("needs improvement") column if you used some but not all of each recommended technique.
3. Place a check mark in the "U" ("unsatisfactory") column if you forgot to include that particular recommended technique.
4. Note whether further practice is indicated, what errors you made, suggestions that will improve your skills, and so on in the section for comments.

RECOMMENDED TECHNIQUE	S	NI	U	Comments
Assist with introducing the tube into the stomach or duodenum, as ordered	☐	☐	☐	_____
Connect the tube to suction equipment and check it regularly for proper function	☐	☐	☐	_____
Check the drainage regularly and note its character	☐	☐	☐	_____
Report unusual signs and symptoms promptly	☐	☐	☐	_____
Record intake and output accurately	☐	☐	☐	_____
Keep the client NPO unless otherwise ordered	☐	☐	☐	_____
Provide oral hygiene at least twice daily	☐	☐	☐	_____
Position the client comfortably	☐	☐	☐	_____
Elevate the head of the bed at least 30°	☐	☐	☐	_____
Be prepared to assist with providing intravenous therapy	☐	☐	☐	_____
Remove the tube properly when therapy is discontinued	☐	☐	☐	_____

B. Examine your techniques when offering nourishment through a feeding tube and complete the following form.

RECOMMENDED TECHNIQUE	S	NI	U	Comments
Assess bowel sounds	☐	☐	☐	_____
Wash your hands	☐	☐	☐	_____
Assess proper tube placement using appropriate methods	☐	☐	☐	_____
Measure capillary blood glucose	☐	☐	☐	_____
Assemble necessary equipment	☐	☐	☐	_____
Warm nourishment to room temperature	☐	☐	☐	_____
Place client in a 30° to 90° sitting position	☐	☐	☐	_____
Measure gastric residual	☐	☐	☐	_____

RECOMMENDED TECHNIQUE	S	NI	U	Comments
If gastric residual is 100 mL or more, wait and recheck it in 30 minutes	☐	☐	☐	_____
Refeed gastric residual	☐	☐	☐	_____
Pour nourishment into a syringe or funnel connected to the feeding tube	☐	☐	☐	_____
Add fresh formula to the syringe before it is empty	☐	☐	☐	_____
Allow nourishment to enter the stomach slowly by gravity	☐	☐	☐	_____
Do not allow the syringe or funnel to become empty while introducing the nourishment	☐	☐	☐	_____
Flush tubing with at least 30 to 60 mL of water after each feeding	☐	☐	☐	_____
Clamp the tube between feedings	☐	☐	☐	_____
Keep the head of the bed elevated for at least 30 to 60 minutes after a feeding	☐	☐	☐	_____
Wash your hands	☐	☐	☐	_____
Record the volume of gastric residual, formula, and water given	☐	☐	☐	_____
Provide oral hygiene at least twice daily	☐	☐	☐	_____

CHAPTER 30

Urinary Elimination

■ Summary

Elimination of excess water and wastes is a normal physiological function of the kidneys and urinary bladder. The urinary system eliminates excess fluid and toxic substances in a waste solution called urine. Illnesses and situations producing stress may interfere with this normal mechanism of elimination. When this function becomes impaired, it can be life threatening.

This chapter reviews the process of urinary elimination and describes nursing skills for assessing and maintaining urinary elimination.

■ Matching Questions

Directions: For items 1 through 5, match the descriptions given in Part B with the types of incontinences in Part A.

PART A

1. _E_ Stress incontinence

2. _d_ Urge incontinence

3. _b_ Reflex incontinence

4. _A_ Functional incontinence

5. _C_ Overflow incontinence

PART B

a. Control over urination is lost because of inaccessibility of a toilet or a compromised ability to use one

b. Loss of urine without any identifiable pattern or warning

c. Urine leaks because the bladder is not completely emptied and remains distended with retained urine

d. Frequent perception of the need to void with short-lived ability to sustain control of the flow

e. The loss of small amounts of urine when intra-abdominal pressure rises

f. Spontaneous loss of urine when the bladder is stretched with urine, but without prior perception of a need to void

Directions: For items 6 through 10, match the nursing approaches in Part B with the types of incontinences in Part A.

PART A

6. ____ Stress incontinence

7. ____ Urge incontinence

8. _A_ Functional incontinence

9. ____ Reflex incontinence

10. ____ Overflow incontinence

PART B

a. Modification of clothing; facilitation of access to a toilet, commode, or urinal; assistance to a toilet according to a preplanned schedule

b. Pelvic floor muscle strengthening; weight reduction

c. Hydration; adequate bowel elimination; maintenance of catheter patency; use of the Credé maneuver

d. Absorbent undergarments; external catheter; indwelling catheter

e. Cutaneous triggering; straight intermittent catheterization

f. Maintenance of fluid intake of at least 2000 mL per day; elimination of bladder irritants, such as caffeine or alcohol; administration of diuretics in the morning

■ Multiple-Choice Questions

Directions: For items 1 through 12, circle the letter that corresponds to the best answer for each question.

1. Urine is formed in the:

    a. Bladder

    b. Ureters

c. Kidneys

d. Urethra

2. The average adult will desire to empty his or her bladder when it contains:

a. 100 to 125 mL of urine

b. 150 to 300 mL of urine

c. 350 to 400 mL of urine

d. 450 to 500 mL of urine

3. The absence of urine is:

a. Anuria

b. Oliguria

c. Polyuria

d. Dysuria

4. The term that indicates the kidneys are not forming urine is:

a. Oliguria

b. Anuria

c. Urinary retention

d. Urinary suppression

5. Urine retained in the bladder after a client voids is called:

a. Overflow urine

b. Residual urine

c. Excess urine

d. Secondary urine

6. Stress incontinence is best described as:

a. The inability to retain urine within the bladder

b. Increased abdominal pressure causing urine to be released

c. The repeated awakening during the night to empty the bladder

d. The voiding of small amounts at frequent intervals

7. The average amount of urine produced every 24 hours by healthy adults is:

a. 1200 mL

b. 1000 mL

c. 1500 mL

d. 500 mL

8. The term used to describe pus in the urine is:

a. Glycosuria

b. Hematuria

c. Pyuria

d. Albuminuria

9. For individuals who have stress incontinence, which of the following techniques is especially helpful to restore continence?

a. The Credé maneuver

b. The cutaneous triggering mechanism

c. Kegel exercises

d. Intermittent straight catheterization

10. The nurse should propose the insertion of a catheter for incontinent clients only when:

a. The client complains of bladder discomfort

b. The benefits for the client outweigh the risks

c. The client is embarrassed by his incontinence

d. The family needs help in dealing with incontinence

11. The catheter that is intended to be inserted and withdrawn following its use for a temporary measure is:

a. An indwelling catheter

b. A Foley catheter

c. A straight catheter

d. A retention catheter

12. The most hazardous problem when external catheters are used is:

a. The blood supply to the tissues of the penis may be restricted

b. The skin may break down because of the collection of moisture

c. The catheter may not fit well and cause urine to leak out

d. The catheter may not be kept as clean as is necessary by the client

■ Alternative Format Questions

1. A clean-catch urine specimen must be refrigerated if analysis will be delayed more than ____ hour(s).

2. Which of the following represents correct condom catheter care? Select all that apply:
   1. Ensure that the tip of the penis fits snugly against the end of the condom
   2. Check the penis for adequate circulation 30 minutes after application
   3. Change the condom catheter every 24 hours
   4. Tape the collection tubing to the leg
   5. Secure the condom to the base of the penis

3. The client with a retention catheter should drink up to _____ mL of fluid per day if permitted to do so.

■ True or False Questions

Directions: For items 1 through 12, decide if the statement is true or false and mark T or F in the space provided.

1. _____ Urine is transported from the kidneys to the bladder via the urethra.

2. _____ The synonym for urination is micturition.

3. _____ Oliguria refers to the absence of urine.

4. _____ Polyuria is the term for blood in the urine.

5. _____ Indwelling catheters should be irrigated routinely.

6. _____ Individuals with indwelling catheters should have an intake of 1000 to 1500 mL daily.

7. _____ Urinary tract infections are one of the most commonly acquired infections in clients who have indwelling catheters.

8. _____ The nurse must insist on sterile techniques when teaching a client self-catheterization.

9. _____ The less skin that is exposed on the client with a urinary diversion, the less the skin will be irritated.

10. _____ A midstream urine specimen is collected under sterile conditions.

11. _____ To ensure accuracy, the second voided specimen should be used when testing for glucose in the urine.

12. _____ Incontinent clients should be instructed to limit their fluid intake.

■ Short Answer Questions

Directions: Read each of the following statements and supply the word(s) necessary in the space provided.

1. List four actions that may be helpful when a male uses a urinal.
   a. _____
   _____
   b. _____
   _____
   c. _____
   _____
   d. _____
   _____

2. Identify eight suggestions that may be developed into a more specific plan for bladder retraining.
   a. _____   e. _____
   b. _____   f. _____
   c. _____   g. _____
   d. _____   h. _____

3. List six factors that influence the amount, contents, and characteristics of urine or its elimination.
   a. _____
   _____
   b. _____
   _____
   c. _____
   _____
   d. _____
   _____
   e. _____
   _____
   f. _____
   _____

4. List five nursing measures that can be utilized when the client needs assistance with urination.

a. _____

_____

b. _____

_____

c. _____

_____

d. _____

_____

e. _____

_____

■ Critical Thinking Exercises

1. Describe adjustments you make when promoting urinary elimination:

a. When the client is an infant or child

b. When the client is pregnant or in the early postpartal period

c. When the client is elderly

2. Plan a teaching program for a client for whom you are caring and complete the following form.

Topic for Teaching	Points to Cover in the Teaching Program
Proper functioning of the urinary system, normal voiding, and normal urine	
Self-catheterization	
Home care, including common urine tests, related to urinary elimination	
The collection of various types of specimens by the client, such as	
Single voided:	
Clean-catch midstream:	
24-hour specimen:	

Performance Checklist

A. This section allows you to examine your techniques for caring for the client who requires assistance with urinary elimination.

1. Place a check mark in the "S" ("satisfactory") column if you used the recommended technique.
2. Place a check mark in the "NI" ("needs improvement") column if you used some but not all of each recommended technique.
3. Place a check mark in the "U" ("unsatisfactory") column if you forgot to include that particular recommended technique.
4. Note whether further practice is indicated, what errors you made, suggestions that will improve your skills, and so on in the section for comments.

RECOMMENDED TECHNIQUE	S	NI	U	Comments
Bring necessary equipment and supplies to the bedside; warm a metal bedpan, if indicated	☐	☐	☐	_____
Wash your hands	☐	☐	☐	_____
Place the bedpan under the client	☐	☐	☐	_____
Roll the client onto the bedpan if he or she cannot assist	☐	☐	☐	_____
Place a urinal between slightly spread legs	☐	☐	☐	_____
Raise the head of the bed slightly, if permitted	☐	☐	☐	_____
Replace top linens, have the signal device and toilet tissue handy, and raise the bed side rails	☐	☐	☐	_____
Provide a receptacle for toilet tissue when a specimen is needed and explain the reason to the client	☐	☐	☐	_____
Leave the client for privacy or remain with the client if indicated	☐	☐	☐	_____
Put on gloves	☐	☐	☐	_____
Remove the bedpan or urinal as it was offered	☐	☐	☐	_____
Cleanse the perineal area as needed	☐	☐	☐	_____
Empty and clean the bedpan or urinal	☐	☐	☐	_____
Replace top bed linens and offer the client equipment and supplies to wash his or her hands	☐	☐	☐	_____
Collect a specimen, if required	☐	☐	☐	_____

B. This section allows you to examine your techniques for inserting a straight catheter for a female.

RECOMMENDED TECHNIQUE	S	NI	U	Comments
Assemble equipment and have additional lighting available	☐	☐	☐	_____
Wash your hands and put on clean gloves	☐	☐	☐	_____
Position and drape the client properly; clean the genital area, if necessary	☐	☐	☐	_____
Remove gloves and wash your hands	☐	☐	☐	_____
Set up the sterile field and don sterile gloves	☐	☐	☐	_____
Lubricate the catheter about 3.75 to 5 centimeters (1.5 to 2 inches) without clogging the eyes of the catheter	☐	☐	☐	_____
Open labia with thumb and fingers and expose the meatus	☐	☐	☐	_____
Clean the area at the meatus with the antiseptic solution	☐	☐	☐	_____
Insert the catheter 7.5 to 10 centimeters (3 to 4 inches)	☐	☐	☐	_____
Keep labia separated until the urine flows freely	☐	☐	☐	_____
Use no force to insert the catheter	☐	☐	☐	_____
If the catheter meets resistance, try these techniques:	☐	☐	☐	_____
Ask the client to take deep breaths	☐	☐	☐	_____
Rotate the catheter in place	☐	☐	☐	_____
Ask the client to wiggle her toes	☐	☐	☐	_____
Withdraw the catheter and discontinue the procedure if it causes continued resistance and discomfort	☐	☐	☐	_____
Hold the catheter securely in place while the bladder empties and drain urine into a receptacle or specimen bottle	☐	☐	☐	_____
Withdraw the catheter slowly	☐	☐	☐	_____
Handle the urine specimen according to agency policy	☐	☐	☐	_____
Work always with gentleness and observe surgical asepsis	☐	☐	☐	_____

C. This section allows you to examine your techniques for inserting a straight catheter for a male.

RECOMMENDED TECHNIQUE	S	NI	U	Comments
Bring supplies to the bedside	☐	☐	☐	_____
Wash your hands	☐	☐	☐	_____
Open supplies and create a sterile field	☐	☐	☐	_____
Put on sterile gloves	☐	☐	☐	_____
Apply gentle traction to the penis by pulling it straight up with your gloved hand	☐	☐	☐	_____

RECOMMENDED TECHNIQUE	S	NI	U	Comments
Instill the contents of the syringe that is pre-filled with lubricant directly through the meatus into the urethra	☐	☐	☐	_____
Gently introduce the catheter while holding the penis almost vertical to the client's body	☐	☐	☐	_____
If resistance occurs, rotate the catheter, ask the client to take some deep breaths, or place more traction on the penis	☐	☐	☐	_____
Continue insertion until only the inflation and drainage ports are exposed and urine flows	☐	☐	☐	_____
Collect a specimen if needed	☐	☐	☐	_____
Gently remove the catheter when urine flow stops	☐	☐	☐	_____
Clean away excess lubricant	☐	☐	☐	_____
Make the client comfortable	☐	☐	☐	_____
Dispose of supplies	☐	☐	☐	_____
Wash your hands	☐	☐	☐	_____

D. This section allows you to examine your techniques for caring for a client with an indwelling catheter.

RECOMMENDED TECHNIQUE	S	NI	U	Comments
Clean the perineal area and around the meatus at least twice a day and after each bowel movement	☐	☐	☐	_____
Use soap and water or an antiseptic of the agency's choice for cleaning the perineal area	☐	☐	☐	_____
Encourage the client to have a generous fluid intake	☐	☐	☐	_____
Keep the tubing free of kinks	☐	☐	☐	_____
Encourage and assist the client to be up and about	☐	☐	☐	_____
Note the volume and characteristics of the urine and report unusual signs and symptoms promptly	☐	☐	☐	_____
Assist the client who can take a shower or tub bath to manage his drainage system properly	☐	☐	☐	_____
Teach the client about the function and care of his drainage system	☐	☐	☐	_____
Empty the balloon completely before removing the indwelling catheter	☐	☐	☐	_____
Continue to observe the client for signs of urinary tract infection	☐	☐	☐	_____
Continue to monitor intake and output	☐	☐	☐	_____

E. This section allows you to examine your techniques for irrigating an indwelling catheter.

RECOMMENDED TECHNIQUE	S	NI	U	Comments
Wash your hands	☐	☐	☐	_____
Gather necessary equipment, including sterile irrigating solution	☐	☐	☐	_____
Clean the area where the catheter and tubing join and disconnect them	☐	☐	☐	_____
Place a cap on the exposed end of the drainage tube	☐	☐	☐	_____
Inject about 30 to 60 mL of solution into the catheter	☐	☐	☐	_____
Allow solution to flow back by gravity into a basin	☐	☐	☐	_____
Repeat the instillation and drainage if the urine appears to contain appreciable debris	☐	☐	☐	_____
Reconnect the catheter and tubing and check for urine flow	☐	☐	☐	_____
Note the amount of solution used for irrigating and the amount returned	☐	☐	☐	_____
Replace sterile solution every 24 hours	☐	☐	☐	_____

F. This section allows you to examine your technique for instructing a client to obtain a clean-catch midstream urine specimen.

RECOMMENDED TECHNIQUE	S	NI	U	Comments
For a Female Client				
Gather the necessary equipment	☐	☐	☐	_____
Ensure the availability of a toilet and privacy	☐	☐	☐	_____
Instruct the client to do the following:	☐	☐	☐	_____
Wash her hands	☐	☐	☐	_____
Remove the lid from the specimen container and rest it upside down	☐	☐	☐	_____
Don't touch the inside of the container	☐	☐	☐	_____
Sit on the toilet and spread her legs	☐	☐	☐	_____
Separate her labia with her fingers	☐	☐	☐	_____
Cleanse each side of the meatus from front to back with a separate antiseptic wipe	☐	☐	☐	_____
Use the final antiseptic wipe to wipe directly down the center	☐	☐	☐	_____
Begin to urinate	☐	☐	☐	_____
Place the open container under the stream of urine and catch some urine in the container	☐	☐	☐	_____

RECOMMENDED TECHNIQUE	S	NI	U	Comments
Remove the container and continue to urinate until finished	☐	☐	☐	_____
Wash her hands	☐	☐	☐	_____
Put the lid on the container without touching the inside of the lid or container	☐	☐	☐	_____
Wipe the closed container dry and bring it to the nurse	☐	☐	☐	_____

For a Male Client

	S	NI	U	Comments
Instruct the client to follow the same steps but clean the penis in the following manner:	☐	☐	☐	_____
If uncircumcised, retract the foreskin	☐	☐	☐	_____
Clean in a circular manner around the tip of the penis toward its base with an antiseptic swab	☐	☐	☐	_____
Repeat with another antiseptic swab	☐	☐	☐	_____
Keep the foreskin retracted until he has collected some urine in the container	☐	☐	☐	_____
Replace the foreskin	☐	☐	☐	_____
Wash his hands	☐	☐	☐	_____
Put the lid on the container without touching the inside of the lid or container	☐	☐	☐	_____
Wash his hands	☐	☐	☐	_____
Wipe the closed container dry and bring it to the nurse	☐	☐	☐	_____

Iatrogenic – Medical tx
Secondary – Pathological

CHAPTER 31

Bowel Elimination

■ Summary

Foods are digested, absorbed, and eliminated by structures in the gastrointestinal tract. Undigestible substances from food and some water are eliminated as stool, or feces. Efficient physiologic function requires that waste products be eliminated through the bowel. Generally, problems encountered are those of either too frequent elimination or those of infrequent elimination. If uncorrected, either situation may lead to death by altering the water and chemical balance in the body.

This chapter reviews the process of intestinal elimination and discusses measures to promote it.

■ Matching Questions

Directions: For items 1 through 8, match the types of constipation given in Part B with the contributing factors listed Part A. (Note: Items in Part B may be used more than one time.)

PART A

1. ____ Spinal cord compression
2. ____ Narcotic analgesia
3. ____ Decreased physical activity
4. ____ Partial intestinal obstruction
5. ____ Inadequate time for defecation
6. ____ Antidepressants
7. ____ Anticonvulsants
8. ____ Inadequate privacy

PART B

a. Primary or simple constipation
b. Secondary constipation
c. Iatrogenic constipation

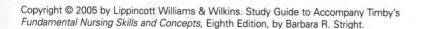

■ Multiple-Choice Questions

Directions: For items 1 through 20, circle the letter that corresponds to the best *answer for each question.*

1. Of the following, which effect would a diet high in fiber and roughage have on normal intestinal elimination?
   a. The production of a smaller stool and the promotion of quicker passage
   b. The production of a larger stool and the promotion of quicker passage
   c. The production of a larger stool and the promotion of slower passage
   d. The production of a smaller stool and the promotion of slower passage

2. Constipation is best described as:
   a. A condition in which the individual is unable to have a daily bowel movement
   b. A condition in which there is a daily bowel movement of a small amount
   c. A condition in which the stool becomes dry and hard and requires straining for elimination
   d. A condition in which the stool is moist and soft and requires a laxative for elimination

3. A typical symptom of fecal impaction is:
   a. The frequent passing of flatus
   b. Liquid fecal seepage from the anus
   c. The passage of small, hard, and dry stool
   d. The lack of an urge to defecate

4. Of the following measures, which is used most often for a client with a fecal impaction:
   a. A large-volume enema
   b. A hypertonic enema
   c. An oil retention enema
   d. A laxative or cathartic

5. The primary reason for using the digital method for clients with a fecal impaction is to:

   a. Relax the anal sphincter
   b. Lubricate the stool
   c. Stimulate the peristalsis
   d. Break up the fecal mass

6. An excessive amount of gas within the intestinal tract is called:

   a. Constipation
   b. Flatulence
   c. Tympanites
   d. Distention

7. The largest percentage of gas in the bowel comes from:

   a. Bacterial fermentation
   b. Spicy foods
   c. Swallowed air
   d. Diffusion from the bloodstream

8. Of the following measures, which one is most helpful for the relief of intestinal distention:

   a. Teach the client to use Valsalva's maneuver
   b. Place the client in a semisitting position
   c. Insert a rectal tube for 20 minutes
   d. Insert an intestinal tube through the nose

9. Diarrhea is best described by its:

   a. Odor
   b. Amount
   c. Frequency
   d. Consistency

10. Of the following, which foods would be the best for a client who has had diarrhea:

    a. Applesauce, coffee, and lettuce
    b. Bananas, bran flakes, and orange juice
    c. Bananas, applesauce, and gelatin
    d. Fried chicken, tomatoes, and tea

11. An action that may help clients with fecal incontinence to establish a pattern of elimination is:

    a. Changing the diet to one of bland and nonirritating foods
    b. Consulting with the physician to give an enema every 2 to 3 days
    c. Consulting with the physician in order to give a laxative daily

    d. Teaching the client to note sensations and ignore the urge

12. Following a large-volume enema, defecation usually occurs within:

    a. 5 to 15 minutes
    b. 10 to 20 minutes
    c. 15 to 25 minutes
    d. 20 to 30 minutes

13. Tap-water enemas that are repeated one after the other can:

    a. Irritate the mucous membrane
    b. Change elimination habits
    c. Result in fluid imbalances
    d. Cause loss of peristalsis

14. Hypertonic enema solutions act by:

    a. Preventing water absorption
    b. Softening the stool
    c. Breaking up fecal impactions
    d. The principle of osmosis

15. The recommended position for the administration of a hypertonic solution enema is:

    a. Left side-lying position
    b. Right side-lying position
    c. Knee-chest position
    d. Prone position

16. The primary purpose of an oil retention enema is to:

    a. Lubricate and soften the stool
    b. Increase the fluid in the bowel
    c. Break up fecal impactions
    d. Increase peristalsis

17. One of the biggest challenges in ostomy care is:

    a. Controlling the embarrassment
    b. Regulating the time of elimination
    c. Regulating the odor from the appliance
    d. Preventing skin breakdown

18. The nurse should assess the intestinal elimination patterns accurately for the elderly client because:

    a. They are easily confused about their patterns of elimination

b. They will need to be taught bowel retraining before discharge

c. They usually have poor knowledge regarding their need for fecal elimination

d. They may be bowel conscious and report problems of constipation erroneously

19. An important teaching responsibility for nurses regarding intestinal elimination is:

a. Explaining the different types of laxatives

b. Teaching the proper use and dangers of abuse regarding enemas and laxatives

c. Explaining the different types and uses of over-the-counter enema preparations

d. Explaining that it is important to have daily intestinal elimination

20. When is the gastrocolic reflex most active:

a. Prior to defecation

b. While sleeping

c. After eating

d. During digestion

■ Alternative Format Questions

1. The nurse is planning care for a client admitted with diarrhea. Which of the following statements should be included in the nursing care plan? Select all that apply:

1. Provide for temporary bowel rest

2. Initiate a clear liquid diet

3. Assess for fecal impaction

4. Resume solid foods by eating bananas, applesauce, and cottage cheese

5. Test for blood in the stool

2. The nurse has spent the last 30 minutes discussing methods to eliminate constipation with a client. Which of the following statements indicate that the client understood the discussion? Select all that apply:

1. "I will need an enema every other day to prevent constipation."

2. "I will drink eight 8-oz glasses of fluid every day."

3. "I will take a half-hour walk in the park every day after dinner."

4. "I will take a whole wheat bagel, carrots, and an apple for lunch tomorrow."

5. "I just don't have enough time to spend in the bathroom. I'm just too busy."

3. The nurse is testing a client's stool for occult blood. After applying two drops of chemical reagent onto the test space, the nurse should wait _____ seconds before observing the color.

■ True or False Questions

Directions: For items 1 through 12, decide if the statement is true or false and mark T or F in the space provided.

1. _____ The internal anal sphincter is under voluntary control.

2. _____ Nervous tension may cause abdominal cramping and diarrhea.

3. _____ Constipation is described as the inability to have daily intestinal elimination.

4. _____ Routine use of laxatives, enemas, or suppositories is often the cause of constipation.

5. _____ The amount of water retained in the stool is dependent upon the undigestible fiber content of the diet.

6. _____ A client with fecal impaction may expel liquid stool around the impacted mass.

7. _____ Eating spicy foods increases the volume of gas in the intestinal tract and lengthens the transit time.

8. _____ Diarrhea is described as frequent intestinal elimination.

9. _____ A hypertonic enema solution causes fluids to move from the feces into the bowel, causing peristalsis.

10. _____ An ileostomy is an opening into the large intestine.

11. _____ A continent ostomy is also referred to as a Kock pouch.

12. _____ The normal aging processes tend to predispose a person to constipation.

■ Short Answer Questions

Directions: Read each of the following statements and supply the word(s) necessary in the space provided.

1. List the conditions that predispose a person to form greater amounts of gas or interfere with its absorption. _____

   _____

   _____

2. List the chief characteristics of constipation. ____

   _____

   _____

3. Identify causes of diarrhea as suggested in this chapter. _____

   _____

   _____

4. Identify nursing measures suggested in this chapter for relieving the effects of diarrhea. _____

   _____

   _____

5. Identify causes of fecal incontinence as suggested in this chapter. _____

   _____

   _____

■ Critical Thinking Exercises

1. Visit a pharmacy and make a list of several of the over-the-counter medications available for alleviating constipation or diarrhea. Choose three medications in either category and compare their actions, side effects, and cautions. Write a teaching plan that you could use for a client who chooses self-medication to relieve his or her problem. You may want to share your plan with your instructor and fellow students.

2. Prepare a teaching plan for a client experiencing the following alterations in bowel elimination:

Topic for Teaching	Points to Cover in a Teaching Plan
The abuse of enemas and laxatives	
Self-administering a cleansing enema when using a hypertonic solution and when using a large volume of solution	
Relieving common problems related to elimination:	
Constipation	
Diarrhea	
Fecal incontinence	
Abdominal distention	
Fecal impaction	
Self-care of a colostomy	
Self-care of an ileostomy	
The collection of a stool specimen	

Performance Checklist

A. This section allows you to examine your techniques for caring for the client who requires a rectal tube.

1. Place a check mark in the "S" ("satisfactory") column if you used the recommended technique.
2. Place a check mark in the "NI" ("needs improvement") column if you used some but not all of each recommended technique.
3. Place a check mark in the "U" ("unsatisfactory") column if you forgot to include that particular recommended technique.
4. Note whether further practice is indicated, what errors you made, suggestions that will improve your skills, and so on in the section for comments.

RECOMMENDED TECHNIQUE	S	NI	U	Comments
Assemble necessary equipment and wash your hands	☐	☐	☐	
Position and drape the client properly	☐	☐	☐	
Lubricate the rectal tube	☐	☐	☐	
Separate the buttocks well and insert the tube about 10 cm (4 inches)	☐	☐	☐	
Provide for a proper method to collect discharge passed through the rectal tube	☐	☐	☐	
Leave the rectal tube in place no longer than 20 minutes	☐	☐	☐	
Reinsert the tube every 3 to 4 hours if discomfort returns	☐	☐	☐	

B. This section allows you to examine your techniques for inserting a rectal suppository.

RECOMMENDED TECHNIQUE	S	NI	U	Comments
Assemble necessary equipment and wash your hands	☐	☐	☐	
Position and drape the client properly	☐	☐	☐	
Don gloves and separate the buttocks so the anus is in view	☐	☐	☐	
Lubricate the suppository and index finger	☐	☐	☐	
Insert the suppository through the anus and beyond the internal sphincter	☐	☐	☐	
Explain to the client that he or she is to retain the suppository for at least 15 minutes	☐	☐	☐	
Assist the client to the toilet, bedpan, or bedside commode	☐	☐	☐	
Instruct the client not to flush the toilet until the stool has been inspected	☐	☐	☐	
Remove gloves and wash your hands	☐	☐	☐	

C. This section allows you to examine your techniques for administering a cleansing enema.

RECOMMENDED TECHNIQUE	S	NI	U	Comments
Assemble necessary equipment and supplies	☐	☐	☐	_____
Have a bedpan, commode, or bathroom ready for the client's use and wash your hands	☐	☐	☐	_____
Auscultate bowel sounds	☐	☐	☐	_____
Pull the privacy curtain	☐	☐	☐	_____
Position and drape the client properly	☐	☐	☐	_____
Wash your hands and put on gloves	☐	☐	☐	_____
Prepare solution and hang container 12 to 20 inches above the anus	☐	☐	☐	_____
Lubricate about 7 to 10 centimeters (3 to 4 inches) of the rectal tube and allow solution to fill the tubing	☐	☐	☐	_____
Lift the buttocks to expose the anus and slowly insert the tube 7 to 10 centimeters (3 to 4 inches) at an angle pointing to the umbilicus	☐	☐	☐	_____
Have the client take several deep breaths	☐	☐	☐	_____
Do not force entry of the tube or place the solution more than 50 centimeters (20 inches) above the level of the client's anus	☐	☐	☐	_____
Introduce the solution slowly over a period of 5 to 10 minutes	☐	☐	☐	_____
To reduce the urge to defecate, have the client take panting breaths or slow the flow rate	☐	☐	☐	_____
Encourage the client to retain the solution for 5 to 15 minutes	☐	☐	☐	_____
Assist the client as necessary to use a bedpan, commode, or a bathroom	☐	☐	☐	_____
Note the character of the stool and leave the client clean and comfortable	☐	☐	☐	_____
Dispose of or clean the equipment	☐	☐	☐	_____

D. This section allows you to examine your techniques for caring for changing an ostomy appliance.

RECOMMENDED TECHNIQUE	S	NI	U	Comments
Obtain necessary equipment and bring it to the bedside	☐	☐	☐	_____
Plan to replace the appliance immediately if the client has localized symptoms	☐	☐	☐	_____
Schedule an appliance change before a meal and before a bath or shower if the client is asymptomatic	☐	☐	☐	_____

RECOMMENDED TECHNIQUE	S	NI	U	Comments
Pull the privacy curtain	☐	☐	☐	_____
Place the client in a supine or dorsal recumbent position	☐	☐	☐	_____
Wash your hands and put on gloves	☐	☐	☐	_____
Unfasten the pouch and discard it appropriately	☐	☐	☐	_____
Gently peel the faceplate from the skin	☐	☐	☐	_____
Wash the stoma and peristomal area with mild soapy water	☐	☐	☐	_____
Suggest the client shower or bathe at this time	☐	☐	☐	_____
Measure the stoma using a stomal guide	☐	☐	☐	_____
Trim the opening of the faceplate 1/8- to 1/4-inch larger than the stoma	☐	☐	☐	_____
Attach a new pouch to the ring of the faceplate	☐	☐	☐	_____
Fold and clamp the bottom of the pouch	☐	☐	☐	_____
Peel the backing from the adhesive on the faceplate	☐	☐	☐	_____
Have the client stand or lie flat	☐	☐	☐	_____
Position the faceplate over the stoma and press into place from the center outward	☐	☐	☐	_____
Dispose of unused materials and store reusable supplies	☐	☐	☐	_____
Remove gloves and wash hands	☐	☐	☐	_____
Document appropriate data per agency policy	☐	☐	☐	_____
Offer the client support as he or she learns to live with the ostomy	☐	☐	☐	_____

E. This section allows you to examine your techniques for irrigating a colostomy.

RECOMMENDED TECHNIQUE	S	NI	U	Comments
Assemble necessary equipment, wash your hands, and put on gloves	☐	☐	☐	_____
Position and drape the client properly	☐	☐	☐	_____
Fill the tubing and cone with irrigating solution	☐	☐	☐	_____
Remove dressings from the stoma or the appliance and place the irrigating sleeve over the stoma; fasten the elastic belt around the client	☐	☐	☐	_____
Lubricate the irrigating cone	☐	☐	☐	_____
Introduce the cone into the stoma gently	☐	☐	☐	_____
Do not force the cone; discontinue the procedure if undue resistance is met	☐	☐	☐	_____

RECOMMENDED TECHNIQUE	S	NI	U	Comments
After the cone is in place, allow solution to enter the colon slowly	☐	☐	☐	_____
Hold the solution container no more than about 30 centimeters (12 inches) above the stoma	☐	☐	☐	_____
Shut off the solution flow temporarily if the client complains of cramping	☐	☐	☐	_____
After the solution is introduced, remove the cone and close the top of the irrigating sleeve	☐	☐	☐	_____
Prepare to receive the return in a bedpan, commode, or toilet	☐	☐	☐	_____
When the return has stopped, remove the belt and sleeve	☐	☐	☐	_____
Clean the stoma and pat it dry	☐	☐	☐	_____
Apply a clean pouch	☐	☐	☐	_____
Remove gloves and wash hands	☐	☐	☐	_____

CHAPTER 32

Oral Medications

■ Summary

Medications, or drugs, are physiologic agents used to treat pathologic conditions. They are substances that chemically change body functions when taken by an individual. The focus of this chapter is the nurse's responsibility for the safe preparation and administration of oral agents.

■ Matching Questions

Directions: For items 1 through 6, match the abbreviations in Part B with the meanings in Part A.

PART A

1. _D_ Immediately
2. _C_ Every other day
3. _F_ Every day
4. _h_ Every 4 hours
5. _G_ Twice a day
6. _b_ Four times a day

PART B

a. tid
b. qid
c. qod
d. stat
e. qh
f. qd
g. bid
h. q 4 h

TRADE
CHEMICAL
BRAND

Directions: For items 7 through 10, match the method of administration in Part B with the route in Part A.

PART A

7. _C_ Oral
8. _d_ Topical
9. _b_ Inhalant
10. _A_ Parenteral

PART B

a. Injection
b. Aerosol
c. Swallowing
d. Application to skin

■ Multiple-Choice Questions

Directions: For items 1 through 12, circle the letter that corresponds to the best answer for each question.

1. The trade or proprietary name for a drug refers to:
   a. The drug's chemical makeup
   b. The manufacturer's name
   c. The drug's generic name
   d. The action of the drug

2. A medication order should never be implemented if the nurse:
   a. Does not know the physician
   b. Does not know the client's history
   c. Questions any part of the order
   d. Did not witness the writing of the order

3. Most health agencies check narcotic supplies:
   a. Once each day by two nurses
   b. Twice each day by a nurse and a pharmacist
   c. At the change of each shift by two nurses
   d. Three times a day by two pharmacists

4. To ensure that medications are prepared and administered correctly, the nurse should:
   a. Use the client's rights
   b. Use the five rights
   c. Give the medication only when requested
   d. Give the medication without question

5. The minimum number of times the nurse should check the label when preparing to give medications is:
   a. Two times
   b. Three times
   c. Four times
   d. Five times

6. If a client is talking on the telephone when the nurse delivers his medication, the correct procedure would be to:
   a. Return the medication to a safe place and record it as refused
   b. Leave it with the client and tell him to take it when he finishes
   c. Ask another nurse to give the medication when he is finished
   d. Wait until he excuses himself and have him take the medication

7. If Mr. S. states that the pill he has been receiving is a different color, the correct procedure for the nurse would be to:
   a. Explain that she will check the situation and return later
   b. Explain that the pharmacy often substitutes, and this medication is the same
   c. Tell Mr. S. that he is probably confused and the medication is correct
   d. Explain that this is the right medication because the physician ordered it

8. The first action to take when a medication error takes place is:
   a. Call the physician
   b. Call the supervisor
   c. Complete an incident report
   d. Check the client

9. Enteric-coated tablets are supposed to dissolve in the:
   a. Esophagus
   b. Stomach
   c. Small intestine
   d. Large intestine

10. Of the following, which is the main reason the nurse should stay with the client until the oral medication is swallowed:
    a. All liquid that is ingested is considered part of the fluid intake
    b. An unopened unit dose drug can be saved if the client refuses it
    c. The nurse is responsible for documenting that the drug was taken
    d. The nurse is the only one who can give the client medications

11. When administering medication via nasogastric tubing that is being used for suction, clamp the tube for at least:
    a. One hour prior to medication administration to prevent complications
    b. One-half hour after instilling medication to allow for absorption
    c. One and one-half hours after instilling the medication to allow for absorption
    d. One-half hour prior to medication administration to prevent complications

12. Elderly clients may have an increased risk of adverse side effects and toxicity to drugs because of:
    a. Poor circulation
    b. Decreased mobility
    c. Decreased gastrointestinal motility
    d. Decreased mental capacity

■ Alternative Format Questions

1. When administering an oral liquid medication, it may be drawn into a sterile syringe without a needle if the volume to be given is less than __5__ mL.

2. A medication is ordered to be given every 4 hours. How many times in a 24-hour period would this medication be given?

   6×3

3. The physician orders 60 mg of a drug. The drug is supplied in tablets containing 20 mg each. How many tablets should be administered?

   3

■ True or False Questions

Directions: For items 1 through 12, decide if the statement is true or false and mark T or F in the space provided.

1. __T__ Safe practice is to follow only a written order for medications.

2. __F__ The nurse may delegate the responsibility of checking and transcribing medication orders to clerical personnel.

3. __F__ TRADE NAME The proprietary name of a drug is usually descriptive of the drug's chemical structure.

4. __T__ The nurse is expected to question any medication order that does not contain all of its parts.

5. __F__ A drug that is ordered to be given four times a day is routinely scheduled at 8 a.m., 12 noon, 4 p.m., and 8 p.m.

6. __F__ FEDERAL LAW State law requires that a record be kept for each narcotic that is administered.

7. __T__ The client has a right to refuse a medication.

8. __F__ The client's right to refuse a medication is one of the five rights.

9. __F__ An incident report must be filed with the client's permanent record if the nurse commits a medication error.

10. __F__ Medications that are not given because the client is off the nursing unit for x-ray studies are considered errors.

11. __F__ Medications may be mixed and administered along with continuous tube feedings.

12. __F__ Enteric-coated tablets may be crushed and mixed with water prior to administration through nasogastric tubing.

■ Short Answer Questions

Directions: Read each of the following statements and supply the word(s) necessary in the space provided.

1. List the parts of a complete medication order. NAME DATE, DOSE, Route, Signature, Frequency

2. Identify items of information the nurse should know about the client before administering medications. Allergies To meds OTC's USED

3. List the five rights pertaining to administering medications. Right PT, Right Dose Right Drugs, Right DATE Right Time, Right Route

4. Identify the steps that should be carried out prior to preparing drugs that will be administered to a client as suggested in this chapter. CHECK ML AGAINST WRITTEN order, CHECK LABEL X3, Check expir dates

5. Identify guidelines the nurse should follow when preparing medications for administration as suggested in this chapter. Good lighting check label 3 x Prepare one if doubt, check drug labels do not flavor containers

■ Critical Thinking Exercises

The following are practice situations for calculating medication dosages. Read each statement carefully, state the formula, and compute the correct dosage for each.

1. A physician orders 50 mg of a drug. It is supplied in tablets containing 100 mg per tablet. How many tablets should be administered?

$\frac{1}{2}$ tab   SSS

2. A physician orders 250 mg of a drug. It is supplied in tablets of 0.5 g per tablet. How many tablets should be administered?

$$\frac{250}{.5} \cdot 1 = \frac{2500}{5} \cdot 1 = 500$$

$\overline{ii}$ tab

3. A physician orders 1 g of a drug. It is supplied in tablets of 500 mg per tablet. How many tablets should be administered?

$$\frac{1 g}{500 mg} \times 1 = \frac{1}{.5} \times 1 =$$

$$\frac{10}{5} \times 1 = 2 \quad \overline{ii} \text{ tab}$$

4. A dosage of ½ gr is ordered. It is supplied in a dosage of 60 mg per tablet. How many tablets should be administered?

Performance Checklist

A. This section allows you to examine your techniques for preparing and administering medication.

1. Place a check mark in the "S" ("satisfactory") column if you used the recommended technique.
2. Place a check mark in the "NI" ("needs improvement") column if you used some but not all of each recommended technique.
3. Place a check mark in the "U" ("unsatisfactory") column if you forgot to include that particular recommended technique.
4. Note whether further practice is indicated, what errors you made, suggestions that will improve your skills, and so on in the section for comments.

RECOMMENDED TECHNIQUE	S	NI	U	Comments
Know the client's medication history	☐	☐	☐	
Know the client's diagnosis, plan of care, and expected results of medication therapy	☐	☐	☐	
Know about each medication to be administered:	☐	☐	☐	
Common average dosage	☐	☐	☐	
Hoped for and undesirable effects	☐	☐	☐	
Reasons for its use	☐	☐	☐	
Symptoms of toxicity	☐	☐	☐	
Common route of administration	☐	☐	☐	
Time your work so that medications are given as near the specified time as possible	☐	☐	☐	
Check the medication order carefully according to agency policy	☐	☐	☐	
Be suspicious when a dosage has been increased or decreased markedly	☐	☐	☐	
Use accepted abbreviations only	☐	☐	☐	
Prepare the medications while using a good light and work alone	☐	☐	☐	
Check the label on the drug container three times	☐	☐	☐	
Do not use medications from containers when the label is difficult to read; do not guess	☐	☐	☐	
Do not return medications to a container or transfer drugs from one container to another	☐	☐	☐	
Do not use a medication that has a sediment, has a change of color, or appears cloudy	☐	☐	☐	
Prepare medications in the order in which they will be given and arrange them accordingly for transporting	☐	☐	☐	

RECOMMENDED TECHNIQUE	S	NI	U	Comments
Transport the medications carefully and safely, using methods recommended by the agency	☐	☐	☐	_____
Protect the needle for injecting drugs to prevent contamination according to agency policy	☐	☐	☐	_____
Do not leave medications out of sight while administering them	☐	☐	☐	_____
Identify clients carefully and accurately before administering medications	☐	☐	☐	_____
Do not give a medication if the client says he or she is allergic to it or if signs or symptoms suggest an unfavorable reaction	☐	☐	☐	_____
Check further if the client believes he or she is receiving a new or different medication	☐	☐	☐	_____
Report immediately when a client refuses a medication or has an unfavorable reaction to it	☐	☐	☐	_____
In case of error, check the client's condition and report the error promptly	☐	☐	☐	_____
Do not give medications prepared by other persons	☐	☐	☐	_____
Observe the five rights of preparing and giving medications: the right drug, dose, route, time, and client	☐	☐	☐	_____

B. This section allows you to examine your techniques for administering oral medications.

RECOMMENDED TECHNIQUE	S	NI	U	Comments
Pour capsules or tablets into the cap of the container	☐	☐	☐	_____
Open prepackaged single-dose medications at the client's bedside	☐	☐	☐	_____
Pour liquids from a bottle opposite the label, to avoid drops on the label, and into an appropriate measuring device	☐	☐	☐	_____
Use an extractor properly when one is available	☐	☐	☐	_____
Read the amount of liquid medication at the bottom of the meniscus	☐	☐	☐	_____
Have medications for the same client in separate containers and offer them to the client separately	☐	☐	☐	_____
Offer fluids generously for certain medications or to swallow capsules or pills, unless contraindicated	☐	☐	☐	_____
Offer no fluids with a liquid used to control a cough	☐	☐	☐	_____

RECOMMENDED TECHNIQUE	S	NI	U	Comments
Use a drinking tube when medications are likely to stain or damage the teeth	☐	☐	☐	_____
Chill a medication that has an objectionable taste, disguise it, or use ice chips as necessary	☐	☐	☐	_____
Stay with the client until all medications are swallowed and leave no medications at the bedside	☐	☐	☐	_____

C. This section allows you to examine your techniques for administering medications through a nasogastric tube.

RECOMMENDED TECHNIQUE	S	NI	U	Comments
Prepare the prescribed medication by dissolving crushed tablets or capsule contents in about 30 mL of warm water	☐	☐	☐	_____
Assemble necessary equipment and the medication at the client's bedside	☐	☐	☐	_____
Drape client properly	☐	☐	☐	_____
Correctly test for placement of the nasogastric tube	☐	☐	☐	_____
Put on clean gloves	☐	☐	☐	_____
Attach the syringe barrel or funnel to the clamped tube	☐	☐	☐	_____
Instill 15 to 30 mL of water by gravity flow	☐	☐	☐	_____
Pour medication in solution into the syringe barrel or funnel	☐	☐	☐	_____
Allow the medication to enter the stomach	☐	☐	☐	_____
Add 30 mL of water to flush the tube before the syringe or funnel is completely empty	☐	☐	☐	_____
After all of the solution has entered, remove the barrel or funnel and clamp the tube for 30 minutes	☐	☐	☐	_____
Have the client remain in a sitting position or on his or her right side with the head slightly elevated for 30 minutes before connecting to suction	☐	☐	☐	_____
Connect the tube for nourishment immediately	☐	☐	☐	_____
Document appropriate data according to agency policy	☐	☐	☐	_____

CHAPTER 33

Topical and Inhalant Medications

■ Summary

Medications may be given by several routes other than oral. The focus of this chapter is the nurse's responsibility for the safe preparation and administration of topical and inhalant medications.

■ Matching Questions

Directions: For items 1 through 5, match the locations in Part B with the routes of administration in Part A.

PART A

1. _e_ Cutaneous
2. _c_ Sublingual
3. _A_ Buccal
4. _b_ Otic
5. _d_ Ophthalmic

PART B

a. Between the cheek and gum
b. Within the ear
c. Under the tongue
d. Within the eye
e. To the skin

■ Multiple-Choice Questions

Directions: For items 1 through 10, circle the letter that corresponds to the best answer for each question.

1. To ensure good absorption when applying an inunction, the nurse should first:
   a. Cleanse the area with soap or detergent and water
   b. Warm the inunction to body temperature
   c. Cleanse the skin with an antiseptic solution
   d. Apply heat to the area for several minutes

2. Of the following, which is <u>contraindicated</u> when applying nitroglycerin to the skin:
   a. Remove any previous application from the skin
   b. Apply the ointment on a clean, nonhairy surface of the skin
   c. Rub the ointment into the skin with your fingers
   d. Cover the area with a square of plastic and tape the sides

3. When giving eardrops to an adult, the ear should be gently pulled:
   a. Upward and forward
   b. Upward and backward
   c. Downward and forward
   d. Downward and backward

   Up + back ADULT

4. When giving eardrops to a child, the ear should be gently pulled:
   a. Upward and forward
   b. Upward and backward
   c. Downward and forward
   d. Downward and backward

   DOWN + BACK CHILD

5. The term for a medication that is administered under the tongue is:
   a. Buccal
   b. Sublingual
   c. Subcutaneous
   d. Transdermal

6. The position of choice when inserting a vaginal medication is:
   a. Sims position
   b. Knee-chest position
   c. Dorsal recumbent position
   d. Horizontal recumbent position

7. The mucous membrane of the eye is called the:

a. Conjunctiva

b. Sclera

c. Cornea

d. Retina

8. If medication must be instilled in both ears, it is appropriate to wait how long between applications:

   a. 5 minutes

   b. 10 minutes

   c. 15 minutes

   d. 20 minutes

9. Chewing, swallowing, smoking, eating, and drinking are contraindicated when which of the following medications is given?

   a. Otic

   b. Ophthalmic

   c. Inunction

   d. Buccal

10. When administering vaginal medications, the applicator is usually inserted into the vagina approximately:

    a. 1 to 2 inches

    b. 2 to 4 inches

    c. 3 to 5 inches

    d. 5 to 10 inches

■ Alternative Format Questions

1. When performing an eye irrigation, the eye irrigating device should be held about _2.5"s_ cm above the eye.

2. Bacitracin topical ointment has a half-life of 6 hours. What percentage of the drug is left in the body at 24 hours?

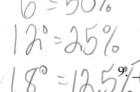

6 hrs — 50%
12 hrs — 25%
24 hrs — 12.

$6^0 = 50\%$
$12^0 = 25\%$
$18^0 = 12.5\%$
$24^0 = 6.25\%$

3. Presume that the full name of the client, the date and time that the order was written, and the physician's signature are present on the physician's order sheet. The following are listed on the medication administration record (MAR). Which of the following order(s) would the nurse question? Select all that apply:

   1. Lasix 40 mg po stat

   2. Ampicillin 500 mg q 6 hr, IVPB

   3. Humulin L (Lente) insulin, sc, q a.m.

   4. Codeine q 4 – 6 hr; po, prn for pain

   5. Nitropaste qd

■ True or False Questions

Directions: For items 1 through 9, decide if the statement is true or false and mark T or F in the space provided.

1. _F_ SYSTEMATIC Topically applied drugs have only a local effect.

2. _T_ It is often necessary to shave body hair prior to applying a transdermal patch.

3. _T_ Solutions, ointments, and equipment used to administer eye medications should be sterile.

4. _T_ The lack of subcutaneous fat in older adults may cause a topical medication to be absorbed more rapidly than in a younger adult.

5. _F_ Bronchodilating drugs cause bradycardia and hypotension in susceptible individuals.

6. _T_ The rebound effect is a phenomenon characterized by rapid swelling of nasal mucosa.

7. _T_ Intense itching, redness with excoriation, and burning on urination are common signs and symptoms of vaginal yeast infections.

8. _T_ The inhalant route is used for medication administration because the lungs provide a massive area of tissue from which drugs may be absorbed.

9. _T_ Cutaneous applications are medications that are incorporated into a transporting agent.

■ Short Answer Questions

Directions: Read each of the following statements and supply the word(s) necessary in the space provided.

1. List the guidelines for giving an inunction. _____

    _____

    _____

2. List the guidelines for applying nitroglycerin ointment.

    _____

    _____

3. List the common routes of topical administration for drugs.

    EPIDERMAL, TRANSMUCOSAL
    RECTAL, VAGINAL

4. Identify six items necessary for teaching self-administration of vaginal medications.

    _____

    _____

    _____

    _____

    _____

    _____

■ Critical Thinking Exercise

Describe the current system for distributing medications in the hospital where you care for clients. What are the checks and balances in this system to protect the client and the nurse from medication errors?

Performance Checklist

A. This section allows you to examine your techniques for administering medications transdermally.

1. Place a check mark in the "S" ("satisfactory") column if you used the recommended technique.
2. Place a check mark in the "NI" ("needs improvement") column if you used some but not all of each recommended technique.
3. Place a check mark in the "U" ("unsatisfactory") column if you forgot to include that particular recommended technique.
4. Note whether further practice is indicated, what errors you made, suggestions that will improve your skills, and so on in the section for comments.

RECOMMENDED TECHNIQUE	S	NI	U	Comments
When Nitroglycerin Paste Is Applied				
Wash your hands	☐	☐	☐	_____
Squeeze the prescribed amount onto the manufacturer's application paper	☐	☐	☐	_____
Place the application paper on a clean, non-hairy area on the chest wall or upper arm	☐	☐	☐	_____
Secure the application paper and cover it appropriately with plastic kitchen wrap	☐	☐	☐	_____
Check blood pressure 30 minutes after application of the drug	☐	☐	☐	_____
Notify proper personnel when a fall in blood pressure and a rise in pulse rate do not occur when nitroglycerin is given	☐	☐	☐	_____
Rotate sites on which ointment is placed	☐	☐	☐	_____
Be careful not to get ointment on your own skin	☐	☐	☐	_____
When a Disk of Ointment Is Used				
Follow the previously mentioned techniques, except for the following differences:	☐	☐	☐	_____
Apply a disk according to directions, usually behind the ear	☐	☐	☐	_____
Monitor the client appropriately	☐	☐	☐	_____

B. This section allows you to examine your technique for administering a nasal medication.

RECOMMENDED TECHNIQUE	S	NI	U	Comments
Compare the MAR with the written medical order	☐	☐	☐	_____
Wash your hands	☐	☐	☐	_____
Identify the client	☐	☐	☐	_____
Position the client in a sitting position or place a rolled towel under the neck	☐	☐	☐	_____
Remove the cap from the medication dropper	☐	☐	☐	_____
Aim the tip of the dropper toward the nares	☐	☐	☐	_____
Squeeze the rubber portion to give the correct number of drops	☐	☐	☐	_____
Instruct the client to breathe through the mouth as the drops are instilled	☐	☐	☐	_____

If the Drug Is a Spray Form

	S	NI	U	
Place the tip of the container just inside the nostril	☐	☐	☐	_____
Occlude the opposite nostril	☐	☐	☐	_____
Instruct the client to inhale as the spray is released	☐	☐	☐	_____
Repeat on the opposite side as required	☐	☐	☐	_____
Advise the client to remain in the sitting position for about 5 minutes	☐	☐	☐	_____
Recap and replace the container where medications are stored	☐	☐	☐	_____
Document the administration on the MAR	☐	☐	☐	_____

C. This section allows you to examine your technique for administering eye medications.

RECOMMENDED TECHNIQUE	S	NI	U	Comments
Compare the MAR with the written medical order	☐	☐	☐	_____
Warm eyedrops and ointments by holding them in the hands	☐	☐	☐	_____
Wash your hands	☐	☐	☐	_____
Position the client supine or sitting with his or her head tilted back	☐	☐	☐	_____
Cleanse the lids and lashes as needed	☐	☐	☐	_____
Instruct the client to look toward the ceiling	☐	☐	☐	_____
Make a pouch in the lower lid by pulling the skin over the bony orbit downward	☐	☐	☐	_____
Bring the medication container to the eye from below the client's line of vision	☐	☐	☐	_____
Instill the prescribed number of drops	☐	☐	☐	_____

RECOMMENDED TECHNIQUE	S	NI	U	Comments
Instruct the client to close the eyes and blink gently	☐	☐	☐	_____
Wipe away excess fluid with a clean tissue	☐	☐	☐	_____
Document medication administration on the MAR	☐	☐	☐	_____

D. This section allows you to examine your technique for teaching the client how to use a metered-dose inhaler.

RECOMMENDED TECHNIQUE	S	NI	U	Comments
Instruct the Client To Do the Following				
Insert the canister into the holder	☐	☐	☐	_____
Shake the canister to distribute the drug within the pressurized chamber	☐	☐	☐	_____
Exhale slowly through pursed lips	☐	☐	☐	_____
Seal lips around the mouthpiece	☐	☐	☐	_____
Compress the canister; slowly inhale	☐	☐	☐	_____
Release the pressure on the canister; continue inhaling	☐	☐	☐	_____
Withdraw the mouthpiece from the mouth	☐	☐	☐	_____
Hold your breath for 10 seconds	☐	☐	☐	_____
Exhale slowly through pursed lips	☐	☐	☐	_____
Wait 1 full minute before another inhalation if one is ordered	☐	☐	☐	_____
Clean the inhaler and check the amount of medication remaining	☐	☐	☐	_____

CHAPTER 34

Parenteral Medications

■ Summary

The parenteral route (route of drug administration other than oral or through the gastrointestinal tract) commonly is used to refer to medications given by injection. This chapter discusses the techniques for administering injections. Preparation and administration follow the principles of asepsis and infection control.

■ Matching Questions

Directions: For items 1 through 4, match the injection routes in Part B with the injection sites in Part A.

PART A

1. ____ Inner aspect of the forearm
2. ____ Upper arm, thigh, abdomen, and back
3. ____ Dorsogluteal, vastus lateralis, and deltoid
4. ____ Blood vessels

PART B

a. intramuscular
b. subcutaneous
c. intravenous
d. intradermal

■ Multiple-Choice Questions

Directions: For items 1 through 12, circle the letter that corresponds to the best answer for each question.

1. When combining drugs from two multiple-dose vials, which procedure best ensures that the second vial will not be contaminated with medication from the first vial:

    a. Change the needle before inserting it into the second vial

    b. Cleanse the rubber stopper of each vial with an antiseptic

    c. Withdraw the exact amount of medication from the first vial

    d. Withdraw the exact amount of medication from the second vial

2. The common site for giving intramuscular injections into the gluteus maximus is the:

    a. Rectus femoris site

    b. Vastus lateralis site

    c. Dorsogluteal site

    d. Ventrogluteal site

3. The common site for giving intramuscular injections into the anterior aspect of the thigh is the:

    a. Rectus femoris site

    b. Vastus lateralis site

    c. Dorsogluteal site

    d. Ventrogluteal site

4. The preferred intramuscular injection site for infants is the:

    a. Vastus lateralis site

    b. Rectus femoris site

    c. Dorsogluteal site

    d. Ventrogluteal site

5. Intramuscular injections into the deltoid muscle should be limited to:

    a. 2.5 mL of solution

    b. 2 mL of solution

    c. 1 mL of solution

    d. 0.5 mL of solution

6. An accepted method for determining the dorsogluteal site for an intramuscular injection is to:

   a. Palpate the greater trochanter at the head of the femur, the anterior superior iliac spine, and the iliac crest

   b. Palpate the posterior iliac spine and the greater trochanter and draw an imaginary line between the landmarks

   c. Divide the thigh into thirds, using the hands, and inject the medication into the middle third

   d. Place the palm of the hand on the greater trochanter and the index finger on the anterior superior iliac spine

7. The primary reason for using the Z-track technique when giving an intramuscular medication is to help:

   a. Avoid striking a major nerve

   b. Seal the medication in the muscle

   c. Hasten the absorption of the medication

   d. Decrease the discomfort of the injection

8. The needle size for subcutaneous injections is usually:

   a. 20 gauge, $\frac{1}{2}$ to $\frac{5}{8}$ inch

   b. 21 gauge, $\frac{1}{2}$ to $\frac{5}{8}$ inch

   c. 22 gauge, $\frac{1}{2}$ to $\frac{5}{8}$ inch

   d. 25 gauge, $\frac{1}{2}$ to $\frac{5}{8}$ inch

9. The strength of insulin prepared by pharmaceutical companies is:

   a. 200 units of insulin per 1 ml

   b. 100 units of insulin per 1 ml

   c. 50 units of insulin per 1 ml

   d. 25 units of insulin per 1 ml

10. A primary concern when giving heparin subcutaneously is to prevent:

    a. Bleeding and bruising

    b. Pain and bruising

    c. Pain and bleeding

    d. Injection of a vein

11. The angle of the syringe and needle for intradermal injections is:

    a. 90°

    b. 45° to 90°

    c. 10° to 45°

    d. 10° to 15°

12. Humulin N is an example of an insulin that is:

    a. Long acting

    b. Intermediate acting

    c. Short acting

    d. Ultrafast acting

■ Alternative Format Questions

1. The physician ordered 750 mg of a certain drug for a client. The drug is stocked in a 10-g multidose vial. The directions on the vial tell the nurse to "add 8.5 mL of sterile water, and each ml will contain 1.0 gram of the drug." How many milliliters of this solution will the nurse administer for the dose ordered?

2. In the apothecary system of measurement, 1 ml is approximately equal to _____ minims.

3. The ventrogluteal site is the preferred site for intramuscular injections because the area has the following characteristics. Select all that apply:

   1. It is usually irritation free

   2. It is safer than other gluteal sites

   3. It provides the greatest thickness of gluteal muscle

   4. It contains consistently less fat than other areas

   5. It is cleaner

   6. It presents no risk of damaging the radial artery

■ True or False Questions

Directions: For items 1 through 11, decide if the statement is true or false and mark T or F in the space provided.

1. ____ Parenteral refers to all oral medications.

2. ____ The smaller the number of the gauge, the larger the lumen of the needle.

3. ____ When combining medications from single-dose and multiple-dose vials, the medication should be withdrawn from the single-dose vials first.

4. ____ The terms *vial* and *ampule* are synonymous.

5. ____ When administering an intramuscular medication, the needle should be introduced slowly to prevent tissue damage.

6. ____ The advantage of prefilled medication cartridges for injection is that the dosage is always correct.

7. ____ Prefilled cartridges are often intended for multiple-dose use and should be checked carefully.

8. ____ When planning to give an injection via the Z-track technique, it is not necessary to change the needle after aspirating the medication into the syringe.

9. ____ Subcutaneous medications may be given at a 90° angle.

10. ____ It is a common practice for one nurse to check the insulin preparation of another nurse.

11. ____ When giving heparin subcutaneously, the plunger of the syringe must be aspirated to make certain the needle is not in a blood vessel.

■ Short Answer Questions

Directions: Read each of the following statements and supply the word(s) necessary in the space provided.

1. Identify four criteria for selecting the appropriate syringe and needle for the administration of parenteral medications.

   a. _____
   _____

   b. _____
   _____

   c. _____
   _____

   d. _____
   _____

2. Identify four activities after a needlestick that are recommended to protect your health.

   a. _____
   _____

   b. _____
   _____

   c. _____
   _____

   d. _____

■ Critical Thinking Exercise

Describe techniques the nurse could use to reduce discomfort associated with injections. State the rationale for their use.

Performance Checklist

A. This section allows you to examine your techniques for removing medications from vials and ampules.

1. Place a check mark in the "S" ("satisfactory") column if you used the recommended technique.
2. Place a check mark in the "NI" ("needs improvement") column if you used some but not all of each recommended technique.
3. Place a check mark in the "U" ("unsatisfactory") column if you forgot to include that particular recommended technique.
4. Note whether further practice is indicated, what errors you made, suggestions that will improve your skills, and so on in the section for comments.

RECOMMENDED TECHNIQUE	S	NI	U	Comments
From a Vial				
Remove the soft metal cover from the rubber stopper	☐	☐	☐	_____
Cleanse the exposed rubber stopper with an alcohol swab	☐	☐	☐	_____
Fill the syringe with the same amount of air as the amount of solution to be withdrawn	☐	☐	☐	_____
Pierce the stopper and instill the air into the vial	☐	☐	☐	_____
Withdraw the desired amount of medication from the vial	☐	☐	☐	_____
Hold the vial straight and at eye level while withdrawing the medication	☐	☐	☐	_____
Withdraw the needle from the vial and prepare to administer the medication	☐	☐	☐	_____
From an Ampule				
Select the appropriate syringe and filter needle	☐	☐	☐	_____
Tap the stem of the ampule until all of the medication is in the well of the ampule	☐	☐	☐	_____
Protect your thumb and fingers with a dry gauze square	☐	☐	☐	_____
Snap the stem from the ampule	☐	☐	☐	_____
Insert the filter needle into the opened ampule, being careful not to touch the outside of the ampule	☐	☐	☐	_____
Remove the medication from the ampule by pulling back on the plunger of the syringe	☐	☐	☐	_____
Remove the needle without touching the edges of the ampule and discard the ampule in a puncture-resistant container	☐	☐	☐	_____

B. This section allows you to examine your techniques for administering intramuscular and subcutaneous injections.

RECOMMENDED TECHNIQUE	S	NI	U	Comments
Intramuscular Injection				
Select proper equipment and supplies and, unless syringe is prefilled, accurately fill the syringe with the drug and 0.2 mL of air	☐	☐	☐	_____
Demonstrate how to locate the proper site for injecting into the dorsogluteal, ventrogluteal, vastus lateralis, rectus femoris, and deltoid muscles	☐	☐	☐	_____
Select an appropriate site for injecting the medication and cleanse the area properly	☐	☐	☐	_____
Use appropriate techniques to reduce discomfort before giving an injection	☐	☐	☐	_____
Spread the tissue taut and quickly thrust the needle for most of its length into the muscle tissue	☐	☐	☐	_____
Aspirate to observe for the presence of blood in the syringe	☐	☐	☐	_____
If blood is present, remove needle and do not inject the medication	☐	☐	☐	_____
Discard the needle, syringe, and medication and prepare fresh medication for injection into another site	☐	☐	☐	_____
Inject the medication slowly, followed by the air bubble	☐	☐	☐	_____
Withdraw the needle quickly while applying pressure against the injection site	☐	☐	☐	_____
Massage the area for a minute or two, unless the manufacturer recommends otherwise	☐	☐	☐	_____
Z-Track Technique				
Select and prepare the site where the medication is to be injected	☐	☐	☐	_____
Grasp the client's muscle with your nondominant hand near the site where the injection is to be made	☐	☐	☐	_____
Pull the skin and underlying tissue laterally about 2.5 cm (1 inch) and hold it there securely	☐	☐	☐	_____
Grasp the syringe with the last three fingers and inject the needle as for an intramuscular injection	☐	☐	☐	_____
Aspirate to observe for blood in the syringe	☐	☐	☐	_____
If no blood is present, inject the medication	☐	☐	☐	_____

RECOMMENDED TECHNIQUE	S	NI	U	Comments
Wait about 10 seconds after injecting the medication before withdrawing the needle	☐	☐	☐	_____
Do not massage the area where the medication was given	☐	☐	☐	_____

Subcutaneous Injection

	S	NI	U	Comments
Observe techniques for giving an intramuscular injection with the following two exceptions:	☐	☐	☐	_____
Select an appropriate site where subcutaneous tissue is abundant	☐	☐	☐	_____
Hold the skin taut over injection site or grasp tissue, depending on the client's size	☐	☐	☐	_____

C. This section allows you to examine your techniques for administering an intradermal injection.

RECOMMENDED TECHNIQUE	S	NI	U	Comments
Select proper equipment and supplies and fill the syringe with the proper medication	☐	☐	☐	_____
Select an area on the inner aspect of the forearm, approximately a hand's breadth above the wrist	☐	☐	☐	_____
Cleanse the intended site of entry with an alcohol swab	☐	☐	☐	_____
Hold the client's arm in your hand and stretch the skin taut with your thumb	☐	☐	☐	_____
Place the needle almost flat against the skin, bevel side up	☐	☐	☐	_____
Inject the needle about $1/8$ inch and test whether the needle is in a vein	☐	☐	☐	_____
Slowly inject the agent while watching for a small wheal or blister	☐	☐	☐	_____
After injecting the agent slowly, withdraw the needle quickly	☐	☐	☐	_____
Do not massage the area where the injection was made	☐	☐	☐	_____
Observe the client for signs of a reaction for at least 30 minutes	☐	☐	☐	_____
Observe the area for signs of a local reaction about 24 to 48 hours after injection	☐	☐	☐	_____

CHAPTER 35

Intravenous Medications

■ Summary

Administering intravenous solutions, discussed in Chapter 15, can be considered a form of intravenous medication administration. It is used for fluid balance and maintenance. However, the focus of this chapter is on the methods for administering intravenous drugs and the techniques for using various venous-access devices, not fluid therapy. The intravenous route includes peripheral and central veins.

■ Matching Questions

Directions: For items 1 through 5, match the terms in Part B with the descriptions in Part A.

PART A

1. ____ Used to administer undiluted medication quickly into a vein.

2. ____ Used to administer a parenteral drug that is diluted in 50 cc of solution over 30 to 60 minutes.

3. ____ Used to administer IV medication without circulatory overload.

4. ____ Used to administer parenteral medication in a large volume of blood.

5. ____ Used to provide the greatest protection against infection when IV medications are required frequently over a very long period of time.

PART B

a. Implanted catheter
b. Secondary infusion
c. Volume-control set
d. Central venous catheter
e. Bolus

■ Multiple-Choice Questions

Directions: For items 1 through 10, circle the letter that corresponds to the best answer for each question.

1. Intravenous medications are usually added to a large volume of solution by the:
   a. Physician
   b. Pharmacist
   c. Manufacturer
   d. Nurse

2. Clients receiving medication via a central venous catheter over an extended period of time are most likely to have which of the following types of catheters:
   a. A percutaneous catheter
   b. An angio-catheter
   c. A tunneled catheter
   d. An implanted catheter

3. Goggles and a respirator mask are recommended when preparing which of the following medications for administration:
   a. Anticoagulant drugs
   b. Parenteral drugs
   c. Intravenous drugs
   d. Antineoplastic drugs

4. A Hickman catheter is an example of:
   a. A percutaneous catheter
   b. An angio-catheter
   c. A tunneled catheter
   d. An implanted catheter

5. An intermittent infusion is one in which IV medication is given:
   a. Over an extended period of time
   b. All at one time
   c. Over a short period of time
   d. At a rate of 1 mL per minute

6. Bolus administration of intravenous medication has the greatest potential for:
   a. Causing life-threatening reactions
   b. Delivering the drug gradually
   c. Backfilling the tubing
   d. Allowing IV fluid to flow slowly

7. The best feature of a medication lock is that it:
   a. Facilitates the administration of medication
   b. Prevents medication errors
   c. Is a venous-access device
   d. Eliminates administration of unneeded IV fluids

8. A secondary infusion involves administering an IV medication that has been diluted in a volume of solution equal to:
   a. 500 to 1000 cc
   b. 250 to 500 cc
   c. 100 to 200 cc
   d. 50 to 100 cc

9. When caring for clients who are at risk for circulatory overload, it would be appropriate to administer IV medications using a:
   a. Volume-control set
   b. Central venous catheter
   c. Continuous infusion set
   d. Bolus administration

10. An advantage resulting from the use of multilumen central venous catheters is:
    a. Unused lumens can be capped with a medication lock
    b. They can be used for short-term intravenous therapy
    c. Incompatible substances can be given simultaneously
    d. They facilitate clearing the catheter of heparin

■ Alternative Format Questions

1. A certain drug was ordered to be given through an IV lock. Place the following activities in the order in which they would most likely be carried out:
   1. Swab port and flush with 1 mL of heparin flush solution
   2. Identify and assess the client
   3. Swab port and flush with 1 mL of sterile normal saline
   4. Instill the medication
   5. Swab port and flush with l mL of sterile normal saline
   6. Wash hands and put on gloves

2. The physician prescribes 25,000 U of heparin in 250 mL of normal saline solution to infuse at 600U/hour. After 6 hours of heparin therapy the client's partial thromboplastin time is subtherapeutic. The physician orders an increase in the infusion to 800 U/hour. The nurse should set the infusion pump to deliver how many milliliters per hour?

3. The client is prescribed 500 mg of IV metronidazole (Flagyl). The mixed IV solution contains 100 mL. The nurse is to run the drug over 30 minutes. The drip factor of the available IV tubing is 15 gtt/mL. What is the drip rate for this drug?

■ True or False Questions

Directions: For items 1 through 9, decide if the statement is true or false and mark T or F in the space provided.

1. _____ Bolus is the term used to designate multiple-dose intravenous medications.

2. _____ A heparin lock is used for continuous intravenous medications.

3. _____ Implanted central venous catheters provide the greatest protection against infection.

4. ____ Antineoplastic drugs can be absorbed accidentally by health care professionals.

5. ____ Implanted ports can sustain about 2,000 punctures over several years.

6. ____ Tunneled catheters are inserted through the skin in a peripheral vein, such as the jugular.

7. ____ Older adults are more likely to experience adverse drug effects because there is more circulating protein-bound drug in the blood.

8. ____ A piggyback solution is a small volume of diluted medication that is connected to and positioned higher than the primary solution.

9. ____ A central venous catheter is a venous-access device that extends to the vena cava.

■ Short Answer Questions

Directions: Read each of the following statements and supply the word(s) necessary in the space provided.

1. List four steps (SASH) the nurse should follow when giving medication through a heparin lock.

   a. S = _____

   b. A = _____

   c. S = _____

   d. H = _____

2. List advantages given in this chapter for using a central venous catheter compared to a peripheral catheter. _____

   _____

   _____

3. List four reasons the intravenous route may be the preferred route of medication administration.

   a. _____

   _____

   b. _____

   _____

   c. _____

   _____

   d. _____

   _____

■ Critical Thinking Exercise

This chapter includes recommendations for avoiding self-contamination when antineoplastic drugs are administered. Discuss how you would explain these precautions:

   a. When the client is a young child

   b. When the client is a teen

Performance Checklist

A. This section allows you to examine your technique for administering IV medication by continuous infusion.

1. Place a check mark in the "S" ("satisfactory") column if you used the recommended technique.

2. Place a check mark in the "NI" ("needs improvement") column if you used some but not all of each recommended technique.

3. Place a check mark in the "U" ("unsatisfactory") column if you forgot to include that particular recommended technique.

4. Note whether further practice is indicated, what errors you made, suggestions that will improve your skills, and so on in the section for comments.

RECOMMENDED TECHNIQUE	S	NI	U	Comments
Compare the medication administration record (MAR) with the written medical order	☐	☐	☐	_____
Observe for documented drug or food allergies	☐	☐	☐	_____
Inspect the current infusion site for swelling, redness, or tenderness	☐	☐	☐	_____
Wash your hands	☐	☐	☐	_____
Identify the client	☐	☐	☐	_____
Clamp the current infusion	☐	☐	☐	_____
Swab the port on the container	☐	☐	☐	_____
Instill the medication into the container	☐	☐	☐	_____
Lower the container and gently rotate it to mix drug and solution	☐	☐	☐	_____
Suspend the solution and release the clamp	☐	☐	☐	_____
Regulate the flow rate	☐	☐	☐	_____
Attach a label to the container indicating the drug, dose, time, and your initials	☐	☐	☐	_____
Record the medication on the MAR	☐	☐	☐	_____
Observe the client and the progress of the infusion at least hourly	☐	☐	☐	_____
Record appropriate data on the required forms for documentation	☐	☐	☐	_____

B. This section allows you to examine your technique for administering an intermittent secondary infusion.

RECOMMENDED TECHNIQUE	S	NI	U	Comments
Compare the MAR with the written medical order	☐	☐	☐	_____
Observe the documented drug or food allergies	☐	☐	☐	_____

RECOMMENDED TECHNIQUE	S	NI	U	Comments
Inspect the current infusion site for swelling, redness, or tenderness	☐	☐	☐	_____
Review drug action and side effects	☐	☐	☐	_____
Remove refrigerated solution at least 30 minutes prior to use	☐	☐	☐	_____
Check the drop factor on the package of secondary tubing, calculate the rate of infusion, and have another nurse check your calculations	☐	☐	☐	_____
Locate and swab the port and insert and tape the needle within the port	☐	☐	☐	_____
Lower the container of the primary solution approximately 10 inches below the height of the secondary solution, using a plastic or metal hanger	☐	☐	☐	_____
Release the clamp on the secondary solution; regulate the rate of flow	☐	☐	☐	_____
Clamp the tubing when the solution has instilled	☐	☐	☐	_____
Rehang the primary container and readjust the flow rate	☐	☐	☐	_____
Leave the secondary tubing in place if another secondary infusion is scheduled within 24 hours	☐	☐	☐	_____
Record the appropriate data on the required forms for documentation	☐	☐	☐	_____

C. This section allows you to examine your technique for using a volume-control set.

RECOMMENDED TECHNIQUE	S	NI	U	Comments
Compare the MAR with the written medical order	☐	☐	☐	_____
Observe for documented food and drug allergies	☐	☐	☐	_____
Review drug action and side effects	☐	☐	☐	_____
Assess the client's fluid status	☐	☐	☐	_____
Inspect current infusion site for redness, swelling, or tenderness	☐	☐	☐	_____
Determine the drop factor on the volume-control set, calculate the rate of infusion, and have another nurse check your calculations	☐	☐	☐	_____
Wash your hands and put on gloves	☐	☐	☐	_____
Close all clamps on the volume-control set; insert spike into IV solution	☐	☐	☐	_____
Seal air vent if the IV solution is in a plastic bag; leave it open if the container is glass	☐	☐	☐	_____

RECOMMENDED TECHNIQUE	S	NI	U	Comments
Release the clamp above the fluid chamber	☐	☐	☐	_____
Fill the calibrated chamber with about 30 cc of IV solution and tighten the clamp	☐	☐	☐	_____
Squeeze and release the drip chamber until it is one-half full	☐	☐	☐	_____
Open lower clamp until the tubing is filled with fluid; reclamp	☐	☐	☐	_____
Open clamp above the calibrated container; fill if with the desired volume	☐	☐	☐	_____
Swab the injection port on the calibrated container	☐	☐	☐	_____
Instill the prepared medication	☐	☐	☐	_____
Rotate the fluid chamber to mix it	☐	☐	☐	_____
Connect the tubing to the client's IV catheter, release the lower clamp, and regulate the drip	☐	☐	☐	_____
Label the fluid chamber with the drug, dose, time, and your initials	☐	☐	☐	_____
Return before the medication is due to finish	☐	☐	☐	_____
Release the upper clamp when the medication is finished	☐	☐	☐	_____
Refill the fluid chamber with the next hour's worth of fluid; readjust the rate	☐	☐	☐	_____
Remove the drug label	☐	☐	☐	_____
Record the appropriate data on the required forms for documentation	☐	☐	☐	_____

CHAPTER 36

Airway Management

■ Summary

The primary function of the respiratory system is to facilitate ventilation so that there is appropriate exchange of oxygen and carbon dioxide at the cellular level. Adequate ventilation is dependent on clear air passages from the nose to the alveoli. This chapter presents information on various skills for promoting and assisting pulmonary function, including caring for the client with an oral airway or a tracheostomy and removing secretions from the respiratory tract.

■ Matching Questions

Directions: For items 1 through 5, match the terms in Part B with the description in Part A.

PART A

1. _____ A type of secretion found in the respiratory tract

2. _____ A secretion raised to the level of the upper airway

3. _____ A surgically created opening into the trachea

4. _____ A technique to loosen retained secretions

5. _____ A collective system of tubes found in the respiratory tract

PART B

a. Sputum

b. Tracheostomy

c. Airway

d. Vibration

e. Mucus

■ Multiple-Choice Questions

Directions: For items 1 through 12, circle the letter that corresponds to the best answer for each question.

1. To avoid the narrowing of respiratory passageways and decreased volume of exchanged gases for clients with lung congestion, the nurse should:
   a. Encourage the client to cough
   b. Encourage the client to exercise
   c. Encourage adequate fluid intake
   d. Encourage adequate nutrition

2. The process of suspending droplets of water in a gas is known as:
   a. Humidification
   b. Atomization
   c. Nebulization
   d. Aerosolization

3. Postural drainage should be performed:
   a. Before breakfast and at bedtime
   b. Before meals and before bedtime
   c. After meals, three times a day
   d. At midmorning and midafternoon

4. The technique used when performing percussion is:
   a. Striking the chest with rhythmic, gentle blows using a cupped hand
   b. Striking the chest with rhythmic, gentle blows using open hands
   c. Using firm, strong, circular movements on the chest with open hands
   d. Using firm, strong, circular movements on the chest with cupped hands

5. The primary purpose for using percussion and vibration over an area of a lung is to:

   a. Move residual air out of the lung

   b. Force the client to take deep breaths

   c. Cause thick secretions to break loose

   d. Prevent the air sacs in the lung from collapsing

6. The points of measurement for determining the appropriate size of oral airway to use are as follows:

   a. The front is parallel with the front teeth, and the back reaches the angle of the jaw

   b. The front is parallel with the front teeth, and the back reaches the back of the throat

   c. The front is parallel with the tip of the nose, and the back reaches the earlobe

   d. The front is parallel with the tip of the chin, and the back reaches the earlobe

7. The best time of the day to collect a sputum specimen is:

   a. After a meal

   b. Between meals

   c. Upon awakening

   d. At bedtime

8. An oral airway should be briefly removed every:

   a. 1 hour

   b. 2 hours

   c. 3 hours

   d. 4 hours

9. Most agencies specify that the inner cannula of a tracheostomy should be cleaned at least every:

   a. 4 hours

   b. 8 hours

   c. 12 hours

   d. 24 hours

10. The catheter for suctioning a tracheostomy on an adult should be inserted no more than:

    a. 10–12.5 cm

    b. 15–20.5 cm

    c. 20–25.5 cm

    d. 25–30.5 cm

11. Clients are most likely to react to the sensation of suffocation with feelings of:

    a. Depression

    b. Anxiety

    c. Hopelessness

    d. Anger

12. The airway is protected by the epiglottis, which:

    a. Seals the airway when swallowing

    b. Keeps the trachea from collapsing

    c. Traps particulate matter

    d. Beats debris upward in the airway so it can be expectorated

■ Alternative Format Questions

1. When collecting a sputum specimen, how many milliliters of sputum is required?

2. The client's nursing diagnosis is Ineffective Airway Clearance. Which of the following assessment data support this diagnosis? Select all that apply:

   1. Persistent, productive cough

   2. Rapid, shallow respirations

   3. Use of accessory muscles

   4. Inspiratory gurgles in the right upper lobe

   5. 70-year-old client

3. An oral airway should be removed and cleaned every _____ hours.

■ True or False Questions

Directions: For items 1 through 9, decide if the statement is true or false and mark T or F in the space provided.

1. ____ Postural drainage should be done before meals and at bedtime.

2. ____ Usually a pressure of 100 to 140 mm Hg is recommended when using a portable machine for suctioning a client's airway.

3. ____ Suctioning should never be done routinely.

4. ____ A good time to collect a sputum specimen is following respiratory therapy treatments.

5. ____ The principles of medical asepsis must be followed when suctioning secretions from a tracheostomy.

6. ____ To ensure a sufficient quantity of specimen for study, it is best to collect at least 10 mL of sputum.

7. ____ Most adults can accommodate an 80-mm oral airway.

8. ____ If an airway is too long, it will depress the epiglottis, thus potentiating the risk of airway obstruction.

9. ____ Because the tracheostomy tube is below the larynx, clients are able to talk.

■ Short Answer Questions

Directions: Read each of the following statements and supply the word(s) necessary in the space provided.

1. List the steps to follow when inserting an oral airway:

2. Identify the approaches for airway suctioning described in this chapter. _____

■ Critical Thinking Exercises

1. Develop a plan for teaching a tracheostomy client how to suction himself or herself.

2. Determine assessment criteria that would indicate the need for suctioning:
   a. When the client is an infant

   b. When the client is an older adult

3. What essential points would you include when explaining how to collect a sputum specimen to a child?

Performance Checklist

A. This section allows you to examine your techniques for using postural drainage.

1. Place a check mark in the "S" ("satisfactory") column if you used the recommended technique.

2. Place a check mark in the "NI" ("needs improvement") column if you used some but not all of each recommended technique.

3. Place a check mark in the "U" ("unsatisfactory") column if you forgot to include that particular recommended technique.

4. Note whether further practice is indicated, what errors you made, suggestions that will improve your skills, and so on in the section for comments.

RECOMMENDED TECHNIQUE	S	NI	U	Comments
Use postural drainage before meals and at bedtime	☐	☐	☐	_____
Administer prescribed medications that dilate respiratory passages before therapy	☐	☐	☐	_____
Be familiar with positions the client cannot safely assume	☐	☐	☐	_____
Have tissues available for the client for expectorating and coughing	☐	☐	☐	_____
Know areas of the lungs to be drained and position the client accordingly	☐	☐	☐	_____
Allow the client to assume positions for 15 to 30 minutes or even 45 minutes if the client is able to tolerate it	☐	☐	☐	_____
Encourage the client to cough and expectorate after each position	☐	☐	☐	_____

B. This section allows you to examine your techniques for caring for a client with a tracheostomy.

RECOMMENDED TECHNIQUE	S	NI	U	Comments
Consider using a face shield and wearing a cover gown and gloves when suctioning a client	☐	☐	☐	_____
Obtain a container of hydrogen peroxide and a flask of normal saline	☐	☐	☐	_____
Remove the cap from each container	☐	☐	☐	_____
Wash your hands	☐	☐	☐	_____
Place the client in a supine or low Fowler's position	☐	☐	☐	_____
Put on a clean glove; remove and discard soiled dressing	☐	☐	☐	_____
Remove glove and wash hands	☐	☐	☐	_____
Open sterile tracheostomy kit	☐	☐	☐	_____
Put on sterile gloves	☐	☐	☐	_____

RECOMMENDED TECHNIQUE	S	NI	U	Comments
Add equal parts sterile normal saline and sterile hydrogen peroxide to basins	☐	☐	☐	_____
Unlock inner cannula by turning counter-clockwise	☐	☐	☐	_____
Put it in the basin with the hydrogen peroxide and normal saline; clean	☐	☐	☐	_____
Rinse in basin with only normal saline and dry	☐	☐	☐	_____
Replace the inner cannula and turn clockwise	☐	☐	☐	_____
Clean around the stoma	☐	☐	☐	_____
Place a sterile stomal dressing beneath the flanges of the outer cannula	☐	☐	☐	_____
Change the ties	☐	☐	☐	_____
Discard all soiled supplies, remove gloves, and wash your hands	☐	☐	☐	_____
Place the client in a safe, comfortable position	☐	☐	☐	_____
Place the "signal device" within easy reach should the client need help	☐	☐	☐	_____
Document tracheostomy care as required by the agency	☐	☐	☐	_____

CHAPTER 37

Resuscitation

■ Summary

Nurses are often the first respondents when clients experience cardiopulmonary emergencies. This chapter reviews the most recent guidelines from the Emergency Cardiac Care Committee and Subcommittees of the American Heart Association for performing basic life-support techniques. Age-related differences for performing cardiopulmonary resuscitation (CPR) are also discussed.

■ Multiple-Choice Questions

Directions: For items 1 through 10, circle the letter that corresponds to the best answer for each question.

1. Of the following, which artery is recommended for checking the pulse of an adult during CPR?
   a. The femoral artery
   b. The radial artery
   c. The carotid artery
   d. The brachial artery

2. Before starting cardiac compressions, it is particularly important to:
   a. Be sure that the victim is not breathing
   b. Be sure that the victim is pulseless
   c. Be sure that the victim's head is tilted back
   d. Be sure that the victim is unconscious

3. Rescue breathing for an adult should be carried out every:
   a. 1 to 1½ seconds for 5 seconds
   b. 5 seconds for 5 seconds
   c. 5 seconds for 1½ seconds
   d. 1 to 1½ seconds for 1 to 1½ seconds

4. When performing CPR on an adult, the ratio of breaths to compressions should be:
   a. Five breaths to every five compressions
   b. One breath to every five compressions
   c. One breath to every 15 compressions
   d. Two breaths to every 15 compressions

5. The depth of chest compressions for an adult receiving CPR should be:
   a. ½ to 1 inch
   b. 1 to 1½ inches
   c. 1½ to 2 inches
   d. 2 to 3 inches

6. A state in which the response pattern of decreased energy reserves results in an individual's inability to maintain breathing adequate to support life describes which of the following nursing diagnoses:
   a. Inability to Sustain Spontaneous Ventilation
   b. Impaired Gas Exchange
   c. Ineffective Airway Clearance
   d. Impaired Cardiopulmonary Tissue Perfusion

7. In order to relieve an airway obstruction for an unconscious victim, you would:
   a. Place your fist in the middle of the abdomen
   b. Begin CPR
   c. Perform the Heimlich maneuver
   d. Administer four back blows immediately

8. Which of the following would indicate that a complete airway obstruction is present:
   a. The victim is unconscious
   b. Hearing an audible, high-pitched sound on inspiration
   c. The victim is not able to speak or cough
   d. The victim grasps his or her throat with his or her hands

9. The method of choice for opening the airway is:

a. The head tilt-chin lift technique

b. The jaw-thrust technique

c. The chest-thrust technique

d. The subdiaphragmatic-thrust technique

10. The recovery position is best described as:

a. A prone position

b. A side-lying position

c. A semi-Fowler's position

d. A Trendelenburg position

■ Alternative Format Questions

1. When performing CPR on an infant, how many breaths per minute should be given?

2. Place the following items in the correct sequence to carry out the chain of survival:

1. Call for emergency assistance

2. Begin advanced life support

3. Begin cardiopulmonary resuscitation

4. Place victim on a flat, firm surface

5. Defibrillate with automated external defibrillator (AED)

6. Recognize the victim's need

3. Basic CPR may be interrupted under which of the following conditions? Select all that apply:

1. The victim continues to have no pulse

2. The rescuer becomes exhausted

3. There is written evidence that the person does not want CPR

4. Advanced life-support measures are administered

5. The victim has a communicable disease

6. A partial airway obstruction is present

■ True or False Questions

Directions: For items 1 through 10, decide if the statement is true or false and mark T or F in the space provided.

1. ____ It is recommended that the carotid artery be used to check for a pulse when performing CPR on an infant.

2. ____ When starting CPR on an infant, only one initial rescue breath should be given.

3. ____ The ratio of breaths to chest compressions is two breaths to 15 compressions.

4. ____ There is always the risk of fracturing ribs when performing CPR.

5. ____ It is not possible to identify, in advance, the type of resuscitation one will allow.

6. ____ Some older adults fear that if they specify that they do not want to be resuscitated, they will receive inferior treatment.

7. ____ Clients who take daily doses of aspirin are more likely to bleed internally when chest compressions are administered.

8. ____ To dislodge an object from an infant's airway, a series of chest thrusts followed by a series of back blows are delivered.

9. ____ Before beginning cardiopulmonary resuscitation, shake the victim and shout his or her name.

10. ____ The decision to cease performing CPR is made by the first respondent.

■ Short Answer Questions

Directions: Read each of the following statements and supply the word(s) necessary in the space provided.

1. Identify the signs that are typical when a victim is choking on a foreign object.

a. _____

_____

b. _____

_____

c. _____

d. _____

e. _____

f. _____

2. Define the ABCs of basic life support.

   a. A is for _____

   b. B is for _____

   c. C is for _____

3. Identify the five criteria for interrupting CPR as presented in this chapter.

   a. _____

   b. _____

c. _____

d. _____

e. _____

■ Critical Thinking Exercises

1. Describe the adjustments that you would make when promoting cardiopulmonary functioning:

   a. When the client is an infant:

   b. When the client is a child:

2. Differences in CPR among infants, children, and adults

   Directions: Review the chart below and fill in the missing information.

Technique	Infant (to 1 year)	Child (1 to 8 years)	Adult (8 years and older)
Rescue Breaths:			
Initial:	2 breaths	2 breaths	2 breaths
Subsequent breaths:	1 every 3 seconds	1 every _____	1 every 5 seconds
Rate:	_____	20/minute	_____
Duration:	1 to 1½ seconds	1 to 1½ seconds	1 to 1½ seconds
Compressions:			
Location:	In the midline, one finger's width below the nipples	_____	Two finger widths above the tip of the sternum
Hand use:	Two or three fingers	Heel of one hand	Two hands
Rate:	At least 100/minute	_____	80–100/minute
Depth:	_____	1 to 1½ inches	1 to 1½ inches or more

Performance Checklist

A. This section allows you to examine your techniques for providing measures to relieve choking.

1. Place a check mark in the "S" ("satisfactory") column if you used the recommended technique.
2. Place a check mark in the "NI" ("needs improvement") column if you used some but not all of each recommended technique.
3. Place a check mark in the "U" ("unsatisfactory") column if you forgot to include that particular recommended technique.
4. Note whether further practice is indicated, what errors you made, suggestions that will improve your skills, and so on in the section for comments.

RECOMMENDED TECHNIQUE	S	NI	U	Comments
Encourage coughing if the choking victim can talk	☐	☐	☐	
If coughing cannot be done to dislodge a foreign object, then:	☐	☐	☐	
Stand behind the victim and allow him or her to lean over your arm with his or her head lower than his or her chest	☐	☐	☐	
Stand behind the victim and place your arms around the victim's abdomen	☐	☐	☐	
Make a fist with one hand and grab it with the other hand	☐	☐	☐	
Place the fist against the victim's abdomen, slightly below the rib cage and above the navel	☐	☐	☐	
Allow the victim to fall forward over your arms	☐	☐	☐	
Press the fist into the victim's abdomen with a forceful upward thrust	☐	☐	☐	
Repeat the maneuver if necessary six to 10 times	☐	☐	☐	
If unsuccessful, begin cardiopulmonary resuscitation as indicated by the client's condition	☐	☐	☐	

B. This section allows you to examine your techniques for administering cardiopulmonary resuscitation to an adult.

RECOMMENDED TECHNIQUE	S	NI	U	Comments
Place the victim on a firm surface, such as the floor or a bed board	☐	☐	☐	
Place one rescuer alongside the client's head and the other on the opposite side near the client's chest	☐	☐	☐	

RECOMMENDED TECHNIQUE	S	NI	U	Comments
Before starting rescue breathing, tilt the victim's head backward, lift it at the neck, and press down on the forehead or thrust the victim's jaw forward to open the airway if the above maneuver does not work	☐	☐	☐	_____
Take a deep breath, pinch the victim's nostrils shut, and forcefully blow your breath into the victim's open mouth	☐	☐	☐	_____
Repeat the above rescue breathing for a total of four times quickly	☐	☐	☐	_____
After the initial two, give one rescue breath every 5 seconds	☐	☐	☐	_____
To give cardiac compressions, place the heel of one hand two finger widths above the tip of the sternum	☐	☐	☐	_____
Place the second hand over the first and interlock your fingers	☐	☐	☐	_____
Exert pressure on the sternum by bringing the shoulders over the hands and keeping the elbows and arms straight	☐	☐	☐	_____
Depress the sternum about 3.75 to 5 centimeters ($1\frac{1}{2}$ to 2 inches) with each compression and then release pressure immediately	☐	☐	☐	_____
Continue with compressions at the rate of 100 per minute and keep the hands properly positioned over the victim always	☐	☐	☐	_____
Check the effectiveness of CPR by noting skin color and pulse	☐	☐	☐	_____
Continue with CPR as long as the victim's heart does not beat spontaneously	☐	☐	☐	_____
Adjust the above techniques correctly when there is only one rescuer	☐	☐	☐	_____

C. This section allows you to examine your techniques for using an AED.

RECOMMENDED TECHNIQUE	S	NI	U	Comments
Obtain the AED, connect cables and pads, and turn on the power	☐	☐	☐	_____
Observe the screen; directions will appear	☐	☐	☐	_____
Kneel at the level of the victim's chest	☐	☐	☐	_____
Peel the paper backing from the electrode pads	☐	☐	☐	_____
Attach one pad to bare skin directly below the right clavicle	☐	☐	☐	_____
Place the second pad lateral to the left nipple with the top of the pad a few inches below the axilla	☐	☐	☐	_____

RECOMMENDED TECHNIQUE	S	NI	U	Comments
Stop CPR to analyze the victim's rhythm — press Analyze button	☐	☐	☐	_____
Do *not* touch the victim at this time	☐	☐	☐	_____
Wait for "shock" or "no shock" message	☐	☐	☐	_____
If shock is indicated, say "Clear" and press the Shock button	☐	☐	☐	_____
If the "No Shock" message appears, check for signs of circulation	☐	☐	☐	_____
If there is still no circulation, resume CPR for 1 minute and check again	☐	☐	☐	_____
If there are still no signs of circulation, analyze the victim's rhythm again	☐	☐	☐	_____
After three "No shock" messages, perform CPR for 1 to 2 minutes	☐	☐	☐	_____
Repeat analyze period every 1 to 2 minutes and continue CPR	☐	☐	☐	_____
If in a moving vehicle, *stop* the vehicle completely before analyzing a rhythm or delivering a shock	☐	☐	☐	_____

CHAPTER 38

Death and Dying

■ Summary

This chapter provides information on many aspects of the dying and grieving experiences. The unique emotional, spiritual, and physical problems of the terminally ill are discussed.

The purposes of this chapter are to assist students with exploring their own attitudes and feelings about death and to identify the nurse's role in helping terminally ill clients die with dignity. The concepts of grief and loss are also explored.

■ Matching Questions

Directions: For items 1 through 5, match the typical emotional responses in Part B with the stages according to Kübler-Ross in Part A.

PART A

1. _____ First stage

2. _____ Second stage

3. _____ Third stage

4. _____ Fourth stage

5. _____ Fifth stage

PART B

a. Bargaining

b. Acceptance

c. Denial and isolation

d. Depression

e. Anger

■ Multiple-Choice Questions

Directions: For items 1 through 10, circle the letter that corresponds to the best answer for each question.

1. An advance directive is:
   a. A statement of the dying person's funeral arrangements
   b. A statement giving the family the right to make final decisions
   c. A statement describing the person's wishes about his or her care when death is near
   d. A statement describing the person's wishes about his or her estate when death is near

2. The third stage of dying according to Kübler-Ross is:
   a. Denial
   b. Anger
   c. Bargaining
   d. Acceptance

3. Anger, according to Kübler-Ross, is considered to be the:
   a. First stage
   b. Second stage
   c. Fourth stage
   d. Fifth stage

4. When the family is physically and emotionally unable to care for the dying member in the home, care must be taken to:
   a. Arrange for financial coverage for the client
   b. Arrange for a special agency for the dying
   c. See that the family is not made to feel guilty
   d. See that the family understands the hospital routine

5. The emphasis of hospice care is:

   a. Helping the individual live until he or she dies

   b. Helping the person with his or her hygiene needs

   c. Teaching the family members to care for the client

   d. Providing counseling for the client and family

6. The nurse can facilitate moving to the stage of acceptance wherein the client can die in peace and dignity by:

   a. Responding to emotional needs

   b. Sustaining realistic hope

   c. Accepting reality

   d. Understanding common fears

7. Of the following, which is considered the last reflex to disappear as death approaches:

   a. Sucking

   b. Gagging

   c. Blinking

   d. Swallowing

8. Of the following pain-relief measures, which would give the dying person the best relief:

   a. Teaching techniques such as imagery and relaxation

   b. Administering medication only when it is absolutely necessary

   c. Administering the pain medication on a routine schedule

   d. Explaining that most pain medications may cause addiction

9. Which of the following signs is the one that is most positive that death has occurred:

   a. The absence of heartbeats

   b. The absence of respirations

   c. The absence of blood pressure

   d. The absence of brain waves

10. A coroner has the right to order an autopsy to be performed if:

    a. The physician requests it

    b. The client was a child

    c. The death was of a suspicious nature

    d. The death happened in the hospital

■ Alternative Format Questions

1. Organ donors must meet certain criteria to be eligible for donation. One of these criteria is age. At how many months of age may an individual be considered to donate a kidney?

2. Place the following stages in the usual order of occurrence experienced by individuals who are terminally ill:

   1. Depression

   2. Anger

   3. Acceptance

   4. Denial

   5. Bargaining

3. Dr. Elisabeth Kübler-Ross identified five stages experienced by terminally ill clients. In which of these stages is an emotional response to feeling victimized by fate a characteristic response?

■ True Or False Questions

Directions: For items 1 through 12, decide if the statement is true or false and mark T or F in the space provided.

1. ____ Denial is an avoidance technique used to separate oneself from situations that are threatening or unpleasant.

2. ____ It is important to understand one's personal feelings about death and dying before providing terminal care.

3. ____ Even though an individual donates his or her organs, in many states the next of kin must sign a permit before the organs are removed from the body.

4. ____ According to Dr. Elisabeth Kübler-Ross, all people go through the five stages of dying in the same order.

5. ____ Each of the five stages of dying lasts for a specified time, and they are sequential.

6. ____ Even though an individual is considered competent, the physician may not allow him to refuse treatment.

7. ____ Sometimes individuals may prolong dying while awaiting a sign that others are prepared to accept the loss.

8. ____ As death approaches, the client's temperature lowers and the skin becomes cold and clammy.

9. ____ Pain can be intensified by fear and anxiety.

10. ____ The death rattle is caused by the client's inability to expectorate sputum.

11. ____ When death is imminent, the client's pain often increases.

12. ____ The physician's signature is required on the death certificate only when the cause of death is suspicious.

■ Short Answer Questions

Directions: Read each of the following statements and supply the word(s) necessary in the space provided.

1. Identify six signs suggested in this chapter that usually clearly indicate that death is imminent.

   a. _____

   b. _____

   c. _____

   d. _____

   e. _____

   f. _____

2. Identify seven suggestions for summoning the family of a dying person.

   a. _____

   b. _____

   c. _____

   d. _____

   e. _____

   f. _____

   g. _____

3. Identify five common physical reactions grieving individuals may experience.

   a. _____

   b. _____

   c. _____

   d. _____

   e. _____

4. List four examples of pathologic grief.

   a. _____

   b. _____

   c. _____

   d. _____

■ Critical Thinking Exercise

Describe adjustments you make when caring for the terminally ill:

   a. When the client is an infant or child

   b. When the client is elderly

Performance Checklist

A. This section allows you to examine your techniques for offering support to someone who is terminally ill.

1. Place a check mark in the "S" ("satisfactory") column if you used the recommended technique.
2. Place a check mark in the "NI" ("needs improvement") column if you used some but not all of each recommended technique.
3. Place a check mark in the "U" ("unsatisfactory") column if you forgot to include that particular recommended technique.
4. Note whether further practice is indicated, what errors you made, suggestions that will improve your skills, and so on in the section for comments.

RECOMMENDED TECHNIQUE	S	NI	U	Comments
Take steps to examine your own feelings about life, death, and dying	☐	☐	☐	_____
Show understanding for the client's feelings and for those of his or her family	☐	☐	☐	_____
Provide a nonjudgmental atmosphere and listen to the client and the family	☐	☐	☐	_____
Show an understanding of how attitudes toward death differ among people	☐	☐	☐	_____
Observe for fear of death and offer appropriate support	☐	☐	☐	_____
Support hope, even when the prognosis is poor, in an appropriate manner	☐	☐	☐	_____
Show an understanding of what to tell the client and family about terminal illness	☐	☐	☐	_____
Respect a rational adult's right to refuse further therapy	☐	☐	☐	_____
Assist the individual to meet his or her spiritual needs during a terminal illness	☐	☐	☐	_____

B. This section allows you to examine your techniques for offering personal care to a client who is terminally ill.

RECOMMENDED TECHNIQUE	S	NI	U	Comments
Nutrition	☐	☐	☐	_____
Intestinal and urinary elimination	☐	☐	☐	_____
Mouth, nose, and eye care	☐	☐	☐	_____
Care of the skin and mucous membranes	☐	☐	☐	_____
Positioning in bed	☐	☐	☐	_____
Environmental considerations	☐	☐	☐	_____
Provision for the proper relief of pain	☐	☐	☐	_____

C. This section allows you to examine your techniques for assisting the family of the client who is terminally ill.

RECOMMENDED TECHNIQUE	S	NI	U	Comments
Strive to meet the various needs of family members when a client is terminally ill	☐	☐	☐	_____
Allow family members to help with care when appropriate	☐	☐	☐	_____
Use appropriate measures when relatives are critical of care	☐	☐	☐	_____
Offer appropriate emotional support when the person dies	☐	☐	☐	_____
Show an understanding of the grieving process	☐	☐	☐	_____

D. This section allows you to examine your techniques for performing postmortem care.

RECOMMENDED TECHNIQUE	S	NI	U	Comments
Transfer any client who shared a room with the deceased temporarily to another room	☐	☐	☐	_____
Notify the nursing administration office and the health agency switchboard	☐	☐	☐	_____
Contact any individuals involved in organ procurement. Inform the designated mortician that the client has died.	☐	☐	☐	_____
Assemble all the equipment for cleaning, wrapping, and identifying the body	☐	☐	☐	_____
Determine that the family and clergyman have spent all the time they want with the body	☐	☐	☐	_____
Place the body supine with the arms extended at the side or folded over the abdomen	☐	☐	☐	_____
Remove hairpins and clips	☐	☐	☐	_____
Close the eyelids by applying gentle pressure	☐	☐	☐	_____
Replace or retain the dentures within the mouth	☐	☐	☐	_____
Use a small towel under the chin to close an open mouth	☐	☐	☐	_____
Remove all medical equipment	☐	☐	☐	_____
Apply gloves and dispose of all contaminated and soiled articles	☐	☐	☐	_____
Cleanse the soiled areas of the body	☐	☐	☐	_____
Apply disposable pads to the perineal area	☐	☐	☐	_____
Attach an identification tag either to the ankle or the wrist and leave the agency identification bracelet intact	☐	☐	☐	_____
Remove or make an inventory of the valuables still attached to the body	☐	☐	☐	_____

RECOMMENDED TECHNIQUE	S	NI	U	Comments
Wrap the body with a shroud	☐	☐	☐	_____
Attach an identification tag to the shroud	☐	☐	☐	_____
Remove gloves and wash hands	☐	☐	☐	_____
Transport the body to the morgue or wait for the arrival of the mortician	☐	☐	☐	_____
Arrange for all valuables to be locked until claimed by the family	☐	☐	☐	_____
Notify housekeeping	☐	☐	☐	_____
Complete the client's permanent record indicating in what manner the body was removed	☐	☐	☐	_____

Answers

Chapter 1

ANSWERS TO MATCHING QUESTIONS

Items 1 Through 4

1. c   2. a   3. d   4. b

Items 5 Through 8

5. d   6. c   7. a   8. b

Items 9 Through 16

9. e   10. i   11. d   12. a   13. f   14. c
15. h   16. j

ANSWERS TO MULTIPLE-CHOICE QUESTIONS

Items 1 Through 12

1. (c) The service of caring for the sick changed with the schism between King Henry VIII of England and the Catholic church when nuns and priests were exiled to Western Europe.
2. (a) Servicemen and their families alike were grateful; the country adored her. To show their appreciation, funds were donated to sustain the great work Florence Nightingale had begun.
3. (b) In her writing and speaking, Henderson proposed that nursing is more than carrying out medical orders. It involves a special relationship and service between the nurse and those entrusted to his or her care.
4. (d) Mildred Montag, a doctoral student, hypothesized that nursing education could be shortened to 2 years and relocated to a vocational school or a junior or community college. The graduate from this type of program would acquire an associate's degree in nursing.
5. (a) See Table 1-2.
6. (c) See Table 1-2.
7. (a) Before the nurse can determine what nursing care a person requires, the client's needs and problems must be determined. This requires the use of assessment skills. The client and family are the primary sources for information.
8. (d) Traditionally, nurses always have been providers of physical care for people unable to meet their own health needs independently. Despite the close relationship that caring involves, the nurse ultimately wants clients to become self-reliant.
9. (b) A counselor is one who listens to a client's needs, responds with information based upon his or her area of expertise, and facilitates the outcome a client desires. Once the client's perspective is clear, the nurse provides pertinent health information without offering specific advice. Nurses promote the right of all individuals to make their own decisions and choices on matters affecting health and illness care.

The role of the nurse is to share information on potential alternatives, allow clients the freedom to choose, and support the decision that is made.

10. (a) A science is a body of knowledge unique to a particular subject. It develops from observing and studying the relation of one phenomenon to another. By developing a unique body of scientific knowledge, it is now possible to predict which nursing interventions are most appropriate for producing desired outcomes.
11. (b) The most recent definition of nursing comes from the American Nurses Association (ANA).
12. (d) Continuing education is any planned learning experience that takes place beyond one's basic nursing program).

ANSWERS TO ALTERNATIVE FORMAT QUESTIONS

1. **Answer: 3, 1, 4, 2**
   Rationale: A theory is an opinion or belief developed by the author that explains a phenomenon. In nursing, theories explain the interactions among the client, health, and nursing. In order of their appearance are Nightingale's Environmental Theory, Henderson's Basic Needs Theory, Orem's Self-Care Theory, and Sister Callista Roy's Adaptation Theory. There is no Reformation Theory in nursing.

Nursing Process:	Data collection
Client Needs Category:	Safe, effective care environment
Cognitive Level:	Analysis

2. **Answer: 3**
   Rationale: There are three paths from which a student may choose to become a registered nurse (RN). An associate's degree nursing program found in junior or community colleges usually requires 2 years of study. A hospital-based diploma program in nursing requires 3 years of study. A collegiate program in nursing is found in colleges and universities and usually requires 4 years of study. Upon successful completion of the program of study, the student receives a diploma or degree and is eligible to take the National Council Licensure Examination for registered nurses (NCLEX-RN).

Nursing Process:	Data collection
Client Needs Category:	Psychosocial integrity
Cognitive Level:	Comprehension

3. **Answer: 1, 2, 5, 6**
   Rationale: In 2002, the federal government attempted to address the shortage of nurses by passing the Nurse Reinvestment Act. This legislation was supposed to authorize funding for programs and incentives to attract students into nursing or to enhance their career choice. The act provides for loan repayment programs and

scholarships for nursing students, funding for public service announcements to encourage more people to enter nursing programs, career ladder programs to facilitate advancement to higher levels of nursing practice, and grants to incorporate gerontology into the curricula of nursing programs among other initiatives. However, before the provisions of the act can be set in motion, Congress must approve appropriations to fund them.

Nursing Process:	Planning
Client Needs Category:	Safe, effective care environment
Nursing Process:	Management of care
Cognitive Level:	Analysis

ANSWERS TO TRUE OR FALSE QUESTIONS

Items 1 Through 7

1. *True.*
2. *False.* In the midst of deplorable health care conditions, Florence Nightingale, an Englishwoman born of wealthy parents, announced that she had been called by God to become a nurse.
3. *True.*
4. *True.*
5. *False.* It may be expected that as the role of the nurse changes in the future, there will be further revisions to the definition of nursing in order to more succinctly describe the scope of nursing practice.
6. *True.*
7. *False.* The nurse provides pertinent health information without offering specific advice.

ANSWERS TO SHORT ANSWER QUESTIONS

1. Criteria used to select applicants include:
   a. Between the ages of 35 and 50
   b. Matronly and plain looking
   c. Educated
   d. Serious disposition, neat, orderly, sober, industrious
   e. Submission of two letters of recommendation attesting to their moral character, integrity, and capacity to care for the sick
2. Refer to Box 1-2.
3. Factors affecting the choice of nursing education programs include:
   a. A person's career goals
   b. Geographic location of schools
   c. Costs involved
   d. Length of programs
   e. Reputation and success of past graduates
   f. Flexibility in course scheduling
   g. Opportunity for part-time versus full-time enrollment
   h. Ease of articulation into the next level of education
4. Factors delaying the decision include:
   a. The date for implementation coincided with a national shortage of nurses.
   b. There was tremendous opposition from nurses without baccalaureate degrees who felt this change threatened their titles and their positions would be jeopardized.
   c. Employers of nurses feared that paying higher salaries to degreed personnel would escalate budgets beyond their financial limits.
5. Refer to Table 1-3 (below).

	Practical/Vocational Nurse	Associate's Degree Nurse	Baccalaureate Nurse
Assess:	Gathers data from person with common health problems with predictable outcomes	Collects data from persons with complex health problems with unpredictable outcomes	Identifies data required to provide an appropriate nursing database
Diagnosis:	Contributes to the development of nursing diagnoses	Uses a classification list to write a nursing diagnostic statement	Conducts clinical tests of approved nursing diagnoses
Plan:	Assists in developing a written plan of care	Develops a written, individualized plan of care with specific nursing orders that reflects the standards for nursing practice	Plans care for healthy or sick individuals or groups in structured health care agencies or the community
Implement:	Performs basic nursing care under the direction of a registered nurse	Identifies priorities; directs others to carry out nursing orders	Applied nursing theory approaches used for resolving health problems of individuals or groups
Evaluate:	Contributes to the revision of the plan of care	Makes revisions in the plan of care	Conducts research that may alter and improve nursing care

Chapter 2

ANSWERS TO MATCHING QUESTIONS
Items 1 Through 5
1. c   2. e   3. a   4. d   5. b
Items 6 Through 11
6. b   7. b   8. a   9. a   10. b   11. a

ANSWERS TO MULTIPLE-CHOICE QUESTIONS
Items 1 Through 15
1. (c) In the distant past, nursing practice involved actions that were based mostly on common sense and the examples set by older, more experienced nurses. Now nurses are planning and implementing client care more independently. Nurses are being held responsible and accountable for providing appropriate client care that reflects current accepted standards for nursing practice.
2. (b) The nursing process is goal directed. It facilitates a united effort between the client and the nursing team in achieving desired outcomes.
3. (b) Data are either objective or subjective. Objective data include information that is observable and measurable, such as the client's blood pressure. Subjective data are information that only the client feels and can describe, such as pain.
4. (c) Diagnosis, the second step in the nursing process, involves identifying problems.
5. (b) The nursing process is dynamic. Considering the health status of any client is constantly changing, the nursing process acts like a continuous loop. Evaluation, the last step in the nursing process, involves data collection, and the process begins again.
6. (a) A characteristic of the nursing process is that it is client centered. The nursing process facilitates a comprehensive plan of care for each client as a unique individual.
7. (c) Assessment, the first step in the nursing process, is the systematic collection and organization of data.
8. (b) Collaborative problems are certain physiologic complications that nurses monitor in order to detect their onset or change in status. Because collaborative problems are beyond the independent scope of nursing practice, their management requires the combined expertise of the nurse and the physician.
9. (a) A nursing diagnostic statement includes three parts: the problem, the etiology, and the signs and symptoms.
10. (b) The etiology is the cause of the problem.
11. (a) Not all of the client's problems may be resolved during a typically short hospitalization. Prioritization involves ranking problems from most to least important. One method, which is frequently used by nurses, is to rank nursing

diagnoses according to Maslow's Hierarchy of Needs.
12. (d) This choice is the best example because the statement shows the expected outcome, or the desired end result, for which one works. Johnny will walk unassisted to the playroom by a specific date. The other choices are not as specific in their terminology or in terms of the date on which they will be accomplished.
13. (a) The best nursing order in this situation states how much fluid (2 ounces), what kind of fluid (clear), and how often it should be given (every 2 hours until 10 P.M.). The other choices are not as specific in their directions and therefore could be misinterpreted.
14. (c) Evaluation is the process of determining if, or how well, a goal has been reached. It helps to determine the effectiveness of the plan of care.
15. (d) When evaluation results show that a goal has not been met, modifications and revisions in the nursing care may be necessary.

ANSWERS TO ALTERNATIVE FORMAT QUESTIONS
1. Answer: 1, 3, 6
Rationale: Subjective data consist of symptoms felt by the client and statements that the client makes regarding his or her health status. Pain is a subjective experience that exists when the client says it does and to the severity the client expresses. The client must tell the nurse that he or she is hungry because the feeling of hunger cannot be observed. Only the client can determine when he or she feels the urge to urinate and, therefore, must communicate this to the nurse.

Nursing Process:	Assessment
Client Needs Category:	Physiological integrity
Cognitive Level:	Analysis

2. Answer: 1, 2, 3, 4, 5
Rationale: A database assessment includes the initial information gathered about the client's physical, emotional, social, and spiritual health. This information is obtained during the admission interview and physical examination and serves as a reference for comparing all future data. All of the items contribute to the database assessment except daily weights. Daily weights are obtained throughout the hospital stay and are compared to the admission weight in order to evaluate progress.

Nursing Process:	Assessment
Client Needs Category:	Physiological integrity
Cognitive Level:	Application

3. Answer: 3, 5, 4, 6, 2, 1
Rationale: Using Maslow's Hierarchy of Needs, the nursing diagnoses are prioritized in the following manner: basic physiologic need—impaired swallowing; safety and security—anxiety, love and belonging—parental role conflict, esteem and self-esteem—powerlessness and caregiver role strain, and finally self-actualization—spiritual distress. Lower-level needs must

be met before higher-level needs.

Nursing Process:	Analysis
Client Needs Category:	Psychosocial integrity
Nursing Process:	Coping and adaptation
Cognitive Level:	Analysis

ANSWERS TO TRUE OR FALSE QUESTIONS

Items 1 Through 10

1. *False.* The information may be gathered in different ways, such as by asking the client or family questions, making observations while examining the client, reading the client's record, and asking other health workers about their observations of the client.
2. *False.* A nursing diagnosis is a statement describing a health problem that has the possibility of being resolved completely through nursing measures.
3. *True.*
4. *False.* Nurses commonly prioritize problems in reference to the hierarchy; however, there may be other methods to do this effectively.
5. *False.* Although the terms *goals* and *outcomes* are sometimes used interchangeably, outcomes are generally more specific.
6. *True.*
7. *False.* Evaluation is the process of measuring how well a goal is reached.
8. *True.*
9. *False.* Subjective data are information that only the client can experience and describe.
10. *True.*

ANSWERS TO SHORT ANSWER QUESTIONS

Items 1 and 2

1. The etiology is immobility.
2. The problem is impaired skin integrity.

Chapter 3

ANSWERS TO MATCHING QUESTIONS

Items 1 Through 6

1. d	2. b	3. e	4. f	5. a	6. c

Items 7 Through 12

7. e	8. f	9. c	10. b	11. d	12. a

ANSWERS TO MULTIPLE-CHOICE QUESTIONS

Items 1 Through 10

1. (a) A tort is litigation in which one citizen asserts that an injury, which may be physical, emotional, or financial, occurred as a consequence of another citizen's actions or failure to act.
2. (d) Many statements of client rights have been established. One that is widely used and distributed has been prepared by the American Hospital Association.
3. (b) An incident report is a written account of an unusual event involving a client, employee, or visitor that has the potential for being injurious.
4. (d) Unintentional torts involve situations that result in an injury, although the person responsible did not purposely mean to cause harm. Cases of unintentional torts involve allegations of negligence or malpractice.
5. (c) Good Samaritan laws, named based on the biblical story of the person who gave aid to a beaten stranger along a roadside, have been enacted in many states. These laws provide legal immunity for passersby who provide emergency first aid to accident victims. None of the Good Samaritan laws provide absolute exemption from prosecution in the event of injury. Nurses and other health care workers are held to a higher standard of care because they have training above and beyond that of average laypeople.
6. (d) The word *ethics* comes from a Greek word that means customs or modes of conduct. Ethics refers to moral or philosophical principles that direct actions as being either right or wrong. Various groups, such as nurses, have identified standards for ethical practice.
7. (d) A code of ethics is a list of written statements describing ideal behavior.
8. (a) A nurse practice act is a form of state legislation that legally defines the unique role of the nurse and differentiates it from other health care practitioners.
9. (d) Each state's board of nursing is the regulatory agency for managing the provisions of its nurse practice acts. The board of nursing develops rules and regulations for the education and licensing of individuals who wish to practice as nurses within the state.
10. (a) Deontology refers to ethical study based on duty or moral obligations; decisions must be based on the ultimate morality of the act itself.

ANSWERS TO ALTERNATIVE FORMAT QUESTIONS

1. **Answer: 24**

Rationale: If the client poses a threat to himself or herself and/or others that is not relieved by the use of alternative measures, restraints may be applied. However, the nurse must obtain a medical order before each and every instance in which restraints are applied. In acute care facilities, the medical order for restraints must be renewed every 24 hours. In addition, once restraints are applied, documentation must demonstrate regular client assessment, provision for fluids, nourishment, and toileting and trial periods of restraint removal.

Nursing Process:	Implementation
Client Needs Category:	Physiological integrity
Cognitive Level:	Application

2. Answer: 1, 2, 3, 6

Rationale: The following techniques communicate a caring and compassionate attitude toward the client and family: greeting the client, smiling, calling the client by name, responding to the call light quickly and in person rather than over the intercom, explaining procedures and routines in terms the client can understand, being a good hostess and seeing to the comfort of visitors by informing them where toilets are located, and stopping to talk with the client during the scheduled mealtime and when not providing a treatment or medication. Finally, the client should be informed when the nurse goes to lunch and returns, and he or she should be told who will care for the client while the nurse is gone. Medications should be placed in the client's hand, the medication should be discussed with the client, his or her questions should be answered, and medication should never be left on the bedside stand. The nurse must be certain to verify the client's identity before administering the medication.

Nursing Process:	Implementation
Clients Needs Category:	Psychosocial integrity
Cognitive Level:	Application

3. Answer: 1, 2, 4

Rationale: The client must be frequently reassessed to determine whether he or she is ready to have the restraints removed. The information should also be documented. Restraints should be tied in knots that can be released quickly and easily. Toileting and range-of-motion exercises should be performed every 2 hours while a client is in restraints. Restraints should never be secured to side rails because doing so can cause injury if the side rail is lowered without untying the restraint. A vest restraint should be positioned so the straps cross in front of the client, not in the back.

Nursing Process:	Implementation
Client Needs Category:	Safe, effective, care environment
Cognitive Level:	Application

ANSWERS TO TRUE OR FALSE QUESTIONS

Items 1 Through 10

1. *True.*
2. *False.* False imprisonment is the unjustifiable restraint or prevention of the movement of a person without proper consent.
3. *True.*
4. *True.*
5. *True.*
6. *False.* The physician is responsible for giving the client information about his or her medical treatment.
7. *True.*
8. *True.*
9. *False.* The person accused of breaking the law is called the defendant.
10. *True.*

ANSWERS TO SHORT ANSWER QUESTIONS

Items 1 and 2

1. Elements that must be proven in a negligence or malpractice case include:
   a. Duty
   b. Breach of duty
   c. Causation
   d. Injury
2. Ethical issues that nurses encounter include:
   a. Telling the truth
   b. Protecting the client's confidentiality
   c. Blowing the whistle on wrongful acts
   d. Allocating of scarce resources
   e. Respecting advance directives
   f. Withholding and withdrawing treatment
   g. Knowing a client's code status

Chapter 4

ANSWERS TO MATCHING QUESTIONS

Items 1 Through 12

1. c	2. a	3. b	4. b	5. d	6. a
7. a	8. c	9. a	10. a	11. a	12. a

ANSWERS TO MULTIPLE-CHOICE QUESTIONS

Items 1 Through 10

1. (c) In the preamble of its constitution, the World Health Organization (WHO) defines health as a state of complete physical, mental, and social well-being and not merely the absence of disease or infirmity.
2. (a) The term *morbidity* refers to the incidence of a specific disease, disorder, or injury. The morbidity rate refers to the number of people affected. Statistics may be compiled on the basis of age, gender, or number per group (e.g., per 1000 people within the population).
3. (d) The state of wellness is a full and balanced integration of physical, emotional, social, and spiritual health. Physical health exists when body organs function normally. Emotional health results when one feels safe. Social health is an outcome of feeling accepted and useful. Spiritual health is a feeling that one's life has purpose.
4. (c) An acute illness is one that comes on suddenly and lasts a relatively short time. Answer (a) describes chronic illness. Answer (b) describes terminal illness. Answer (d) describes primary illness.
5. (c) An idiopathic illness is one for which there is no known explanation for its development. Treatment of idiopathic illness generally focuses on relieving the signs and symptoms of the disease.
6. (b) One method for administering nursing care is the functional method. When this approach is used, each nurse on a client care unit is assigned specific tasks.

7. (c) Providing nursing care by the case method involves assigning one nurse to administer all the care a client needs for a designated period of time. The case method is most often used in home health and public health nursing.

8. (c) In team nursing, many nursing staff members divide client care and all the work until it is completed. The personnel are organized and directed by a nurse called the "team leader." The team leader usually supervises the team.

9. (b) A new way of administering nursing care is called nurse-managed care or case management. It is similar to the principles practiced by a successful business.

10. (a) The term *continuity of care* refers to a continuum of health care. The goal is to avoid causing a client, whether healthy or ill, to feel isolated, fragmented, or abandoned during the transfer from one type of health care services to another.

ANSWERS TO ALTERNATIVE FORMAT QUESTIONS

1. **Answer: 2, 6**

   Rationale: When providing care to a client, the nurse should consider family members to be all the people whom the client views as family. Family members may also include those people who provide for the physical and emotional needs of the client. The traditional definition of a family has changed and may include people not related by blood or marriage, those of a different racial background, and those who may not live in the same house as the client. Family members are defined by the client, not by the nurse.

Nursing Process:	Data collection
Client Needs Category:	Health promotion and maintenance
Cognitive Level:	Analysis

2. **Answer: 1, 3, 5, 6**

   Rationale: Illness in one family member can affect all family members, even children. Each member of a family may have several roles to perform. A middle-aged woman, for example, may have the roles of mother, wage earner, wife, and housekeeper. Families move through certain predictable life cycles (such as the birth of a baby, a growing family, adult children leaving home, and grandparenthood). The impact of illness on the family may depend on the stage of the life cycle as family members take on different roles and the family structure changes. Illness produces stress in families; changes in eating and sleeping patterns are signs of stress. When one family member can't fulfill a role because of illness, the roles of the other family members are affected.

Nursing Process:	Implementation
Client Needs Category:	Health promotion and maintenance
Cognitive Level:	Analysis

3. **Answer: 3, 4, 5**

   Rationale: Many community services exist for Alzheimer's clients and their families. Encouraging use of these resources may make it possible for the client to stay at home and to alleviate the spouse's exhaustion. The nurse can also support the caregiver by urging her to talk about the difficulties she's facing in caring for a spouse. Friends and church members may be able to help provide care to the client, allowing the caregiver a time for rest, exercise, or an enjoyable activity. A family meeting to tell the children to participate more would probably be ineffective and may evoke anger or guilt. Counseling may be helpful, but it wouldn't alleviate the caregiver's physical exhaustion and wouldn't address the client's immediate needs. A long-term care facility is not an option until the family is ready to make that decision.

Nursing Process:	Implementation
Client Needs Category:	Psychosocial integrity
Cognitive Level:	Analysis

4. **Answer: 65**

   Rationale: Medicare (a federal program that finances health care costs of persons 65 years and older, permanently disabled workers of any age and their dependents, and those with end-stage renal disease) is funded primarily through withholdings from an employed persons' income. Medicare has two parts:

   Part A covers acute hospital care, rehabilitative care, hospice, and home care services.

   Part B is purchased for an additional fee and covers physician services, outpatient hospital care laboratory tests, durable medical equipment, and other selected services.

   Although Medicare is primarily used for older Americans, it does not cover long-term care and limits coverage for health promotion and illness prevention. It also does not cover prescription medications, which are significant expenses for older adults and those with chronic illnesses.

Nursing Process:	Data collection
Client Needs Category:	Health promotion and maintenance
Cognitive Level:	Knowledge

ANSWERS TO TRUE OR FALSE QUESTIONS

Items 1 Through 10

1. *False.* A chronic illness is an illness that comes on slowly and lasts a relatively long time.
2. *False.* Functional nursing is the least-practiced method of giving nursing care in this country.
3. *False.* Physical health is a state in which body organs function normally. Health is a state of complete physical, mental, and social well-being.
4. *True.*
5. *True.*

6. *False.* Spiritual well-being is characterized as feeling that one's life is purposeful.
7. *True.*
8. *True.*

9. *False.* A resource is a possession that is valuable because its supply is limited and it has no substitute. Therefore, health is considered a resource.
10. *True.*

EXAMPLE OF AN ANSWER TO THE CRITICAL THINKING QUESTION

Method of Administration	Characteristics	Individual Responsible	Advantage/ Disadvantage	Health Care Setting
Primary Nursing				
Team Nursing				
Functional Nursing				
Nurse-Managed Care				

Chapter 5

ANSWERS TO MATCHING QUESTIONS

Items 1 Through 6

1. d   2. f   3. c   4. e   5. b   6. a

Items 7 Through 12

7. d   8. c   9. a   10. d   11. b   12. c

Items 13 Through 20

13. c   14. f   15. a   16. g   17. b   18. e
19. h   20. d

ANSWERS TO MULTIPLE-CHOICE QUESTIONS

Items 1 Through 8

1. (c) Homeostasis is the term used to describe a relatively stable state of physiologic equilibrium or balance. It literally means "staying the same." Although it sounds contradictory, staying the same requires constant physiologic activity.

2. (b) The autonomic nervous system, which is subdivided into the sympathetic and parasympathetic nervous systems, is composed of peripheral nerves that affect physiologic functions that are largely automatic and beyond voluntary control.

3. (d) The parasympathetic nervous system tends to restore equilibrium after the danger is no longer present. It does so by inhibiting the physiologic stimulation of the sympathetic nervous system. The sympathetic nervous system prepares the body for the "fight or flight" response.

4. (b) Behaving in a manner that is characteristic of a younger age is the coping mechanism known as regression.

5. (a) The general adaptation syndrome (GAS) refers to the collective physiologic processes that take place in response to a stressor.

6. (d) The Social Readjustment Rating Scale was developed by Holmes and Rahe (1967). It is used to predict a person's potential for developing a stress-related disorder.

7. (b) Powerlessness is an example of a psychologic stressor.

8. (a) Rapid heart rate, rapid breathing, and dry mouth are examples of physical signs and symptoms of stress.

ANSWERS TO ALTERNATIVE FORMAT QUESTIONS

1. **Answer: 2, 4, 6**

   Rationale: When a situation occurs that the mind perceives as dangerous, the sympathetic nervous system prepares the body for flight or flight. It accelerates the physiologic functions that ensure survival through enhanced strength or rapid escape. The person becomes active, aroused, and emotionally charged. Therefore, the heart rate, perspiration, and blood glucose level increase.

Nursing Process:	Assessment
Client Needs Category:	Physiologic integrity
Cognitive Level:	Application

2. **Answer: 1, 5, 4, 3, 2**

   Rationale: By offering appropriate interventions to people with severe or accumulated stressors, nurses can help prevent or minimize stress-related illnesses. Prevention takes place on three levels. Primary prevention involves eliminating the potential for illness before it occurs. In order to do this, the nurse must first identify the actual stressor. Secondary prevention includes screening for risk factors and providing a means for early diagnosis of disease. The nurse does this by assessing the client's response to stress and preventing additional stress. Tertiary prevention minimizes the consequences through aggressive rehabilitation or appropriate management of stress. This is accomplished by supporting the client's psychological coping strategies and assisting the client to build or maintain a network of social supports.

Nursing Process:	Planning
Client Needs Category:	Coping and adaptation
Cognitive Level:	Analysis

3. **Answer: 3, 5, 6**

   Rationale: Although homeostasis is associated primarily with a person's physical status, emotional, social, and spiritual components also affect it. Holism implies that entities in all of these areas contribute to the whole of a person. The relationship between the mind and body can potentially sustain health as well as cause illness. Fear is a psychological stressor. Abandonment and isolation are social stressors. Other spiritual stressors are listed in Table 5-1 from the text.

Nursing Process:	Application
Client Needs Category:	Health promotion and maintenance
Cognitive Level:	Comprehension

ANSWERS TO TRUE OR FALSE QUESTIONS

Items 1 Through 10

1. *True.*
2. *False.* Forgetfulness is a cognitive symptom of increased stress.
3. *True.*
4. *False.* The general adaptation syndrome refers to the collective physiologic process that takes place in response to a stressor.
5. *True.*
6. *True.*
7. *False.* Irritability, withdrawal, and depression are common *emotional* signs and symptoms of stress.
8. *True.*
9. *False.* Bruxism is a term that refers to "tooth grinding."
10. *False.* Accusing a person of a race different from one's own of being prejudiced is an example of projection.

ANSWERS TO SHORT ANSWER QUESTIONS

1. List the stages of the general adaptation syndrome:
   a. Alarm
   b. Stage of resistance
   c. Stage of exhaustion
2. The reticular activating system is an area of the brain through which a network of nerves passes. It is the communication link between the body and the mind. Information is processed on both a conscious and subconscious level. The cortex processes the information and generates behavioral and physiologic responses by activating the hypothalamus.
3. List and describe the three levels of prevention related to stressors:

Level	Description
a. Primary level	Eliminates the potential for illness before it occurs
b. Secondary level	Includes screening for risk factors and early diagnosis of disease
c. Tertiary level	Provides aggressive rehabilitation to minimize the consequences of disease and provide appropriate management

Chapter 6

ANSWERS TO MATCHING QUESTIONS

Items 1 Through 5

1. b   2. d   3. e   4. c   5. a

Items 6 Through 10

6. c   7. e   8. a   9. d   10. b

ANSWERS TO MULTIPLE-CHOICE QUESTIONS

Items 1 Through 9

1. (b) Transcultural nursing, a term coined by Madeline Leininger in the 1970s, refers to providing nursing care within the context of another's culture. Culturally sensitive care requires planning care within the client's health belief system to achieve the best health outcome.

2. (a) Currently, there are approximately 270 Native American tribes in the United States, with the Navajos being the largest surviving group.

3. (b) See Table 6-3.

4. (c) See Table 6-3.

5. (a) Lactase is a digestive enzyme that converts lactose, the sugar in milk, into the simpler sugars glucose and galactose. A lactase deficiency causes an intolerance to dairy products.

6. (d) All choices are correct.

7. (c) See Table 6-4.

8. (a) See Table 6-5.

9. (d) The health practices that are unique to a particular group of individuals are sometimes referred to as "folk medicine." Folk medicine has come to mean those methods of disease prevention or treatment that are outside the mainstream of conventional practices. Folk medicine is often provided by laypeople rather than formally educated and licensed individuals.

ANSWERS TO ALTERNATIVE FORMAT QUESTIONS

1. **Answer: 1, 2, 3**

Rationale: Nonverbal cues may have different meanings in different cultures. In one culture, eye contact shows respect and attentiveness; in another, eye contact is a sign of disrespect. The nurse should always respect the client's cultural beliefs and ask if there are cultural or religious requirements. This may include food choices or restrictions, body coverings, or time for prayer. The nurse should attempt to understand the client's culture. The nurse should never impose his or her beliefs on the client. Culture also influences a client's experience of pain. In one culture pain may be expressed, whereas in another, it must be stoically endured.

Nursing Process:	Planning
Client Needs Category:	Psychosocial integrity
Cognitive Level:	Analysis

2. **Answer: 1, 3, 4**

Rationale: Culture, the values, beliefs, and practices of a particular group, incorporates the attitudes and customs learned through socialization with others. It includes, but is not limited to, language, communication style, traditions, religion, art, music, dress, health beliefs, and health practices. A group's culture passes from one generation to the next; it is learned from birth; shared by members of a group; influenced by environment, technology, and resources; and is dynamic and ever changing.

Nursing Process:	Planning
Client Needs Category:	Psychosocial integrity
Cognitive Level:	Comprehension

3. **Answer: 1, 4**

Rationale: The nurse knows that religious practices in certain cultures impose certain rules and restrictions. Nurses can jeopardize the client's compliance with health care regimens if there is disregard for cultural or religious preferences. It is usual for Catholics to request baptism for the infant and to place a religious medal on the infant's blanket for spiritual comfort and for the infant's salvation.

Nursing Process:	Implementation
Client Needs Category:	Psychosocial integrity
Cognitive Level:	Application

ANSWERS TO TRUE OR FALSE QUESTIONS

Items 1 Through 10

1. *False.* Assuming that all people who affiliate themselves with a particular group behave alike or hold the same beliefs is always incorrect. Diversity exists even within cultural groups.

2. *True.*

3. *True.*

4. *True.*

5. *True.*

6. *False.* When it is possible to choose from several translators, select one who is the same gender as the client and approximately the same age. Some clients may feel embarrassed to relate personal information to someone with whom they have little in common.

7. *False.* If the client speaks some English, speak slowly, using simple words and short sentences. Lengthy or complex sentences are barriers to communicating with someone who is not skilled in English. If the client appears confused by a question, repeat it slowly, without changing the words. Rephrasing tends to compound the client's confusion as it forces him or her to translate yet another group of unfamiliar words.

8. *True.*

9. *False.* Praying and doing penance, relying on spiritual healers, and eating foods that are "hot" or "cold" are common health practices among Latinos.

10. *True.*

ANSWERS TO SHORT ANSWER QUESTIONS
Items 1 and 2
1. You may choose any of the examples cited in Box 6-1.
2. You may choose any of the examples cited under the topic "Culturally Sensitive Nursing."

Chapter 7

ANSWERS TO MATCHING QUESTIONS
Items 1 Through 6
1. e   2. c   3. a   4. f   5. b   6. d
Items 7 Through 12
7. f   8. d   9. e   10. b   11. c   12. a

ANSWERS TO MULTIPLE-CHOICE QUESTIONS
Items 1 Through 10
1. (d) The nurse is promoting independence in Miss H. by explaining how to prepare her insulin injection. Just to give the client a syringe, needle, and an orange is not helpful; the client needs to know how to use them correctly. Nurses provide skills or services that assist clients to cope with health problems that will not improve. Clients are expected to become actively involved and to retain as much independence as possible.
2. (c) The desired outcome of a therapeutic nurse-client relationship is one of moving toward restoring health.
3. (a) The relationship between a client and a nurse usually begins with a period of getting acquainted. The client explains health problems that are interfering with the quality of his or her life. The nurse uses this information to formulate an understanding of the services being sought.
4. (c) Verbal communication is communication that uses words. It includes speaking, reading, and writing.
5. (b) Nonverbal communication is the exchange of information without using words. It is what is *not* said. People communicate nonverbally through facial expressions, posture, mode of dress, grooming, and movements. Crying, laughing, and moaning are also considered nonverbal communication because they do not use words.
6. (d) A common obstacle to effective communication is to ignore the importance of silence.
7. (a) To promote effective communication, the nurse should avoid "pat" answers that offer false reassurance. These are often misinterpreted by clients as a lack of interest.
8. (c) Kinesics refers to body language, those collective nonverbal techniques like facial expressions, posture, gestures, and body movements.
9. (a) Touch is a tactile stimulus produced by making personal contact with another individual. Task-oriented touch involves the personal contact that is required when performing nursing procedures.

10. (a) Giving attention to what clients say provides a stimulus for meaningful interaction. It is best to position oneself at the person's level and make frequent eye contact. It is important that the nurse avoid giving signals that indicate impatience, boredom, or the pretense of listening.

ANSWERS TO ALTERNATIVE FORMAT QUESTIONS
1. **Answer: 1, 2, 5**
   Rationale: A relationship is established between the nurse and the client when nursing services are provided. Nurses provide services or skills that assist clients to promote, maintain, or restore health; to cope with disorders that will not improve; or to die with dignity. Nurses encourage and expect clients for whom they care to become actively involved and to retain as much independence as possible. In order to protect their clients, nurses are legally and ethically required to be knowledgeable and safe caregivers.

Nursing Process:	Assessment
Client Needs Category:	Safe, effective care environment
Cognitive Level:	Comprehension

2. **Answer: 6, 4**
   Rationale: Proxemics describes the use and relationship of space to communication. Personal space describes interactions occurring within 6 inches to 4 feet of the individual. Physical assessment requires direct physical contact with the client, while interviewing is usually a private conversation for the purpose of gathering pertinent information about the client's health.

Nursing Process:	Assessment
Client Needs Category:	Psychosocial integrity
Cognitive Level:	Application

3. **Answer: 1, 2, 3, 6**
   Rationale: An advance directive is a legal document that is used as a guideline for instituting life-sustaining medical care for a client with an advanced disease who is no longer able to indicate his or her own wishes. An advance directive includes the living will, which provides instructions for the physician to administer selected life-sustaining treatment(s), and a durable power of attorney for health care, which names another person to act in the client's behalf for medical decisions in the likelihood that the client is not able to act for himself or herself. The nurse provided an explanation in terms the client could understand when informed of the client's lack of knowledge of this legal document and observed the client's individuality with her explanation. The advance directive allows the client to choose medical treatment(s) that are compatible with the client's values and thereby promotes the client's physical, emotional, and spiritual well-being.

Nursing Process:	Assessment
Client Needs Category:	Safe, effective care environment
Cognitive Level:	Application

ANSWERS TO TRUE OR FALSE QUESTIONS
Items 1 Through 10

1. *False.* Intimate space is reserved for making love, confiding secrets, and sharing confidential information.
2. *True.*
3. *False.* Begin an initial contact with an exchange of names. Avoid addressing older adults in familiar terms such as "gramps" or "granny" because they convey disrespect and may be offensive to the client.
4. *False.* Nursing acts are prompted by a concern for the well-being of everyone.
5. *False.* Identifying the problem, describing desired outcomes, and answering questions honestly are *client* responsibilities within the nurse-client relationship.
6. *True.*
7. *True.*
8. *False.* The introductory phase of the nurse-client relationship is the period of getting acquainted. The working phase involves mutually planning the client's care.
9. *True.*
10. *True.*

ANSWERS TO SHORT ANSWER QUESTIONS
Items 1 Through 3

1. Silence may be used to:
   a. Encourage participation in verbal discussions
   b. Relieve a client's anxiety by providing a personal presence
   c. Provide a brief period of time to process information
   d. Provide for introspection when needing to explore feelings
   e. Provide an opportunity for prayer
2. Principles providing a basis for a therapeutic relationship include:
   a. Treating each client as a unique person
   b. Respecting the client's feelings
   c. Promoting the client's physical, emotional, social, and spiritual well-being
   d. Encouraging the client to participate in problem solving and decision making
   e. Accepting that the client has the potential for growth and change
3. Touch is a tactile stimulus produced by making personal contact with another individual. Task-oriented touch is the personal contact required to do nursing procedures or provide nursing care. Affective touch is used to demonstrate concern or affection. Affective touch is generally used when the client is lonesome, uncomfortable, anxious, frightened, or near death. In these situations, hugging, patting on the shoulder, or taking hold of the client's hand may be examples of affective touch.

Chapter 8

ANSWERS TO MATCHING QUESTIONS
Items 1 Through 17

1. a	7. c	13. c
2. b	8. c	14. a
3. c	9. a	15. a
4. b	10. b	16. a
5. b	11. a	17. c
6. a	12. c	

Items 18 Through 27

18. b 19. c 20. a 21. b 22. a 23. a
24. b 25. c 26. b 27. a

ANSWERS TO MULTIPLE-CHOICE QUESTIONS
Items 1 Through 15

1. (b) The cognitive domain involves processing information by listening or reading facts and descriptions.
2. (d) The psychomotor domain involves learning by doing.
3. (a) When preparing reading materials for the visually impaired, choose large-size print in black ink on white paper. Letters and words are more distinct when they are set in large print with a typestyle that promotes visual discrimination. Black print on white paper provides maximum contrast and makes the letters more legible. Glossy paper reflects light, causing glare that makes reading more difficult.
4. (c) Hearing loss is generally in the higher-pitch ranges. Select words that do not begin with F, S, or K. These letters are formed with high-pitched sounds and are, therefore, difficult for the hearing-impaired person to discriminate.
5. (a) When caring for older adults, it is important to reduce noise and distractions in the environment.
6. (d) Learning is motivated by potential rewards or punishment.
7. (c) The term *literacy* refers to the ability to read and write.
8. (d) Evaluation, the last step in the nursing process, enables nurses to determine whether goals have been met. When teaching a skill to a client, the best means of evaluating whether the skill has been learned is to observe the client doing the skill. In addition, talking about and doing the skill will assist the client to retain approximately 90% of what was learned.
9. (c) Demonstrating how to do a task involves talking about it and doing it. Learners retain 90% of what they talk about as well as what they do.
10. (a) Informal teaching is unplanned and occurs spontaneously at the client's bedside. Formal teaching requires a plan.
11. (d) When the capacity and motivation for learning exist, the final component of learning readiness must be determined. Readiness refers to the

client's physical and psychological well-being. For example, a person who is in pain, depressed, or having difficulty breathing is not in the best condition for learning to take place.

12. (b) Learning a neuromuscular skill is in the psychomotor domain.

13. (b) The following behaviors are associated with the cognitive domain: list, label, identify, summarize, locate, and select.

14. (a) Teaching may be formal if the preplanned information is presented at a scheduled time. Informal teaching occurs spontaneously at the client's bedside.

15. (b) Optimum learning takes place when an individual has a purpose for acquiring new information. The desire for new learning may be to satisfy intellectual curiosity, to restore independence, to prevent complications, or to facilitate discharge and return to the comfort of home. Other, less-desirable reasons for learning are to please others and to avoid criticism.

ANSWERS TO ALTERNATIVE FORMAT QUESTIONS

1. **Answer: 1, 3, 5, 6**
   Rationale: Clients who are hearing impaired may benefit from using flash cards, which can be read easily, or a magic slate to write instructions or responses. Written communication may substitute for spoken communication. The letters "f," "s," "k," and "sh" are formed with high-pitched sounds and are therefore difficult for the client with a hearing impairment to discriminate. Speaking in a normal tone of voice may not be helpful; one should lower the voice pitch because hearing loss is usually in the higher pitch range. Turning on the ceiling lights will not impact the client's ability to hear. Rephrasing may provide additional clues to facilitate the client's understanding. Standing in front of the client may facilitate lipreading for clients who do this as a means of coping with their hearing loss.

Nursing Process:	Planning
Client Needs Category:	Psychosocial integrity
Cognitive Level:	Application

2. **Answer: 1, 4, 6**
   Rationale: When teaching the client about enalapril maleate (Vasotec), the nurse should tell him or her to avoid salt substitutes, as these products may contain potassium that can cause light-headedness and syncope. Facial swelling or difficulty breathing should be reported immediately; the drug may cause angioedema, which would require discontinuation of the drug. The client should also be advised to change position slowly to minimize orthostatic hypotension The nurse should tell the client to report light-headedness, especially in the first few days of therapy, so dosage adjustments can

be made. The client should report signs of infection, such as sore throat and fever, because the drug may decrease the white blood cell count. White blood cell and differential counts should be performed before treatment, every 2 weeks for 3 months, and periodically thereafter.

Nursing Process:	Planning
Client Needs Category:	Physiological integrity
Cognitive Level:	Application

3. **Answer: 2, 3, 5**
   Rationale: Dizziness, headache, and hypotension are all common adverse effects of lisinopril and other ACE inhibitors. Lisinopril may cause diarrhea, not constipation. Lisinopril is not known to cause hyperglycemia or impotence.

Nursing Process:	Implementation
Client Needs Category:	Physiological integrity
Cognitive Level:	Application

ANSWERS TO TRUE OR FALSE QUESTIONS

Items 1 Through 10

1. *True.*
2. *False.* Literacy refers to the ability to read and write. Approximately 21% of American adults are illiterate (unable to read or write). Another 27% possess minimal literacy skills (functionally illiterate). Because many of these people are not apt to volunteer this information or they have developed elaborate mechanisms to compensate for their learning deficits, literacy may be difficult to assess.
3. *True.*
4. *False.* Health teaching is no longer an optional nursing activity. Many nurse practice acts require it, part of ANA standards requires it, and legal documentation is required in the client's record.
5. *True.*
6. *False.* Ceiling lights tend to diffuse light rather than concentrate it on a small area where the client needs to focus.
7. *True.*
8. *False.* The desire for new learning may be to satisfy intellectual curiosity, restore independence, prevent complications, or facilitate discharge and return to the comfort of home. Other, less-desirable reasons for learning are to please others and to avoid criticism.
9. *True.*
10. *False.* Because teaching and learning involve language, the nurse must modify teaching approaches if the client cannot speak English. Language barriers do not justify omitting health teaching.

ANSWERS TO SHORT ANSWER QUESTIONS
Items 1 and 2

1. Refer to Table 8-1. You may choose any three of those listed for gerogogic learners.
2. Some of the *most* important factors are:
   a. Style of learning
   b. Developmental stage
   c. Capacity to learn
   d. Motivation for learning
   e. Readiness to learn
   f. What the client wants to know
   g. What the client needs to know

Chapter 9

ANSWERS TO MATCHING QUESTIONS
Items 1 Through 10

1. f	2. d	3. e	4. h	5. b	6. g
7. i	8. a	9. j	10. c		

ANSWERS TO MULTIPLE-CHOICE QUESTIONS
Items 1 Through 11

1. (a) The medical record is a written, chronological account of a person's illness or injury and the health care provided, from the onset of the problem through discharge or death.
2. (c) Another purpose of the client's health record is to ensure safety and continuity in the client's care. Sharing of information prevents duplication and helps to reduce the chance of error or omission.
3. (d) Clients' records are admissible as evidence in courts of law in this country. They are the basis for proving or disproving allegations concerning a client's care. Therefore, it is essential that entries on the records be objectively written, accurate, complete, and legible.
4. (b) A traditional record is organized according to the source of information.
5. (c) The problem-oriented record is organized according to a client's specific health problem.
6. (d) There are four major parts to a problem-oriented record (POR). These are the database, the problem list, the initial plan, and the progress notes and follow-up.
7. (d) Narrative charting involves writing information about the client and his or her care in a chronological order. It is used primarily in traditional records. Each person involved in a client's care, such as the doctor, nurse, physical therapist, and so on, writes information on separate forms in the client's chart. This adds bulk to the medical record and tends to fragment the information.
8. (b) PIE charting is very similar to a SOAP format of charting. "PIE" stands for "problem, intervention, and evaluation." However, when using the PIE method for charting, assessments are documented on a separate form.
9. (b) Historically, clients were not allowed to see their health care records. Certain federal laws have now changed that practice. Health agencies have developed guidelines by which clients may read their records.
10. (a) 3:30 P.M. is equal to 1530 in military time. To convert to military time, add 12 to every hour after noon. Therefore, by adding 12 to 3:30, you get 1530 hours.
11. (a) It is important to write or print clearly when recording a client's care. Illegible entries on the record become questionable information in a court of law. The entry loses its value for exchanging information if it is unreadable.

ANSWERS TO ALTERNATIVE FORMAT QUESTIONS

1. **Answer: 1, 2, 4**
   Rationale: The client must be frequently reassessed to determine whether he is ready to have the restraints removed. The information should also be documented. Restraints should be tied in knots that can be released quickly and easily. Toileting and range-of-motion exercises should be performed every 2 hours while a client is in restraints. Restraints should never be secured to side rails because doing so can cause injury if the side rail is lowered without releasing the restraint. A vest restraint should be positioned so that the straps cross in front of the client, not in the back. Documentation must reveal the appropriate assessments and nursing interventions for this client.

Nursing Process:	Implementation
Client Needs Category:	Safe, effective care environment
Cognitive Level:	Application

2. **Answer: 2, 3, 5**
   Rationale: Conveying information and providing communication can alleviate fears and strengthen the individual's sense of control. Encouraging verbalization of feelings helps build a therapeutic relationship based on trust and reduces anxiety. Telling the daughter not to worry ignores her feelings and discourages further communication. Appropriate documentation would reveal that this discussion took place and what the outcome was.

Nursing Process:	Implementation
Client Needs Category:	Psychosocial integrity
Cognitive Level:	Analysis

3. **Answer: 1, 3, 6**
   Rationale: The nurse should objectively document her assessment findings. A detailed description of physical findings of abuse in the medical record is essential if legal action is pursued. All women suspected to be victims of abuse should be counseled on a safety plan, which consists of recognizing escalating violence within the family and formulating a plan to exit quickly. The nurse should not report this suspicion of abuse because the client is a competent adult who has the right to self-determination. Nurses do, however, have a duty to

report cases of actual or suspected abuse in children and the elderly. Contacting the client's husband without her consent violates confidentiality. The nurse should respond to the client in a nonthreatening manner that promotes trust, rather than ordering her to break off her relationship. Providing the client with telephone numbers of local shelters and safe houses offers her the opportunity to put her safety plan into action.

Nursing Process: Implementation
Client Needs Category: Psychosocial integrity
Cognitive Level: Analysis

ANSWERS TO TRUE OR FALSE QUESTIONS
Items 1 Through 12

1. *True.*
2. *False.* Entries on the health record are made by all health practitioners according to their areas of expertise. It is impossible for all health care workers to meet at the same time in order to exchange information on a personal basis. Therefore, the written record becomes central to sharing information.
3. *False.* The traditional record is organized according to the source of information. The problem-oriented record is organized according to the client's specific health problems.
4. *True.*
5. *False.* Planning, regardless of the way it is recorded, *should always be done* with the client.
6. *False.* PIE charting is very similar to a SOAP format of charting. However, when using the PIE method for charting, assessments are documented on a separate form.
7. *False.* Charting by exception is a method of documenting care, but it limits the amount of writing to information that is abnormal or deviates from written standards. A checklist is a form that can be used to document routine types of care, such as bathing and mouth care.
8. *True.*
9. *True.*
10. *True.*
11. *True.*
12. *False.* The information on the Kardex should be written in pencil because it is constantly being updated or changed.

ANSWERS TO SHORT ANSWER QUESTIONS
Items 1 Through 5

1. Analysis
2. Evaluation
3. Subjective information
4. Revision
5. Objective information

Chapter 10

ANSWERS TO MATCHING QUESTIONS
Items 1 Through 7

1. b   2. f   3. h   4. g   5. a   6. e
7. c

ANSWERS TO MULTIPLE-CHOICE QUESTIONS
Items 1 Through 10

1. (b) Skilled nursing care involves 24-hour nursing care. A person needing skilled care requires the continuous skills, judgment, and knowledge of a registered nurse. Examples of skilled care include wound care, suctioning, tube feeding, and administration of intravenous fluids.
2. (c) When the nurse is responsible for handling the client's valuables and clothing, *the agency's policies must be carefully observed.* It is best to have a second nurse or a representative from the hospital's administrative staff present when a nurse receives valuables for safekeeping. An inventory is sometimes made. The nurse and the client may cosign the inventory. One copy is given to the client and the other copy is attached to the chart.
3. (d) Referral is often a part of good discharge planning. The nurse should begin to anticipate what kind of care the client will require before it is time for him or her to leave. Planning, coordination, and communication take time in order to ensure that clients receive continuity of care.
4. (b) Preparing a client for discharge actually should begin when he or she is admitted. The purpose of his or her stay is to help him or her reach an improved state of wellness, and this process begins at the time of admission.
5. (c) The client cannot be forcefully detained when he or she is a rational adult.
6. (b) The nurse responsible for the client's care should be sure the physician is notified and aware of the client's wishes to leave. Unsuccessful attempts to locate the doctor should be noted on the client's record. The hospital's nursing supervisor may also be notified.
7. (b) Cleaning a client's room and equipment after discharge is ordinarily a housekeeping responsibility.
8. (b) Early planning helps ensure that continuity of care is maintained. The term means that the client's care remains uninterrupted despite changes in caregivers, thus avoiding any loss in the progress that has already been made.
9. (a) Discharge is a process that occurs when a client leaves a health agency. It consists of obtaining a written medical order for discharge, completing discharge instructions, notifying the business office, helping the client leave the health agency, writing a

summary of the client's condition at the time of discharge, and requesting that the room be cleaned.

10. (b) Intermediate care facilities provide health-related care and services to individuals who, because of their mental or physical condition, require institutional care but not 24-hour nursing care.

ANSWERS TO ALTERNATIVE FORMAT QUESTIONS

1. Answer: 1, 3, 5, 6

Rationale: When assisting a newly admitted client to undress, the nurse provides privacy by closing the door to the room and pulling the curtains around the bed. The client who requires assistance should be seated on the edge of the bed, which is already in the lowest position. If the client is weak or tired, assist him or her to lie down. While the client is lying down, gently unfasten and pull off his or her shoes. These activities provide for the client's safety while undressing.

Release fasteners, zippers, buttons, and ask the client to lift the hips to facilitate easy removal of the clothing without causing added discomfort. During the hospital stay, clients wear hospital gowns for comfort and convenience while in bed. Placing a blanket over the client provides for privacy and comfort because he or she may become chilled otherwise.

Nursing Process:	Implementation
Client Needs Category:	Safe, effective care environment
Cognitive Level:	Application

2. Answer: 1, 2, 3, 6

Rationale: Discharge instruction includes client teaching related to medications that will be self-administered, demonstration of skills involved in self-care, and providing opportunities for return demonstrations. Discharge instructions also include informing the client about follow-up activities and referrals such as physical therapy and rehabilitation. The client must also be given information about signs and symptoms that require immediate attention from the health care provider.

Nursing Process:	Planning
Client Needs Category:	Physiological integrity
Cognitive Level:	Analysis

3. Answer: 1, 2, 4, 5

Rationale: When assessing a client who has a rash, the nurse should first find out when the rash began; this information can identify where the rash is in the disease process and assists with the correct diagnosis. The nurse should also ask about allergies because rashes related to allergies can occur when a person changes medication, eats new foods, or comes into contact with allergens in the air such as pollen. It is also important for the nurse to ask how the client has been treating the rash because use of topical ointments or oral medications may make the rash worse. The nurse should ask about recent travel outside the United States because such travel exposes the client to foreign environments, which may

contribute to the onset of the rash. Although the client's smoking and drinking habits can be important to know, this information will not provide further insight into the rash or its cause.

Nursing Process:	Assessment
Client Needs Category:	Physiological integrity
Cognitive Level:	Analysis

ANSWERS TO TRUE OR FALSE QUESTIONS
Items 1 Through 10

1. *True.*
2. *True.*
3. *False.* Preparing an identification bracelet for the client is one of the first components of the admission routine.
4. *False.* When the nurse learns that a client will be arriving, the room should be prepared. The client should feel that everyone on the nursing unit is prepared and ready for his or her admission.
5. *True.*
6. *False.* Some hospitals provide booklets with general information for newly admitted clients. Many clients are anxious when they are admitted. Anxiety interferes with the ability to remember. A booklet acts as a reminder for what was explained. Booklets should never take the place of a nurse's explanations.
7. *False.* Losing personal items belonging to a client can have serious legal implications for the nurse and the health agency. It is best to have a second nurse or a representative from the hospital's administrative staff present when a nurse receives valuables for safekeeping. An inventory is sometimes made. Problems occur when, in the course of hospitalization, other valuable items are brought in without subsequent documentation.
8. *True.*
9. *False.* A step-down unit is a special area in the hospital for clients who are recovering from serious conditions and require less-intensive nursing care.
10. *True.*

ANSWER TO SHORT ANSWER QUESTIONS
Refer to "Nursing Guidelines for Transferring a Client." You may choose any of the actions listed.

Chapter 11

ANSWERS TO MATCHING QUESTIONS
Items 1 Through 5
1. b   2. f   3. d   4. e   5. a
Items 6 Through 10
6. c   7. f   8. e   9. a   10. d
Items 11 through 14
11. e   12. d   13. a   14. b

Items 15 Through 24

15. d 16. f 17. h 18. c 19. o 20. j
21. a 22. g 23. n 24. b

ANSWERS TO MULTIPLE-CHOICE QUESTIONS

Items 1 Through 24

1. (c) Body temperature normally remains within a fairly constant range as a result of a balance between heat production and heat loss. This process is regulated by a thermostat-like arrangement in the brain's hypothalamus.

2. (b) When the Fahrenheit scale is used, water freezes at 32°F and boils at 212°F.

3. (d) The vital signs normally fluctuate in circadian rhythm. The body temperature is ordinarily lowest from midnight to dawn.

4. (c) The client's temperature is 101.8°F. To convert centigrade to Fahrenheit, multiply by $^9/_5$ and add 32. To change Fahrenheit to centigrade, subtract 32 and multiply by $^5/_9$.

5. (c) Persons having strong emotional experiences, such as fear and anxiety, are likely to have a higher-than-average temperature. Conversely, persons experiencing apathy and depression are likely to have a lower-than-average body temperature.

6. (c) A person is considered to be in danger when the temperature reaches beyond 41°C (105.8°F).

7. (b) A body temperature below the average normal is called hypothermia.

8. (c) Death usually occurs when the temperature falls below approximately 84°F (28.8°C).

9. (a) Cold body temperatures are best measured with a tympanic thermometer.

10. (a) Tall, slender persons usually have a slower pulse rate than short, stout persons. The rate for women is slightly faster, by about 7 to 8 beats per minute, than it is for men.

11. (d) A rapid pulse rate is called tachycardia.

12. (c) An irregular pattern of heartbeats and consequently an irregular pulse rhythm is called an *arrhythmia*. It may also be called *dysrhythmia*.

13. (d) The term *palpitation* means that a person is aware of his or her own heart contraction without having to feel the pulse. The pulse rate is usually rapid when palpitations are noted.

14. (d) A rapid and weak pulse is called a thready pulse. This type of pulse is noted when the blood volume is small, making the pulse difficult to feel and, once felt, very easily stopped with pressure.

15. (d) The best area to obtain an apical pulse on an adult is at site D. The heartbeats are best heard at the apex, or lower tip of the heart. This area is located slightly below the left nipple in line with the middle of the clavicle.

16. (a) The difference between the apical and radial pulse rates is called the *pulse deficit*.

17. (c) The process of exchanging oxygen and carbon dioxide between the blood and the body is called *internal respiration. External respiration* is the process of exchanging oxygen and carbon dioxide between the lungs and the blood.

18. (b) The respiratory center in the medulla and specialized sensing tissue in the carotid arteries are very sensitive to the amount of carbon dioxide in the blood.

19. (c) The relationship between the pulse and respiratory rates is fairly consistent in normal persons. The ratio is one respiration to approximately four or five heartbeats.

20. (b) *Hypoventilation* is a term that describes a less-than-normal amount of air entering the lungs.

21. (d) Blood is pushed forward into the arteries during systole. Systole is the phase during which the heart works. The pressure increases during this time. This is called the *systolic pressure*.

22. (a) Blood pressure falls in relation to position changes from lying to sitting or standing. The normal difference in systolic pressure tends to be no greater than 10 mm Hg lower than it was in a reclining position.

23. (a) The difference between the systolic and diastolic blood pressure measurements is called the pulse pressure. It is computed by subtracting the smaller figure from the larger.

24. (b) If the blood pressure cuff is too small, the blood pressure reading will be falsely high.

ANSWERS TO ALTERNATIVE FORMAT QUESTIONS

1. **Answer: "X" at the 5th intercostal space at the midclavicular line.**

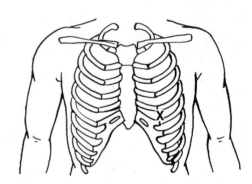

Rationale: The apical pulse is found at the apex of the heart in the 5th intercostal space at the midclavicular line, slightly below the left nipple.

Nursing Process:	Assessment
Client Needs Category:	Physiologic integrity
Cognitive Level:	Application

2. **Answer: 4, 1, 2, 5, 3**
Rationale: The sounds described are the five phases of Korotkoff sounds. Phase I begins with the first faint but clear tapping sound that follows a period of silence as pressure is released from the blood pressure cuff. Phase II is characterized by a change from tapping sounds to swishing sounds. Phase III is characterized by a change to loud distinct sounds as blood flows freely through

the artery. Phase IV sounds are muffled and have a blowing quality, resulting from a loss in the transmission of pressure from the deflating cuff to the artery. Phase V is the point at which the last sound is heard, known as the second diastolic pressure measurement.

Nursing Process:	Assessment
Client Needs Category:	Physiologic integrity
Cognitive Level:	Analysis

3. **Answer: 38.3°C**
   Rationale: Use the following formula:
   $C = (F - 32) / 1.8$ $C = (101 - 32) / 1.8$ $69 / 1.8$
   $C = 38.33$

Nursing Process:	Evaluation
Client Needs Category:	Physiologic integrity
Cognitive Level:	Analysis

ANSWERS TO TRUE OR FALSE QUESTIONS

Items 1 Through 12

1. *False.* Obtaining the apical-radial pulse rate requires two persons. One listens at the apex of the heart while the other feels the pulse at the client's wrist. They use one watch placed conveniently between them, decide on a specific time to start counting, and count for a full minute.
2. *True.*
3. *True.*
4. *True.*
5. *True.*
6. *False.* When the nurse assesses for blood pressure changes from lying to upright positions, the client should be lying for at least 3 minutes.
7. *False.* The mercury type of sphygmomanometer uses a mercury gauge. The aneroid type does not use mercury but contains a needle that moves about a dial.
8. *False.* The diastolic pressure cannot be measured using the palpation technique.
9. *True.*
10. *True.*
11. *True.*
12. *True.*

ANSWERS TO SHORT ANSWER QUESTIONS

Items 1 Through 3

1. Circumstances in which nursing judgment should be used are:
   a. A change in vital signs is noted and a trend is developing.
   b. Findings are very different from previous recordings.
   c. The vital signs are not in keeping with the client's condition.
   d. The vital signs could possibly be fraudulent.
2. Refer to Figure 11-18.
3. Refer to Figure 11-12.

Chapter 12

ANSWERS TO MATCHING QUESTIONS

Items 1 Through 7

1. d   2. f   3. h   4. a   5. g   6. e
7. c

Items 8 Through 13

8. d   9. f   10. a   11. e   12. g   13. b

ANSWERS TO MULTIPLE-CHOICE QUESTIONS

Items 1 Through 10

1. (d) The synonym for rales is crackles.
2. (c) *Inspection* is purposeful observation. Using the term broadly, inspection refers to a technique in which the nurse uses many senses collectively to scan the client. Using the term more strictly, inspection refers to a technique in which the nurse simultaneously focuses vision and attention looking for minute details.
3. (b) *Palpation* uses the sense of touch to gather information. The examiner feels or presses on the body.
4. (d) *Percussion* is most often used to examine the lungs and abdomen.
5. (c) Clients can be taught to use some assessment methods for detecting certain early signs of disease. Nurses should instruct female clients in the use of inspection and palpation for performing breast self-examinations.
6. (c) Because the trachea is large and close to the mouth, the sound is loud and coarse.
7. (c) Bronchovesicular sounds are heard on either side of the center of the chest and back. They are equal in length during inspiration and expiration with no noticeable pause.
8. (c) A wheal is the skin lesion that is elevated, irregular in shape, and has no free fluid.
9. (b) A wart is an example of a skin lesion called a papule.
10. (a) When using percussion to examine a client, an empty, moderately loud, resonant sound is a normal finding for the lung.

ANSWERS TO ALTERNATIVE FORMAT QUESTIONS

1. **Answer:**

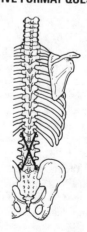

Rationale: Lordosis is characterized by an accentuated curve of the lumbar area of the spine.

Nursing Process:	Assessment
Client Needs Category:	Health promotion and maintenance
Cognitive Level:	Application

2. **Answer:**

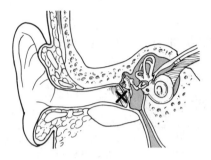

Rationale: The tympanic membrane separates the external and middle ear and may appear red and bulging in a client with otitis media.

Nursing Process:	Assessment
Client Needs Category:	Physiological integrity
Cognitive Level:	Application

3. **Answer:**

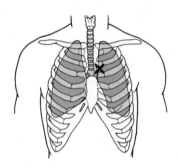

Rationale: The pulmonic area is best heard at the second intercostal space, just left of the sternum.

Nursing Process:	Assessment
Client Needs Category:	Health promotion and maintenance
Cognitive Level:	Application

4. **Answer: 3, 5, 2, 1, 6, 4**

Rationale: Effective client teaching is organized and logical. It is age appropriate and is of value to the client; it must be easily adapted to the client's routine of self-care activities.

The nurse teaches the client as follows: Examine the breasts monthly, about 1 week after the menstrual period. Postmenopausal women should select a specific date each month for examining their breasts. Begin the examination in the shower. Use the right hand to examine the left breast and the left hand to examine the right breast. Place the hand on the side that will be examined behind the head. Glide the flat portion of the fingers over all aspects of each breast in a circular fashion. Determine whether there are any lumps, hard knots, or thickened areas. Next, stand in front of the mirror. Look at both breasts with the arms relaxed at the side, with the hands pressing on the hips, and with the hands elevated above the head. Look for dimpling in the skin or retraction of either nipple. Lie down for the remainder of the examination. Put a pillow or folded towel under the shoulder on the side where the first breast will be examined; reverse the pillow before examining the second breast. Again, place the arm behind the head. Press the flat surface of the fingers in small circular motions from the outer margin of the breast toward the nipple, feeling for changes in any area of the breast. Feel upward toward the axilla of each arm. Complete at least three revolutions about the breast. Squeeze the nipple gently between the thumb and index finger to determine whether there is any clear or bloody discharge. Repeat the examination on the opposite breast axilla. Report any unusual findings or changes to a physician. Breast self-examination is combined with a clinical examination and mammography to ensure early diagnosis and treatment of cancerous tumors.

Nursing Process:	Implementation
Client Needs Category:	Health promotion and maintenance
Cognitive Level:	Application

ANSWERS TO TRUE OR FALSE QUESTIONS

Items 1 Through 10

1. *True.*
2. *False.* The physician also obtains a medical history. Although the data gathered by the physician and the nurse are similar in content, the nurse uses the information differently. Duplication in many areas can be avoided if the nurse is present when the physician obtains the medical history.
3. *False.* Although the client may have weighed himself recently at home, it is best to weigh him or her again. The recorded measurements are extremely important in assessing trends in future weight loss or gain and are used to calculate dosages of some drugs.
4. *True.*
5. *False.* A diseased area of the skin is generally referred to as a lesion. A fissure is a groove or crack in the skin or mucous membrane.
6. *True.*
7. *True.*
8. *False.* When doing a visual assessment, the nurse should check the six cardinal positions.
9. *False.* Bronchial sounds are heard over the upper portion of the sternum and are harsh and loud.
10. *True.*

ANSWERS TO SHORT ANSWER QUESTIONS

Items 1 Through 3

1. The recommended techniques for obtaining the client's height and weight are:

a. Check to see that the scale is calibrated to "0."
b. Ask or assist the client to remove his or her robe and shoes if he or she is wearing them.
c. Place a paper towel on the scale.
d. Assist the client onto the scale.
e. Slide the weight until the scale balances; read and record the weight.
f. Ask the client to stand straight in order to measure the height.
g. Move the measuring bar down until it lightly touches the top of the client's head.
h. Read and record the height.
i. Record the height and weight on the client's record.

2. The purposes of a physical assessment are:
a. It is an excellent way to evaluate an individual's current health status. It is also a time when health practitioners can carry out client teaching.
b. It helps detect signs and symptoms of early illness.
c. Findings contribute to the informational database guiding the nursing care that the client may need.
d. To evaluate responses to medical and nursing interventions.

3. Techniques to use during assessment are:
a. Touch—sharp, dull, vibration, and temperature
b. Taste—sweet, salty, sour, and bitter
c. Smell—coffee, lemon, vanilla, or peppermint

Chapter 13

ANSWERS TO MATCHING QUESTIONS
Items 1 Through 5
1. g   2. d   3. a   4. e   5. c
Items 6 Through 13
6. b   7. f   8. c   9. e   10. a   11. g
12. h   13. d

ANSWERS TO MULTIPLE-CHOICE QUESTIONS
Items 1 Through 12
1. (d) The suffix *-gram* describes the actual image or results of the test. By combining a root word that refers to a part of the body with a word ending that has a common meaning, the nurse can interpret the definition of medical terms.
2. (a) The suffix *-centesis* describes a procedure involving the puncture of a body cavity. A thoracentesis is a puncture of the pleural cavity, which lies in the thorax.
3. (d) A *paracentesis* is a procedure that involves puncturing the skin and subsequently the abdominal cavity so that body fluid may be withdrawn.
4. (a) The Queckenstedt test is done during a lumbar puncture. This is used to determine the presence or absence of an obstruction of the flow of cerebrospinal fluid.

5. (c) Electroencephalography is an examination that records an image of the electrical activity in the brain. It is abbreviated EEG.
6. (b) The dorsal recumbent position is used most often to examine the rectum and vagina.
7. (d) The lithotomy position is used to examine the vagina with a speculum. It is also used when the internal female reproductive organs are palpated, and when male or female bladder inspections are done with a cystoscope.
8. (d) In some cases, a signed consent form may be required before certain tests or examinations may be performed. In order to be legally sound, consent must contain three elements: capacity, comprehension, and voluntariness.
9. (d) A cystoscopy refers to an examination that involves inspection of the urinary bladder.
10. (c) The modified standing position is most commonly used to examine the prostate gland.
11. (b) A Class III result on the cellular portion of the Pap smear indicates that the sample on the smear is suggestive of cancer cells, but it is not definite.
12. (a) A #1 result on the identifiable microorganisms portion of the Pap smear indicates that the sample contained normal microorganisms.

ANSWERS TO ALTERNATIVE FORMAT QUESTIONS
1. **Answer: 1, 2, 3, 6**
Rationale: Having the client who is able to understand the procedure and voluntarily give consent for the procedure provides legal protection for the health care providers and must be obtained before the procedure begins. Measuring weight, blood pressure, respiratory rate, and abdominal girth provides baseline data for postprocedural comparison. Emptying the bladder prior to the test prevents accidental puncture of the bladder. Measuring vital signs periodically throughout the procedure allows assessment of the client's response. The client is in a sitting position in order for the fluid to pool in the lower abdomen. The fluid withdrawn is measured, described, and sent to the lab.

Nursing Process:	Implementation
Client Needs Category:	Physiologic integrity
Cognitive Level:	Application

2. **Answer: 3, 1, 6, 2, 5, 4**
Rationale: In order to complete blood glucose testing in an efficient and effective manner, the client would gather the necessary equipment and supplies; he or she must ensure that the monitor is calibrated correctly for the test strips prior to proceeding with the test. Washing hands with soap and warm water reduces the risk of microorganisms residing on the skin and therefore reduces the risk of infection. The warmth of the water dilates capillaries, increasing blood flow to the test site and thus ensuring an adequate sample.

Selecting a nontraumatized site reduces infectious potential and discomfort. Once the site is pierced, the sample must be collected promptly to ensure accuracy of the measurement. Once the sample is collected, the strip must be placed properly in the meter for accurate results. When the meter beeps, the test is complete, and the numbers displayed indicate the test result.

Nursing Process:	Implementation
Client Needs Category:	Physiologic integrity
Cognitive Level:	Application

3. **Answer: 70**

Rationale: Screening guidelines for this age group are relaxed because cervical cancer in women 70 or older is almost entirely confined to women who have not been previously screened or who have deviated from screening guidelines in the previous 10 years.

Nursing Process:	Evaluation
Client Needs Category:	Physiological integrity
Cognitive Level:	Knowledge

ANSWERS TO TRUE OR FALSE QUESTIONS

Items 1 Through 15

1. *True.*
2. *False.* Many examinations and tests require special preparation in order to obtain accurate results. The requirements for certain tests are usually located in a reference manual at each nursing unit. The nurse should refer to these written instructions each time a client is undergoing a test *rather than rely on memory.*
3. *True.*
4. *False. Draping* is a term that refers to covering a body part in such a manner that it does not interfere with access to the area being examined. Draping avoids exposing the client unnecessarily. If the client feels chilled, a sheet or blanket may be used to cover him or her.
5. *True.*
6. *False.* The atomic structure of some chemical elements, such as iodine, can be altered in such a way that it gives off radiation. It is then referred to as a *radionuclide.*
7. *True.*
8. *True.*
9. *True.*
10. *False.* Unless alcohol evaporates before the finger stick, it can alter the results.
11. *True.*
12. *True.*
13. *False.* Glucose is the type of sugar present in the blood as a result of eating carbohydrates. Normal blood levels are maintained by the body's production of glucagons and insulin, hormones that regulate glucose metabolism.
14. *True.*
15. *True.*

ANSWERS TO SHORT ANSWER QUESTIONS

Items 1 Through 3

1. Items to record on the client's record include:
   a. The date and time
   b. Pertinent preexamination assessments and preparation
   c. The type of examination or test
   d. Who performed the test and where it was done
   e. The client's responses during and after the procedure
   f. The type of specimen that was collected (e.g., tissue, fluid, blood)
   g. A description of the specimen (e.g., size, appearance, volume, color) and the site from which it was taken
   h. The disposition of the specimen
2. Factors to be considered when procedures are done on older adults are:
   a. Unless separate age-specific norms are available, test findings from older adults may be misinterpreted.
   b. Prescription drugs may affect test results.
   c. Before giving multiple daily medications (with a small amount of water) to older adults who are fasting for a procedure, the physician should be consulted.
   d. Older adults may not be able to tolerate having food and fluids withheld for long periods of time.
   e. Dehydration may cause blood values to seem elevated.
   f. Intensive and repeated bowel preparation for some tests may cause exhaustion.
   g. A bedside commode and assistance to use it are a frequent need for older adults.
   h. A bed alarm that sounds when the client gets out of bed may be a necessary safety precaution for older adults who need assistance to the bathroom or bedside commode.
   i. Coordination of tests and examinations diminish waiting time and extensive preparation and provide increased periods of rest.
   j. It may be appropriate to warm blankets, slippers, and robes if the older adult has to wait in drafty or air-conditioned hallways.
   k. After the procedure, food, fluid, and an opportunity to use the toilet should be provided; then a period of rest should be given before beginning other nursing activities.
3. Client responsibilities prior to outpatient procedures include the following:
   a. If you have questions, call (provide a number for the client to call).
   b. Do *not* eat or drink anything for at least 8 to 12 hours prior to the test.
   c. Follow all dietary restrictions or recommendations for the procedure.
   d. Check with your physician about taking regular medications on the day of the procedure.
   e. Bathe or shower as usual.
   f. Dress casually and comfortably in layers.
   g. Ask a friend or family member to bring you to the examination and take your home after it.
   h. Come to the test or examination location at least one-half hour before the scheduled time.

i. Check in at the information or appointment desk when you arrive.
j. Bring insurance information and forms with you.
k. Bring a list of medications you take and a list of your allergies.

Chapter 14

ANSWERS TO MATCHING QUESTIONS

Items 1 Through 5

1. d   2. f   3. b   4. g   5. e

Items 6 Through 8

6. c   7. d   8. b

Items 9 Through 13

9. c   10. g   11. a   12. d   13. f

ANSWERS TO MULTIPLE-CHOICE QUESTIONS

Items 1 Through 16

1. (b) Nutrition is defined as the process whereby the body uses food.
2. (d) A calorie is the amount of heat necessary to raise the temperature of 1 gram of water 1°C.
3. (c) Most average adults need between 1800 and 3000 calories per day according to the National Research Council of the National Academy of Sciences.
4. (a) Proteins are the source of amino acids.
5. (d) Fats have a higher energy value than other nutrients; they yield 9 calories per gram.
6. (c) The U.S. Department of Health and Human Services in its publication *Healthy People 2010: National Health Promotion and Disease Prevention Objectives* (1999), has recommended that Americans reduce their present fat intake to no more than 30% of their daily calories.
7. (c) Minerals, such as calcium, sodium, potassium, and chloride, are chemical substances. When these substances are dissolved in the body, they are called electrolytes.
8. (a) Those who arbitrarily select to become vegetarians may need to learn how to combine plant sources to ensure that they are consuming adequate amounts of all the essential amino acids.
9. (c) Regurgitation occurs quite commonly among infants after eating.
10. (a) A retired widow would be at the greatest risk for inadequate nutritional intake.
11. (d) Transfats are unsaturated fats that have been hydrogenated and remain solid at room temperature.
12. (b) Fortified food are foods that have been enhanced with extra amounts of nutritional substances that are normally present in food.
13. (d) The normal range of measurement for the triceps skin fold in adult males is 12.5–7.3 mm.
14. (a) Minerals are noncaloric substances in food that are essential to all cells.
15. (a) The term *dysphagia* means difficulty swallowing.
16. (c) Good sources of carbohydrates include cereals and grains, such as rice, wheat and wheat germ, oats, barley, corn and cornmeal; fruits and vegetables; molasses, maple and corn syrups, honey, and common table sugar.

ANSWERS TO ALTERNATIVE FORMAT QUESTIONS

1. **Answer: 30%**
   Rationale: Generally Americans eat more fat than people in most other countries. The relationship between fat consumption and disorders such as obesity, heart disease, hypertension, and some cancers is well documented. In an effort to improve health, the U.S. Department of Health and Human Services is continuing its initiative, *Healthy People 2010: National Health Promotion and Disease Prevention* (1999). Among the goals is that at least 50% of people 2 years of age and older consume no more than 30% of their daily calories from fat.

Nursing Process:	Planning
Client Needs Category:	Health promotion and maintenance
Cognitive Level:	Application

2. **Answer: 1, 2, 4, 6**
   Rationale: Placing the client in a sitting position, giving short simple prompts to eat, and limiting distracting stimuli increase client safety for focusing attention on the process of eating and swallowing. This also reduces the risk of aspiration of food. Should choking occur, suctioning can be done immediately when the proper equipment is at the bedside.

Nursing Process:	Planning
Client Needs:	Safe, effective care environment
Cognitive Level:	Application

3. **Answer: 24.2**
   Rationale: Use the formula $BMI = kg \div m^2$

   Step 1 — Convert 160 pounds to kilograms ($160 \div 2.2 = 72.2$ kg)

   Step 2 — Divide height in inches by 39.4 (inches in 1 meter) = meters ($69 \div 39.4 = 1.75$ meters)

   Step 3 — Square the answer in Step 2 = m^2 ($1.75 \times 1.75 = 3$)

   Step 4 — Divide weight in kilograms by m^2 ($72.7 \div 3 = 24.2$) BMI = 24.2

Nursing Process:	Assessment
Client Needs Category:	Health promotion
Cognitive Level:	Analysis

ANSWERS TO TRUE OR FALSE QUESTIONS

Items 1 Through 10

1. *False.* Most eating habits are learned in early life and vary from culture to culture.
2. *False. Anorexia* is the loss of appetite or lack of desire

for food. *Cachexia* is a condition in which there is a general wasting away of body tissue.
3. *True.*
4. *True.*
5. *False.* Protein complementation is the act of combining two or more plant sources in the same meal.
6. *True.*
7. *False.* Many deficiency diseases have been associated with diets in which specific foods, rich in a source of *a vitamin,* have been lacking.
8. *False.* Fat-soluble vitamins are stored in reserve in the body for future needs.
9. *True.*
10. *True.*

ANSWERS TO SHORT ANSWER QUESTIONS

Items 1 Through 2

1. According to the food pyramid, the food groups and their daily servings are:
   a. Bread, cereal, rice, pasta—6 to 11 servings
   b. Vegetables—3 to 5 servings
   c. Fruits—2 to 4 servings
   d. Milk, yogurt, cheese—2 to 3 servings
   e. Meat, poultry, fish, eggs, beans, nuts—2 to 3 servings
   f. Fats, oils, sweets—Use sparingly
2. Facts that appear on a nutritional label are:
   a. Serving size
   b. Number of servings in a container
   c. Number of calories per serving
   d. Number of calories from fat
   e. Total fat
   f. Amount of saturated fat
   g. Cholesterol
   h. Amount of sodium
   i. Total carbohydrate
   j. Dietary fiber
   k. Sugars
   l. Protein
   m. Vitamins and minerals, if any
   n. Percent of daily value based on 2000- and 2500-calorie diet
   o. Number of calories per gram for fat, carbohydrate, and protein
   p. Percent of daily value supplied by each nutrient present in each serving contained in the container

Chapter 15

ANSWERS TO MATCHING QUESTIONS

Items 1 Through 6

1. c   2. d   3. f   4. a   5. e   6. b

Items 7 Through 12

7. c   8. e   9. b   10. f   11. d   12. a

Items 13 Through 19

13. f   14. c   15. g   16. a   17. c   18. d
19. b

ANSWERS TO MULTIPLE-CHOICE QUESTIONS

Items 1 Through 35

1. (c) The human body is composed of approximately 45% to 75% water. The amount varies according to an individual's age, gender, and body fat composition.
2. (d) The infant would have the most body water.
3. (a) The total amount of water that adults consume each day is about 1200 to 1500 mL. An additional 700 to 1000 mL per day is extracted from the foods eaten. As a result of metabolism, about 200 to 400 mL per day is added to the total fluid intake to bring it to about 2100 to 2900 mL per day.
4. (b) Most of the water is lost through the kidneys. Some moisture is lost in the stool and in obvious perspiration from areas where skin contains abundant sweat glands. A certain amount of water is lost in a form that cannot usually be seen or felt. This is called insensible water loss. It occurs from the lungs during expiration and through the skin.
5. (b) Body fluid is located in two general compartments: inside and outside cells. The fluid inside the cells is referred to as intracellular fluid.
6. (c) Osmosis is a process that regulates the distribution of water from one compartment to another. Under the influence of osmosis, water moves through a semipermeable membrane from an area where the fluid is more dilute to another area where the fluid is more concentrated.
7. (c) One of the simplest methods for objectively assessing fluid balance is to compare the amount of a client's fluid intake with fluid output.
8. (a) When an individual is healthy, the amount of fluid that is taken in should approximate the same amount that is lost.
9. (b) In some cases, to ensure accurate assessment of fluid loss, the nurse may be required to measure liquid stool or weigh wet linens, diapers, or dressings saturated with blood or other secretions. The weight of wet items is compared to the weight of a similar dry item. An estimate of output is based on the knowledge that 1 pint (475 mL) of water weighs about 1 pound (0.47 kg).
10. (c) The skin may appear warm, flushed, and dry when the client is experiencing fluid deficit. It may appear cool, pale, and moist in fluid excess.
11. (b) *Fluid imbalance* is a general term describing any of several conditions in which the body water is not in proper volume or location within the body. One of the locations in which fluid levels is likely to become imbalanced is the blood, or the area of intravascular fluid. When fluid is excessive in this location, the term *hypervolemia* is used to describe

it. This term means that there is a high volume, or amount, of water present in the blood.

12. (d) Fluid imbalance can occur when fluid becomes trapped in interstitial areas. This is called *third spacing*. It often occurs when there is a loss of proteins from the plasma of blood.

13. (c) Intravenous solutions are selected and ordered by the physician. They are considered to be a form of medication. The specific type of solution, volume, and rate of administration are part of the medical order. The nurse must exercise extreme caution that the correct solution is infused. This is a priority concern because any substance that is instilled directly into the circulatory system produces a rapid effect, because of its almost instant distribution throughout the body.

14. (d) Intravenous fluids fall into two basic categories. They are either a crystalloid or a colloid solution. A crystalloid solution is a mixture of water and uniformly dissolved crystals, such as salt and sugar.

15. (b) Crystalloid solutions are further subdivided into isotonic, hypotonic, and hypertonic solutions on the basis of the amount of dissolved crystals present in the solution. A hypotonic solution contains fewer crystals than are normally found in plasma. When infused intravenously, the water in the solution will enter through the semipermeable membrane of blood cells. The blood cells will become larger as they fill with water.

16. (c) A hypertonic solution has a higher amount of dissolved crystals than plasma. It will draw water into the intravascular compartment from the more dilute areas of water within the cells and interstitial spaces. This can help relieve edema because cells and tissues shrink and dehydrate from fluid loss.

17. (c) Normally, the pressure in the client's vein is higher than atmospheric pressure. The solution is placed on a standard at a level of 45 to 60 cm (18 to 24 inches) above the level of the vein. At this height, gravity is sufficient to overcome the pressure within the vein and allow the solution to infuse.

18. (d) For most intravenous infusions for adults, an 18-, 20-, or 22-gauge needle is used. A size 18- or 20-gauge needle should be selected when colloid solutions are infused because a smaller needle may become plugged with the suspended proteins.

19. (c) Superficial veins are more easily located and are more accessible for puncturing. Veins in the arms and hands are used in preference to veins in the foot or leg. Use veins in the arm or hand on the client's nondominant side. In general, when the arm is used, it is *best* to select a vein as low as possible on the back of the hand or the lower forearm.

20. (c) A common time frame for changing an intravenous solution is every 24 hours or when it is finished.

21. (b) A common practice is to change the dressing over the venipuncture site once in every 24 to 72 hours.

22. (a) Swelling in the area of the venipuncture site and coolness of the skin are two of the signs of infiltration. The other signs of infiltration include slowing or stopping of the flow and discomfort.

23. (c) The first nursing action when discontinuing an intravenous infusion is to clamp the tubing and remove the tape that held the dressing and venipuncture device in place.

24. (b) Dextran is a plasma expander.

25. (d) A scalp vein is often used for an infant.

26. (c) Nonelectrolytes are chemical compounds that remain bound together when dissolved in a solution and, therefore, cannot conduct electricity. Glucose is an example of a nonelectrolyte.

27. (a) Electrolytes are chemical compounds that dissolve and separate into individual molecules, each carrying either a positive or negative electrical charge. In general, these separated molecules are called *ions*. More specifically, a *cation* is an ion with a positive electrical charge. An *anion* is an ion with a negative electrical charge.

28. (c) Electrolytes are distributed in different proportions in extracellular and intracellular tissue. Their proportions remain relatively constant because of the movement and relocation of various ions through the processes of diffusion and active transport. *Diffusion* is the process in which ions move from an area of greater concentration to an area of lesser concentration through a semipermeable membrane.

29. (b) Active transport is a process requiring energy in order to move molecules through a semipermeable membrane from an area of low concentration to one that is higher. Diffusion acts passively, with no release of energy.

30. (d) Potassium is a cation. It is the most abundant cation in intracellular fluid.

31. (b) Chloride is an anion. It is the major anion in extracellular fluid.

32. (b) Heparin lock is another name for a sealed chamber that provides a means for administering IV medications or solutions periodically.

33. (c) The term *parenteral nutrition* refers to a technique for providing nutrients, such as protein, carbohydrates, fats, vitamins, minerals, and trace elements, intravenously rather than by the oral, enteral, or intestinal routes.

34. (a) Peripheral parenteral nutrition is an isotonic or hypotonic nutrient solution that provides temporary nutritional support when oral intake is expected to resume in 7 to 10 days.

35. (c) An emulsion is a mixture of two liquids, one of which is insoluble in the other, but when combined is distributed throughout as small droplets within the other. A lipid emulsion is a mixture of water and fats in the form of soybean or safflower oil, egg yolk, phospholipids, and glycerin.

ANSWERS TO ALTERNATIVE FORMAT QUESTIONS

1. **Answer: 125**

   Rationale: Use this formula:

   Total volume in mL / total hours = mL per hour

   1000 mL / 8 hours = 125 mL per hour

Nursing Process:	Planning
Client Needs Category:	Physiological integrity
Cognitive Level:	Analysis

2. **Answer: 42**

   Rationale: Use this formula:

   Total volume in mL /

   Total time in minutes × gtt factor = gtt per minute

   250 mL ÷ 60 minutes = 4.16 mL per minute

   Multiply by the drip factor:

   4.16 × 10 gtt = 41.6 gtt per minute
   or 42 gtt per minute

Nursing Process:	Implementation
Client Needs Category:	Physiological integrity
Cognitive Level:	Analysis

3. **Answer: 8**

   Rationale: Use this formula:

   Dose on hand / Quantity on hand = Dose desired / X

   25,000 U / 250 ml = 800 U per hour / X

   Cross multiply to solve for X and divide each side of the equation by 25,000 U

   X = 8 mL per hour

Nursing Process:	Implementation
Client Needs Category:	Physiological integrity
Cognitive Level:	Application

ANSWERS TO TRUE OR FALSE QUESTIONS

Items 1 Through 20

1. *False.* A *cation* is an electrolyte with a positive charge. An *anion* is an electrolyte with a negative charge.
2. *False. Diffusion* is a process in which dissolved substances move passively through a semipermeable membrane from an area of higher concentration to an area of lower concentration. *Osmosis* is the movement of water through a semipermeable membrane from an area of lower concentration of dissolved substances to one of higher concentration.
3. *True.*
4. *False.* The extracellular fluid is subdivided into intravascular fluid and interstitial fluid.
5. *True.*
6. *False.* Most of the water in the body is lost through the kidneys. Insensible water loss is the water that is lost through the skin and lungs.
7. *True.*
8. *False.* When the amount of a liquid is not known, a calibrated pitcher should be used to measure the volume. The nurse should avoid estimating an amount. Too often the estimate is inaccurate.
9. *False.* Fluid output is the sum of all the liquid eliminated from the body. Fluid output is determined by measuring urine, emesis, drainage from tubes, and fluid drained following irrigation.
10. *True.*
11. *False.* The skin may appear warm, flushed, and dry when the client is experiencing fluid deficit. It may appear cool, pale, and moist in fluid excess.
12. *False.* The consumption of salty food can affect the intake and retention of fluids.
13. *True.*
14. *False.* Sodium is the most common electrolyte in the extracellular fluid.
15. *True.*
16. *False.* A glass container of solution requires vented tubing. Because a plastic bag collapses upon itself while the solution infuses, unvented tubing can be used.
17. *True.*
18. *False.* An angiocath is a flexible catheter threaded *over* a needle into a vein. An intracath is a flexible catheter threaded *through* a needle into a vein.
19. *True.*
20. *False.* Cross-matching is a laboratory test that determines whether blood specimens of the donor and the recipient are compatible. *Typing* is the laboratory test that identifies the proteins on red blood cells.

ANSWERS TO SHORT ANSWER QUESTIONS

Items 1 Through 5

1. Factors to be considered when selecting a vein for intravenous infusion are:
   a. Superficial veins are more easily located and more accessible.
   b. Veins in the arms and hands are preferred to veins in the foot and lower leg. The circulation may be reduced in the lower extremities.
   c. The client is less likely to be inconvenienced if the veins on the nondominant side are used.
   d. Choices may be limited because of other factors, such as injury to or surgery on the upper extremities.
   e. Compromise of joint movement should be avoided.
   f. The veins far down on the arm and hand should be used first so that if problems arise, there are others available farther up the forearm.
   g. A vein should be selected that is fairly straight.
   h. Thin-walled and scarred veins should be avoided.
   i. Insertion of the needle into a valve of the vein should be avoided.
   j. Larger veins should be used for hypertonic solutions, those containing irritating medications, those administered rapidly, and those that are thick and sticky.
   k. The future need for veins should be considered and care should be exercised in the selection.
2. Steps for cleansing the venipuncture site include:
   a. Use Betadine or alcohol to cleanse the skin.
   b. Start at center of site and cleanse in a circular motion outward 2 to 4 inches.
   c. Allow the antiseptic to dry.

3. The signs of complications that may occur when a client is receiving intravenous fluids are:
   a. *Circulatory overload:* Check for signs and symptoms of dyspnea, noisy respirations, and coughing, possibly caused by administration that is too rapid.
   b. *Infiltration:* Check for swelling of the tissues, pallor and coldness of the skin at the site, complaints of burning sensations, and slowing or stopping of the flow.
   c. *Phlebitis:* Check for redness, warmth, and swelling. The client may complain of pain or burning in the area of the venipuncture site.
   d. *Infection:* Check for all of the previously mentioned signs in addition to purulent drainage from the venipuncture site.
   e. *Air embolism:* Check for a sudden drop in blood pressure, tachycardia, cyanosis, and a diminished level of consciousness. Air embolism is caused by air entering the circulatory system.
4. Techniques for promoting vein distention are:
   a. Apply a tourniquet or blood pressure cuff tightly about the arm.
   b. Have the client make a fist and pump the fist intermittently.
   c. Tap the skin over the vein several times.
   d. Lower the client's arm to promote distal pooling of blood.
   e. Stroke the skin in the direction of the fingers.
   f. Apply warm compresses for 10 minutes; then reapply the tourniquet.
5.

Blood Product	Purpose for Administration
a. Platelets	Restore or improve ability to control bleeding
b. Granulocytes	Improve ability to overcome infection
c. Plasma	Replace clotting factors; increase intravascular fluid volume
d. Albumin	Pull third-spaced fluid by increasing colloidal osmotic pressure
e. Cryoprecipitate	Treat blood-clotting disorders

Chapter 16

ANSWERS TO MATCHING QUESTIONS
Items 1 through 6
1. d   2. e   3. b   4. c   5. g   6. a
Items 7 through 10
7. c   8. e   9. b   10. f

ANSWERS TO MULTIPLE-CHOICE QUESTIONS
Items 1 Through 14
1. (b) The primary concern for nurses is that hygiene be carried out in a manner that promotes health. The other choices may or may not be of concern for the nurse.

2. (d) The main component of the integumentary system is the skin.
3. (a) Many bacteria in the mouth become lodged between the teeth. The toothbrush cannot reach these areas well. Therefore, flossing several times a day is recommended. Flossing helps to break up groups of bacteria between the teeth.
4. (b) Soak the client's feet before trimming brittle, thick toenails.
5. (d) If the hair is tangled, use a wide-tooth comb and comb starting at the ends of the hair rather than from the crown downward.
6. (a) Sudoriferous glands in the skin regulate body temperature.
7. (c) Immersion of the buttocks and perineum in a small basin of continuously circulating water is called a sitz bath.
8. (b) Many substances may be used for mouth care. Milk of magnesia reduces oral acidity, dissolves plaque, increases the flow of saliva, and soothes oral lesions.
9. (d) The accumulation of cerumen within the ear may cause reduced or absent sound from a hearing aid.
10. (a) The temperature of the water for a tub bath should be between 105° and 110°F.
11. (c) The skin consists of the epidermis, dermis, and subcutaneous layers. The epidermis, or outermost layer, contains dead skin cells that form a tough protein called keratin, which serves to protect the underlying layers and structures within the skin.
12. (a) The teeth begin to erupt at about 6 months of age and continue to do so for 2 or 2½ more years.
13. (d) Gingivitis is an inflammation of the gums.
14. (c) A partial bath consists of washing those areas of the body that are subject to the greatest soiling or sources of body odor, such as the face, hands, and axillae. Partial bathing may be done at a sink or with a basin at the bedside.

ANSWERS TO ALTERNATIVE FORMAT QUESTIONS
1. **Answer: 1, 6, 2, 3, 4, 5**
   Rationale: This procedure follows the steps of the nursing process. Assessment, consulting the Kardex to verify the type of bath to be given, ensures continuity of care. Identifying the client ensures that the correct procedure is performed on the correct person. Planning, involving cleaning the tub prior to use, reduces the risk of spreading microorganisms. Implementation, assisting the client to the bathing area, shows concern for the client's safety. Evaluation of the procedure upon completion reveals that the client remains uninjured. Documentation is usually carried out upon completion of the task according to agency requirements.

Nursing Process:	Implementation
Client Needs Category:	Safe, effective care environment
Cognitive Level:	Application

2. **Answer: 2, 3, 4**

Rationale: Tinea capitis is a fungal infection of the scalp. It appears as a ring or cluster of papules or vesicles that itch and become scaly, cracked, and sore. It is spread by contact with the person or grooming items. Growth of the fungus is promoted when the skin is damp or with skin-to-skin contact, found in skin folds that are warm, moist, and dark.

Nursing Process:	Implementation
Client Needs Category:	Physiological integrity
Cognitive Level:	Application

3. **Answer: 2, 4**

Rationale: Lemon and glycerin swabs are used for mouth care in clients who are unconscious or postseizure. They increase salivation and refresh the mouth. Glycerin may absorb water from the lips and cause them to become dry and cracked if used for more than a few days. They are not known to reduce acidity or dissolve plaque.

Nursing Process:	Evaluation
Client Needs Category:	Safe, effective care environment
Cognitive Level:	Analysis

ANSWERS TO TRUE OR FALSE QUESTIONS

Items 1 Through 12

1. *False.* Some clients wear eyeglasses in addition to their contact lenses. For this reason, the nurse should not assume that a client who wears eyeglasses does not use at least one contact lens.
2. *False.* Generally, routine hygiene measures are documented on a checklist.
3. *True.*
4. *False.* Consult with the client to determine personal preferences. This promotes cooperation between the client and nurse and allows client participation in decision making.
5. *True.*
6. *False.* Tap water is most often used to cover dentures when they are not in the mouth; you may add mouthwash or denture cleanser to the water.
7. *True.*
8. *False.* Preparations made with oil should be used on dry hair. Alcohol is suggested for loosening some tangles.
9. *True.*
10. *False.* Sebaceous glands located within the hair follicles release an oily substance called sebum.
11. *True.*
12. *True.*

ANSWERS TO SHORT ANSWER QUESTIONS

Items 1 Through 4

1. The functions of the skin are as follows:
   a. Protects the body
   b. Helps regulate body temperature
   c. Assists with fluid and chemical balance
   d. Has nerve endings that are sensitive to pain, temperature, touch, and pressure
   e. Produces vitamin D with the help of sunlight, and the vitamin D is then absorbed from the skin into the body
2. The characteristics of healthy nails are:
   a. Thin
   b. Pink coloration
   c. Smooth texture
   d. A free white margin extending from the end of each nail
   e. Intact skin around the nail
3. Adults normally have 32 teeth.
4. The benefits of bathing are:
   a. It cleans and refreshes.
   b. Warm water and massage associated with washing and drying aid in relaxation.
   c. It stimulates circulation.
   d. It reduces the chance for infection.
   e. It may help self-image and morale.
   f. It eliminates body odor.

Chapter 17

ANSWERS TO MATCHING QUESTIONS

Items 1 Through 6

1. f   2. d   3. a   4. c   5. b   6. e

Items 7 through 11

7. c   8. e   9. d   10. a   11. b

ANSWERS TO MULTIPLE-CHOICE QUESTIONS

Items 1 Through 20

1. (b) For sleep to occur, the individual must be relaxed.
2. (d) Phenomena that cycle on a daily basis are referred to as circadian rhythms.
3. (c) Sleep is a basic human need characterized by a state of arousable unconsciousness.
4. (a) REM sleep is the phase in which most dreaming occurs.
5. (d) If the onset of sleep is delayed more than 20 to 30 minutes, get out of bed and do something else, such as reading.
6. (c) Blue and colors with blue tints, such as mauve and light green, promote relaxation.
7. (c) Most people are comfortable when the room temperature is 68° to 74°F (20° to 23°C).
8. (b) The REM phase of sleep is referred to as paradoxical sleep because the EEG waves appear similar to those produced during periods of wakefulness, but it is the *deepest* stage of sleep. REM is active sleep. Darting eye movements occur.
9. (a) Refer to Table 17-1.
10. (c) In the absence of bright light, the pineal gland secretes melatonin. Light triggers the suppression of melatonin.

11. (d) The photoperiod is the number of daylight hours to which a person is accustomed.

12. (b) The symptoms of seasonal affective disorder begin during the darker winter months and disappear in the spring.

13. (d) Tryptophan is found in protein foods, dairy products, and legumes.

14. (b) Narcolepsy is a sleep disorder characterized by the sudden onset of daytime sleep.

15. (a) Newborns sleep approximately 16 to 20 hours per day.

16. (d) Five- and 6-year-olds spend 20% of their sleep in REM sleep.

17. (d) In severe cases of sleep apnea, clients wear a special breathing mask that keeps the alveoli inflated at all times.

18. (d) Parasomnias are non-life-threatening activities that cause arousal or partial arousal, usually during transitions in NREM periods of sleep.

19. (a) Restless leg syndrome is also known as nocturnal myoclonus.

20. (a) Sundown syndrome in older adults is characterized by disorientation as the sun sets.

ANSWERS TO ALTERNATIVE FORMAT QUESTIONS

1. **Answer: 1, 3, 4, 5**
   Rationale: Initially, ingestion of alcohol makes one feel sleepy and relaxed. However, as the normal process of alcohol metabolism occurs, chemicals are released that have the effects mentioned. Alcohol may or may not cause wakefulness in some individuals.

Nursing Process:	Assessment
Client Needs Category:	Physiological integrity
Cognitive Level:	Comprehension

2. **Answer: 1, 3, 5, 6**
   Rationale: To reduce gastric reflux, the nurse should instruct the client to sleep with his upper body elevated; lose weight, if obese; avoid constrictive clothing; avoid caffeine and spicy foods; remain upright for 2 hours after eating; and eat small frequent meals.

Nursing Process:	Implementation
Client Needs Category:	Physiological integrity
Cognitive Level:	Application

3. **Answer: 3, 5**
   Rationale: Barbiturate hypnotics when taken over a prolonged period of time cannot be stopped abruptly. They should first be tapered off by thirds and then taken every other night before stopping completely. There is no evidence that a client cannot taper off the sleeping pills or that discontinuing them on a weekend is more effective.

Nursing Process:	Implementation
Client Needs Category:	Physiological integrity
Cognitive Level:	Application

ANSWERS TO TRUE OR FALSE QUESTIONS
Items 1 Through 10

1. *True.*
2. *True.*
3. *True.*
4. *False.* NREM sleep usually precedes REM sleep, the phase during which most dreaming occurs.
5. *False.* The indoor lighting to which most shift workers are exposed is not bright enough to adequately suppress melatonin. Consequently, many shift workers fight to stay awake. According to recent research, most individuals who work night shifts never completely adapt to the reversal of day and night activities no matter how long the pattern is established.
6. *True.*
7. *True.*
8. *True.*
9. *False.* Tranquilizers are drugs that produce a relaxing and calming effect. *Hypnotics* are drugs that induce sleep.
10. *False.* Sleep apnea is highest among older adults, especially obese men who snore.

ANSWERS TO SHORT ANSWER QUESTIONS
Items 1 Through 3

1. Components of phototherapy used to relieve the symptoms of seasonal affective disorder include the following actions:
   a. Initiate a schedule of full-spectrum light exposure in October or November.
   b. Remove eyeglasses or contact lenses that have ultraviolet filters.
   c. Sit within 3 feet of a light source for 2 hours.
   d. Glance at light periodically; the client may do other things such as read.
   e. Repeat exposure to light after sundown.
   f. Expose client to light 3 to 6 hours per day.
   g. Continue light exposure until spring.

2. Tips for client teaching to promote sleep include:
   a. Taking diuretics early in the morning.
   b. Exercising regularly during the day but not late in the evening.
   c. Not napping during the day.
   d. Avoiding alcohol, nicotine, and caffeine.
   e. Eating dairy products and other proteins daily.
   f. Modifying temperature and ventilation to your preference.
   g. Using the bedroom just for sleeping.
   h. Maintaining personal sleep rituals.
   i. Using earplugs and eyeshades for sleep.
   j. Maintaining consistent sleep routines.
   k. If not asleep in 20 to 30 minutes, getting out of bed and doing something else.
   l. Avoiding using sleep medications unless ordered by a physician.
   m. Following labeled directions on any medications.

3. Tips for client teaching related to facilitating the use of progressive relaxation include the following suggestions:
   a. Select a quiet, dimly lit, private room.
   b. Assume a comfortable lying or sitting position.
   c. Avoid talking.
   d. Close your eyes and focus on breathing.
   e. Inhale deeply through the nose and exhale slowly through the mouth.
   f. Tighten a group of muscles (e.g., left arm or right foot) and hold for 5 seconds.
   g. Relax those muscles and focus on the pleasurable feeling.
   h. Continue doing Steps f and g until all muscle groups have been exercised and relaxed.
   i. During the exercises, focus on how relaxed you feel and notice the feeling of weightlessness you experience.
   j. Count from 10 to 1 as you begin to move about ending this period of progressive relaxation.

Chapter 18

ANSWERS TO MATCHING QUESTIONS

Items 1 Through 10

1. j	2. e	3. h	4. i	5. b	6. f
7. c	8. g	9. d	10. a		

ANSWERS TO MULTIPLE-CHOICE QUESTIONS

Items 1 Through 12

1. (b) Class B fire extinguishers contain carbon dioxide.
2. (d) When a fire occurs, the first measure the nurse should follow is to evacuate the people in the room with the fire. Remembering the shortened version of the steps as *RACE* will help the nurse: *R*escue the people first before *A*, giving the alarm; *C*, confining the fire; and *E*, extinguishing the fire.
3. (c) When an accident does occur, check the client's condition immediately. Note his or her condition and be ready to describe it accurately.
4. (b) After the client has been properly cared for and the physician has been notified, prepare an incident or accident report. All information related to the accident is entered on the form. It is signed by the person completing the form.
5. (c) A *thermal burn*, which is the most common type of skin injury, is caused by flames, hot liquids, or steam. Burns may also result from contact with caustic chemicals, electric wires, or lightning.
6. (a) Asphyxiation is a term that means the inability to breathe.
7. (d) The body is quite susceptible to electrical shock because it is composed of water and electrolytes, both of which are good conductors of electricity. A conductor is a substance that facilitates the flow of electrical current.
8. (b) Falls, more than any other injury discussed thus far, are the most prevalent accident experienced by older adults, and they have the most serious consequences for this age group.
9. (d) The National Fire Protection Association recommends using the acronym RACE, which stands for: R = rescue; A = alarm; C = confine (the fire); and E = extinguish, to identify the essential steps in fire rescue proceedings.
10. (a) Macroshock, if it occurs, is the harmless distribution of low-amperage electricity over a large area of the body. Macroshock is experienced as a slight tingling.
11. (c) There are Class A, B, C, and ABC fire extinguishers. Class A extinguishers are used for paper, wood, and cloth fires.
12. (a) Although physical restraints prevent falls, they create concomitant risks for constipation; incontinence; and infections such as pneumonia, pressure sores, and a progressive decline in the ability to perform activities of daily living.

ANSWERS TO ALTERNATIVE FORMAT QUESTIONS

1. **Answer: 1, 3, 4, 5**
   Rationale: Poisoning is an injury caused by ingesting, inhaling, or absorbing a toxic substance. Poisonings are more common in homes, and many children treated for accidental poisoning will have a repeat episode. Installing child-resistant latches and cupboard doors and drawers helps to keep toxic substances locked away from children. Tamper-proof lids on prescription drug containers make it difficult for a child to gain access to a potentially toxic substance; never keeping medications in your purse keeps these substances away from curious children. Keeping plants out of reach or outside reduces access to potentially toxic plant leaves, berries, and sap. Never store toxic substances in containers intended for food or previously used for food. This practice invites the child to ingest a toxic substance.

Nursing Process:	Planning
Client Needs Category:	Health Promotion and Maintenance
Cognitive Level:	Application

2. **Answer: 3, 5, 4, 2, 6, 1**
   Rationale: Maintaining breathing and cardiac function supports life. Identifying the substance, quantity ingested, and time and date of occurrence determines whether the substance was corrosive, the size of the dose, the potential severity of the effect, and whether the substance might still be in the stomach. This information allows emergency management personnel to follow the decision tree used for treating victims of poisoning. Because the substance was corrosive, the next intervention would be to dilute the substance with water or milk, prevent vomiting, hydrate the client, and treat any symptoms present.

Nursing Process:	Analysis
Client Needs Category:	Safe, effective care environment
Cognitive Level:	Application

3. Answer: 2, 4, 5

Rationale: The first food given to the newborn is breast milk or formula. Between the ages of 4 and 6 months, rice cereal can be introduced, followed by pureed or strained fruits and vegetables. Meats must be ground or finely chopped before they are given to an infant to prevent choking. Infants generally are not given whole milk until they reach 1 year of age. Fruit drinks provide fluid but have little nutritional benefit.

Nursing Process:	Implementation
Client Needs Category:	Health promotion and maintenance
Cognitive Level:	Application

ANSWERS TO TRUE OR FALSE QUESTIONS

Items 1 Through 10

1. *True.*
2. *False.* It is best to place *moist* blankets on the threshold to contain smoke.
3. *True.*
4. *True.*
5. *False.* Victims of cold-water drownings are more apt to be resuscitated because of their lowered metabolism, which conserves oxygen, than those who succumb in warm water.
6. *False.* Poisonings are more prevalent in homes than in health care institutions. More often than not, accidental poisonings occur among toddlers and usually involve the ingestion of substances that are located in the bathroom or kitchen. This is not to imply that poisonings never occur in health care institutions. One could consider medication errors in which the wrong medication or dose is administered to the wrong client a form of poisoning.
7. *False.* Educating children is not the only way to prevent childhood poisoning, although it certainly is one component.
8. *True.*
9. *True.*
10. *False.* Among older adults, hospitalizations are twice as lengthy for those who fall when compared to those who do not fall, and about half of those who are hospitalized for falling eventually are transferred to a nursing home.

ANSWERS TO SHORT ANSWER QUESTIONS

Items 1 Through 5

1. Applying a restraint without just cause or a medical order could result in being sued for false imprisonment. Consulting with a doctor or a nursing supervisor helps collaborate that this is the most reasonable action to protect the client.
2. Methods for helping to prevent falls are:
   a. Place adjustable beds in low position when clients may be getting in and out of bed.
   b. Have the client use a sturdy step stool when the bed is high and not adjustable.
   c. Use tub and shower stools and sturdy handrails in bathrooms.
   d. Have clients in wheelchairs use wide doorways, ramps, and elevators so that they are not tempted to try to walk stairways.
3. The risk factors for accidental falls are:
   a. Advancing age
   b. Impaired mobility
   c. Confusion
   d. Diarrhea or urinary frequency
   e. Impaired vision
   f. Sedating medications
   g. Postural hypotension
   h. Weakened state
4. When a fire occurs, the nurse should:
   a. Evacuate the people in the room with the fire.
   b. Close the door to the room with the fire.
   c. Notify the switchboard using the proper code and location for the fire. Do not hang up until the operator repeats the information.
   d. Close all room doors and fire doors.
   e. Turn off oxygen in the vicinity of the fire. Use a manual resuscitation mask for clients who need continuous ventilation.
   f. Place moist towels or bath blankets at the threshold of doors where smoke is leaking.
   g. Use the appropriate fire extinguisher if it is a minor fire.
5. When using a fire extinguisher, the nurse should:
   a. Free the extinguisher from its enclosure.
   b. Remove the pin that locks the handle.
   c. Aim the nozzle near the edge, not the center, of the fire.
   d. Move the nozzle side to side.
   e. Avoid skin contact with the contents of the fire extinguisher.
   f. Return the extinguisher to the maintenance department for replacement or refilling.

Chapter 19

ANSWERS TO MATCHING QUESTIONS

Items 1 Through 5

1. c   2. d   3. b   4. e   5. a

Items 6 Through 10

6. e   7. c   8. a   9. b   10. d

ANSWERS TO MULTIPLE-CHOICE QUESTIONS

Items 1 Through 10

1. (b) Pain perception occurs when the pain threshold is reached. Passing the pain threshold results in awareness of discomfort. Pain thresholds tend to be the same among healthy people, but individuals tolerate pain differently. Pain tolerance is influenced by learned behaviors specific to gender, age, and culture.

2. (a) *Acute pain* is physical discomfort of short duration. Short duration is defined as existing less than 6 months; for most, it is shorter than this. *Chronic pain* is physical discomfort that usually lasts longer than 6 months.

3. (d) *Referred pain* is pain perceived in another location some distance from the body part that is diseased or injured. For example, although heart pain is usually felt in the chest, it may be felt in the arms, neck, and even jaw.

4. (b) The exact nature in which acupuncture and acupressure work has not been definitely determined. The gate-control theory is used by some to explain their effectiveness. Others believe that acupuncture and acupressure may stimulate the production of endogenous opioids, chemicals produced by the body that have pain-relieving qualities.

5. (c) *Biofeedback* consists of a training program that helps a person become aware of certain body changes. The individual then learns to alter these physical responses.

6. (d) A placebo is an inactive substance given as a substitute for drug therapy. Studies have shown that placebos can be effective pain relievers when not used on a continuous basis and when the client has confidence in his health caretakers. It is wrong to assume that a client who has pain relief with placebos is a malingerer or is imagining his or her pain.

7. (c) TENS has several advantages. It is a nonnarcotic, noninvasive agent without toxic effects. It is contraindicated for pregnant individuals because its effect on the unborn has not been determined.

8. (b) The equianalgesic dose would be 30 mg of morphine sulfate by mouth every 3 to 4 hours.

9. (d) The term *equianalgesic* dose of a medication refers to the adjusted oral dose of the medication that provides the same level of relief as the parenteral dose.

10. (b) Nondrug interventions are most likely to be used for clients with chronic pain or for those clients for whom acute pain management techniques are unsuccessful or contraindicated.

ANSWERS TO ALTERNATIVE FORMAT QUESTIONS

1. **Answer: 15**
   Rationale: To convert morphine gr $\frac{1}{4}$ to milligrams, use the following calculations:

   $$1 \text{ mg} = \frac{1}{60} \text{ gr or } 60 \text{ milligrams} = 1 \text{ gr}$$
   $$\text{If } 60 \text{ mg} = 1 \text{ gr}$$
   $$\text{Then } \times \text{ mg} = \frac{1}{4} \text{ gr } (0.25 \text{ gr})$$
   $$\times = \frac{(60 \times 0.25)}{1}$$
   $$\times = 15 \text{ mg}$$

Nursing Process:	Implementation
Client Needs Category:	Physiologic integrity
Cognitive Level:	Analysis

2. **Answer: 0.5**
   Rationale: To calculate the correct dose use the following formula:

   $$\text{Amount to administer (X)} = \frac{\text{desired dose}}{\text{dose on hand}} \times \frac{\text{quantity on}}{\text{hand}}$$
   $$X = \frac{50}{100} \times 1$$
   $$X = .5 \text{ mL}$$

Nursing Process:	Implementation
Client Needs Category:	Physiologic integrity
Cognitive Level:	Analysis

3. **Answer: 2, 3, 4**
   Rationale: Chronic pain is prolonged, usually recurring or persisting over 6 months or longer. It interferes with functioning. Suffering usually increases with time, and the client requires more and more medication to achieve an acceptable pain level. Chronic pain is usually nonspecific, generalized, and unrelated to the healing process.

Nursing Process:	Assessment
Client Needs Category:	Physiological integrity
Cognitive Level:	Application

ANSWERS TO TRUE OR FALSE QUESTIONS

Items 1 Through 12

1. *False.* Pain threshold is the point at which the sensation of pain becomes noticeable. *Pain tolerance* is the ability of the individual to endure pain.

2. *False.* Phantom limb pain is pain that is felt in a missing arm or leg. Discomfort in a location distant from the diseased or injured part of the body is known as *referred pain.*

3. *True.*

4. *False.* Pain has cultural implications. In some cultures, people learn to bear pain bravely and behave as though it is hardly present, even when it is severe. However, a person from another culture may learn to express emotions and to show great concern and anxiety about pain.

5. *True.*

6. *False.* The body does not adapt to pain as it does to heat, cold, noise, and odors.

7. *True.*

8. *False.* Client-controlled analgesia infusers are used in hospitals primarily to relieve acute pain following surgery.

9. *False.* The initial dose is slightly higher to establish an acceptable serum level of the drug and provide reduction in pain.

10. *True.*

11. *True.*

12. *True.*

ANSWER TO SHORT ANSWER QUESTIONS

Items 1 Through 2

1. The advantages to both the client and the nurse when a client-controlled analgesia is used are:

a. Pain relief is rapidly experienced because the drug is delivered directly into the bloodstream.
b. Pain is maintained within a constant tolerable level.
c. Less total drug is actually used because small doses continuously control the pain.
d. The client avoids the additional discomfort of multiple injections into muscle or subcutaneous tissue.
e. Anxiety is reduced because the client's pain does not intensify while waiting for the nurse to administer medication.
f. Drug side effects, such as sedation and respiratory depression, are avoided with lower doses.
g. Complications associated with immobility, such as blood clots and pneumonia, are reduced because the client ambulates or moves about more.
h. The client takes an active role in his or her treatment.
i. The client's sense of control and independence is preserved.
j. Use of a PCA infuser frees the nurse to carry out other adjunctive pain-relieving measures.

2. Five components of pain assessment are:
a. Onset or the time or circumstances under which pain became apparent
b. Quality or the degree of suffering
c. Intensity or the magnitude of the pain
d. Location or the anatomical site
e. Duration or the amount of time the pain lasts

Chapter 20

ANSWERS TO MATCHING QUESTIONS

Items 1 Through 10

1. d	2. e	3. h	4. a	5. j	6. g
7. c	8. i	9. f	10. b		

Items 11 Through 14

11. d	12. c	13. a	14. b

ANSWERS TO MULTIPLE-CHOICE QUESTIONS

Items 1 Through 10

1. (a) The client's responses to oxygen therapy are most accurately determined by pulse oximetry. Observations of the client are also important for judging responses prior to and concurrent with oxygen therapy.
2. (b) Oxygen becomes progressively toxic at high concentrations. Signs of oxygen toxicity include a dry cough, which may eventually become moist as lung damage occurs; chest pain felt beneath the sternum; nasal stuffiness; nausea and vomiting; and restlessness.
3. (d) An oxygen tank should be cracked before the humidifier and gauge are attached. To *crack* a tank means to briefly open the valve and release oxygen to clear the outlet of dust and other debris.

4. (a) If the client has a chronic lung ailment, 2 to 3 liters per minute are prescribed.
5. (c) For a client with a chronic lung condition, high levels of oxygen may decrease or even stop respirations because his or her body is accustomed to higher-than-normal carbon dioxide levels. If the chronically high carbon dioxide level falls too low, it no longer acts as one of the normal stimulants of respirations.
6. (d) The Venturi mask allows air to enter the mask and exhaled carbon dioxide to leave the mask at special ports. It can supply up to 40% oxygen.
7. (a) The lung collapses because of the loss of negative pressure within the pleural space. The atmospheric air, which is higher in pressure, moves into and remains within the pleural space. The lung is no longer able to completely expand during each inhalation.
8. (d) The water-seal drainage system is designed to prevent atmospheric air from reentering the pleural space by partially filling one of the chambers in the drainage device with water. As the air and blood drain from the pleural space via the catheters, the lung will gradually reexpand.
9. (b) Because oxygen is being delivered constantly to the lower airway, clients with transtracheal oxygen usually achieve adequate oxygenation with lower liter flows.
10. (c) Oxygen is drying to the mucous membranes. Therefore, oxygen is humidified, in most cases, when 4L/min is administered for an extended period of time.

ANSWERS TO ALTERNATIVE FORMAT QUESTIONS

1. **Answer: 1, 3, 5, 6**
Rationale: Pneumothorax is air in the pleural space. Signs and symptoms include chest pain, dyspnea, shoulder or neck pain, irritability, palpitations, light-headedness, hypotension, cyanosis, and unequal breath sounds. A chest x-ray will reveal the collapse of the affected lung.

Nursing Process:	Analysis
Client Needs Category:	Physiological integrity
Cognitive Level:	Analysis

2. **Answer: 1, 3, 4**
Rationale: Among the common therapies used to treat pulmonary hypertension are oxygen, diuretics, and vasodilators. Additional therapies may include fluid restriction, digoxin, calcium channel blockers, beta-adrenergic blockers, and bronchodilators. Aminoglycosides and sulfonamides are antibiotics used to treat infections, if present. Antihistamines are indicated for allergies, pruritus, vertigo, nausea, vomiting, and cough suppression.

Nursing Process:	Implementation
Client Needs Category:	Physiological integrity
Cognitive Level:	Analysis

3. **Answer: 2, 3, 5**
   Rationale: Typical assessment findings for clients with COPD include dyspnea on exertion, a barrel chest, and clubbed fingers and toes. Clients with COPD usually have an increased respiratory rate with a prolonged expiratory phase. Unless an infection is present, fever is not associated with COPD.

Nursing Process:	Assessment
Client Needs Category:	Physiological integrity
Cognitive Level:	Application

ANSWERS TO TRUE OR FALSE QUESTIONS

Items 1 Through 10

1. *False. Hypoxia* is defined as a deficiency in the amount of oxygen in inspired air; it is also a term that has come to mean a condition in which cells and tissues are receiving an inadequate supply of oxygen. *Hypoxemia* is a condition in which there is a less-than-adequate level of oxygen in the blood.
2. *False.* Oxygen supports combustion but is not flammable.
3. *False.* A nonrebreathing mask, which provides the client with the highest concentration of oxygen, is most often used for persons suffering with smoke inhalation or carbon monoxide poisoning.
4. *False.* Lung collapse is caused by the loss of negative pressure within the pleural space. The atmospheric air, which is higher in pressure, moves into and remains within the pleural space, and the lung can no longer completely expand during each inhalation.
5. *True.*
6. *False.* Do not empty the water-seal drainage collection container routinely. Emptying the collection chamber increases the risk that air will enter the pleural space when the equipment is disconnected.
7. *True.*
8. *False.* An advantage of the nasal cannula is that it does not interfere with eating, drinking, or talking.
9. *False.* The respiratory center of clients with chronic pulmonary diseases adapt to elevated levels of carbon dioxide in the blood. The stimulus to breathe comes from sensing a low level of oxygen. If high percentages of oxygen are administered to chronic lung disease clients, respirations slow and the client may even stop breathing.
10. *True.*

ANSWERS TO SHORT ANSWER QUESTIONS

Items 1 Through 5

1. Nursing guidelines for the safe use of oxygen are as follows:
   a. Post "Oxygen in Use" signs whenever oxygen is stored or in use.
   b. Prohibit the burning of candles during religious rites.
   c. Check that electrical devices have three-pronged plugs.
   d. Inspect electrical equipment for the presence of frayed wires or loose connections.
   e. Avoid petroleum products, aerosol products like hair spray, and products containing acetone like nail polish remover where oxygen is used.
   f. Secure portable cylinders to rigid stands.
2. Common signs of inadequate oxygenation are:
   a. Restlessness
   b. Rapid, shallow breathing
   c. Rapid heart rate
   d. Sitting up to breathe
   e. Nasal flaring
   f. Use of accessory muscles
   g. Hypertension
   h. Confusion, stupor, coma
   i. Cyanosis of the skin, lips, and nail beds
3. Evaluation components are as follows:
   a. Respiratory rate is 12 to 24 breaths per minute at rest.
   b. Breathing is effortless.
   c. Heart rate is <100 bpm
   d. The client is alert and oriented.
   e. Skin and mucous membranes are normal color.
   f. SaO_2 is $\geq 90\%$.
   g. FIO_2 and the delivery device correspond to the medical order.
4. Actions taken when administering oxygen from a tank include:
   a. Being sure the tank contains oxygen and not some other gas.
   b. Cracking the tank to remove dust and debris before attaching the gauges.
   c. Attaching a humidifier to the tank and filling it with water.
   d. Stabilizing the tank at the bedside on a rigid standard with belts.
5. Methods of administering oxygen include:
   a. Nasal catheter
   b. Nasal cannula
   c. Various masks
   d. Tent
   e. Into a tracheostomy

Chapter 21

ANSWERS TO MATCHING QUESTIONS

Items 1 through 5
1. c	2. e	3. b	4. a	5. d

Items 6 through 10
6. d	7. b	8. e	9. a	10. c

ANSWERS TO MULTIPLE-CHOICE QUESTIONS

Items 1 Through 16

1. (a) Microorganisms, or what most people call germs, are everywhere, but they cannot be seen without a microscope. Many are harmless; they are called

nonpathogens. Those that cause infections or contagious diseases are called *pathogens.*

2. (c) Following generations of reproduction, many microorganisms have gradually changed. One example of an adaptive change is the ability to become spore forming.

3. (d) The port of entry is the part of the body where organisms enter. Examples include any break in the skin or mucous membranes, mouth, nose, and genitourinary tract.

4. (b) The vehicle of transmission is the means by which organisms are carried about. Examples include hands, equipment (e.g., bedpan), instruments, china and silverware, linen, and droplets.

5. (b) Soaps and detergents can be considered antimicrobial agents. An antimicrobial agent is a chemical that kills or suppresses the growth or reproduction of microorganisms.

6. (a) *Antiseptics* are chemical agents used to reduce the growth of microorganisms on living tissue. This category of antiinfective agents only prevents or inhibits the growth and reproduction of microorganisms. They do not completely destroy all microbes; therefore, their use is not a form of sterilization.

7. (c) A *disinfectant* is a bactericidal substance. A bactericide is a substance that is capable of destroying or killing microorganisms, but not necessarily spores. These antimicrobials are not intended for use on people.

8. (d) Nosocomial infections are infections acquired after being admitted to a health care agency.

9. (d) Hand washing is the most frequently used medical aseptic practice in health care agencies. It is the most effective way to prevent nosocomial infections.

10. (b) The care given to cleaning contaminated supplies and equipment throughout the time a person is a client in a health care agency is called *concurrent disinfection.* When the client is discharged, all the contaminated supplies and equipment are cleaned a final time in order to get them ready for use by another client. This is called *terminal disinfection.*

11. (c) Dry heat, or hot-air sterilization, uses equipment similar to a home baking oven. It is a good way to sterilize sharp instruments and reusable syringes because moist heat damages cutting edges and the ground surfaces of glass.

12. (c) Surgical asepsis is based on the underlying principle that equipment and areas that are free of microorganisms must be protected from contamination.

13. (a) A sterile field is a work area that is free of microorganisms. The inner surface of a wrapper that holds sterilized equipment is often used as a sterile field much like a tablecloth would be used. The nurse must open the sterile package in such a way as to keep the inside of the wrapper and its contents sterile. This may be done by positioning the wrapped package so that the outermost triangular edge can be moved away from the nurse.

14. (c) A sterile package should be opened by unfolding the wrapper on the far side of the package first and the nearest side last. The risk of contamination is increased by reaching over a sterile area.

15. (b) Opened wrappers are considered sterile within 1 inch of the edge. The sterile margin of a peeled package is its inner edge.

16. (b) Talking, coughing, and sneezing over a sterile area must be avoided. Microorganisms are present in the moisture from respiratory secretions. These droplets can fall onto sterile areas, causing contamination.

ANSWERS TO ALTERNATIVE FORMAT QUESTIONS

1. **Answer: 6, 1, 5, 2, 3, 4**
   Rationale: Turn on water and dispense the paper towel before washing hands to prevent contamination of clean hands. Rinse the bar soap before lathering to prevent transfer of microorganisms from wet bar soap sitting in a container to hands. Lather hands with soap and rub them together to create friction to loosen microorganisms. Rinse hands under running water from wrists to fingers to avoid transferring microbes to cleaner areas. Dry hands well. Use clean, dry paper towel to turn off faucet and avoid recontaminating hands.

Nursing Process:	Implementation
Client Needs Category:	Safe, effective care environment
Cognitive Level:	Application

2. **Answer: 1, 4, 5**
   Rationale: A discussion that provides accurate information in response to the client's concerns increases the client's knowledge and helps to decrease anxiety. The incubation period for hepatitis A is 25 to 30 days. Keeping her out of school is not appropriate. The mode of transmission for hepatitis A is from the stool of an infected person to the oral route of a susceptible person. Signs and symptoms include low-grade fever, loss of appetite, dark urine, and yellowing of the skin and sclera. Hand washing is an excellent preventive measure when done after using the toilet and before eating. Demonstrate this for the mother who can then teach her daughter. Temporary passive immunity can be gained from an injection of immune serum globulin when exposed to hepatitis A.

Nursing Process:	Implementation
Client Needs Category:	Health promotion and maintenance
Cognitive Level:	Application

3. **Answer: 1, 2, 4, 5**
   Rationale: Masks cover the nose and mouth and help prevent the spread of microorganisms by droplet and

airborne transmission. Particulate filter respirators are used by health care personnel caring for clients with tuberculosis. The minimum specification for this type of mask is N95. It is effective in blocking particulate aerosols that are free of oil. These masks must bear a label indicating approval by the National Institute for Occupational Safety and Health (NIOSH). They are custom fitted for each person to obtain a face-seal leakage of less than 10%. They must be refitted if the user gains or loses 10 pounds. Although they are disposable, they may be reused. Used particulate filter respirators are discarded in a waterproof container.

Nursing Process:	Implementation
Client Needs Category:	Safe, effective care environment
Cognitive Level:	Application

ANSWERS TO TRUE OR FALSE QUESTIONS

Items 1 Through 10

1. *False.* A microbe that requires free oxygen in order to exist is called an *aerobic microorganism.* Anaerobic microorganisms depend on an environment without oxygen for survival.
2. *True.*
3. *True.*
4. *False.* The *reservoir* is a place on which or in which microorganisms grow and reproduce. A person or animal on which or in which microorganisms live is called the *host.*
5. *False.* Medical asepsis (clean technique) refers to the practices that help confine or reduce the number of microorganisms, especially pathogens.
6. *False.* Hand washing is the single most effective way to prevent nosocomial infections.
7. *False.* Antibiotics have saved many clients' lives. However, they are only useful in reducing or destroying the growth of bacteria, one type of microorganism. Even so, not *all* bacteria are affected by all antibiotics.
8. *False.* Rinse items first under *cool,* running water. Hot water causes many substances to coagulate (that is to thicken or congeal), making them difficult to remove.
9. *True.*
10. *False.* Objects may be soaked in a 70% solution of ethyl alcohol for 10 to 20 minutes. This is *not* considered a reliable sterilization method; its action should be regarded more as that of an antimicrobial agent.

ANSWERS TO SHORT ANSWER QUESTIONS

Items 1 Through 5

1. The conditions most microorganisms need to grow and survive are:
   a. Warmth
   b. Air
   c. Water
   d. Darkness
   e. Nourishment

2. The factors that can result in reduced resistance to the entry of disease-causing organisms are:
   a. Poor nutrition
   b. Poor personal hygiene
   c. Broken skin or mucous membranes
   d. Aging
   e. Illness
   f. Suppressed immune system
3. The guidelines for safe and effective practices of medical asepsis when soap or detergents and water are used to clean supplies and equipment are:
   a. Wear waterproof gloves if items are heavily contaminated.
   b. Disassemble equipment immediately after use.
   c. Rinse items first under cool, running water.
   d. Rinse catheters and rectal tubes immediately after use to remove lubricant or body excretions.
   e. Use water and soap or detergent for cleaning purposes.
   f. Use a brush with stiff bristles to loosen dirt as necessary.
   g. Force sudsy water through the openings of reusable needles and other hollow channels.
   h. Rinse items well under running water after cleaning with soap or detergent and water.
   i. Air-dry equipment.
   j. Treat gloves, brushes, sponges, cleaning cloths, and water used for cleaning as reservoirs for microorganisms.
   k. Avoid splashing or spilling water on yourself or on the floor or other equipment during the entire procedure.
   l. Consider hands heavily contaminated after cleaning equipment. Even when wearing gloves during cleaning, hand washing should be performed.
4. The body is capable of producing additional specialized cells and chemicals that are responsible for inhibiting the growth and spread of microorganisms. Biologic defense mechanisms are anatomic or physiologic methods that stop microorganisms from causing an infectious disease. Mechanical defense mechanisms are physical barriers such as intact skin, coughing, sneezing, or vomiting that prevent microorganisms from entering the body or expel them before they multiply. Chemical defense mechanisms include enzymes, gastric acid, and antibodies that destroy or incapacitate microorganisms.
5. Hand washing should be performed:
   a. When arriving and leaving work
   b. Before and after contact with each client
   c. Before and after equipment is handled
   d. Before and after gloving
   e. Before and after specimens are collected
   f. Before preparing medications
   g. Before serving trays or feeding clients
   h. Before eating
   i. After toileting, hair combing, or other hygienic practices
   j. After cleaning a work area

Chapter 22

ANSWERS TO MATCHING QUESTIONS
Items 1 Through 5

1. d   2. e   3. a   4. c   5. b

ANSWERS TO MULTIPLE-CHOICE QUESTIONS
Items 1 Through 10

1. (a) An *infection* is a condition that results when microorganisms cause injury to their host.
2. (c) Infection control refers to physical measures that attempt to curtail the spread of infectious or contagious diseases.
3. (c) Hand washing is the single most effective means of preventing the spread of microorganisms.
4. (a) Gloves are required when an infectious disease is transmissible by direct contact or contact with blood or body substances.
5. (d) Standard precautions are infection-control measures to be used when caring for all clients in hospitals, regardless of their infectious status. Standard precautions combine what were previously referred to as "universal precautions and body substance isolation."
6. (c) To control the spread of most communicable diseases in a health agency, the client is placed in a private room. In this way, no other client is in direct contact with the infected or susceptible person.
7. (b) Rubella is an example of a disease requiring droplet precautions.
8. (a) Diarrhea is an example of a disease requiring contact precautions.
9. (b) Tuberculosis is an example of a disease requiring airborne precautions.
10. (b) The current list of body fluids with the potential for containing these infectious viruses includes blood and all body fluids except sweat.

ANSWERS TO ALTERNATIVE FORMAT QUESTIONS

1. **Answer: 4, 5**
   Rationale: Standard precautions include wearing gloves for any known or anticipated contact with blood, body fluids, tissue, mucous membranes, or skin that is not intact. If the task may result in splashing or splattering of blood or body fluids to the face, a mask and goggles or face shield should be worn. If the task may result in blood or body fluids to the body, a fluid-resistant gown or apron should be worn. Hands should be washed before and after client care and after removing gloves. A gown, mask, and gloves aren't necessary for client care unless contact with body fluids, tissue, mucous membranes, or skin that is not intact is expected. Nurses have an increased, not decreased, risk of occupational exposure to blood-borne pathogens. HIV isn't transmitted in sputum unless blood is present.

Nursing Process:	Implementation
Client Needs Category:	Safe, effective care environment
Cognitive Level:	Application

2. **Answer: 3, 2, 6, 1, 5, 4**
   Rationale: To remove soiled personal protective equipment, properly untie the waist tie if the gown is tied in front at the waist. Remove soiled gloves and wash your hands. Remove the soiled mask, touching only the ties. Then, remove the soiled gown by grasping it along the inside of the neck and pulling it down off the shoulders, rolling it up with the soiled part inside the roll. Finally, remove the protective eyewear. Discard all equipment in the appropriate receptacle. Wash your hands. Apply lotion. Removing garments in this order ensures that the most contaminated items are removed without contaminating the health care worker.

Nursing Process:	Implementation
Client Needs Category:	Safe, effective care environment
Cognitive Level:	Analysis

3. **Answer: 2, 4, 5**
   Rationale: A parent can assess infection-control measures by appraising steps taken by the facility to prevent the spread of potential diseases. Placing diapers in covered receptacles, covering the diaper-changing tables with disposable papers, and ensuring that there are available sinks for personnel to wash their hands after activities are all indicators that infection-control measures are being followed. Gloves should be readily available to personnel and should be kept in every room—not an office. Toys typically are shared by numerous children; however, this contributes to the spread of germs and infections. All soiled clothing and cloth diapers should be placed in sealed plastic bags prior to being sent home.

Nursing Process:	Implementation
Client Needs Category:	Safe, effective care environment
Cognitive Level:	Application

ANSWERS TO TRUE OR FALSE QUESTIONS
Items 1 Through 10

1. *False.* In the most recent guidelines from the CDC in 1996, two major categories of infection-control practices were recommended. They are standard precautions and transmission-based precautions. Standard precautions combine universal precautions and body substance isolation. Transmission-based precautions replace the previous categories, referred to as STRICT Isolation, CONTACT Isolation, RESPIRATORY Isolation, TUBERCULOSIS Isolation, ENTERIC Precautions, and DRAINAGE/SECRETION Precautions. The new transmission-based precaution categories are Airborne, Droplet, and Contact precautions.

2. *True.*
3. *True.*
4. *False.* Droplet spread is the physical transfer of microorganisms between material released from the nose and mouth of an infected person when he or she coughs, sneezes, and talks and a susceptible host.
5. *True.*
6. *True.*
7. *True.*
8. *False.* Gloves do not provide a total and complete barrier to microorganisms. Leakage occurs approximately 2% of the time and increases with the stress of their use.
9. *True.*
10. *False.* Hepatitis B is only one of several diseases that can be spread by blood. So regardless of having received the vaccine, whenever there is a possibility for contact with blood or body fluids that can potentially spread blood-borne viruses, gloves should be worn.

ANSWERS TO SHORT ANSWER QUESTIONS

Items 1 and 2

1. Standard precautions include the following:
   a. Wear gloves when touching blood, body fluids, secretions, excretions, mucous membranes, and skin that is not intact.
   b. Perform hand washing immediately when there is direct contact with blood, body fluids, secretions, excretions, and contaminated items; after removing gloves; and between client contacts.
   c. Wear a mask and eye protection or a face shield when there is chance of splashes or sprays of blood, body fluids, secretions, and excretions.
   d. Wear a cover gown when there is a chance of sprays or splashing clothing with blood, body fluids, secretions, and excretions.
   e. Remove soiled protective items promptly when potential contact with pathogens is no longer present.
   f. Clean and reprocess all equipment before reuse.
   g. Discard all single-use items in appropriate containers.
   h. Handle, transport, and process soiled linen in a manner that prevents contamination of self, others, and the environment.
   i. Prevent injury with used sharp devices by handling them appropriately.
   j. Place clients who contaminate the environment and cannot or do not assist with appropriate hygiene or environmental cleanliness in a private room.
2. Methods of contracting AIDS are:
   a. Contact with the blood, semen, or vaginal secretions of an HIV-infected person during unprotected vaginal, anal, or oral sexual intercourse
   b. Contact with the blood, semen, or vaginal secretions of an HIV-infected person during medical, dental, and nursing procedures in which these fluids enter through an open cut or splash into a caregiver's eyes or nose
   c. Contact with the blood of an HIV-infected person by sharing needles, receiving a transfusion of contaminated blood or blood cell components, receiving plasma or clotting factors that have not been heat-treated, and being exposed to contaminated ear-piercing or tattooing equipment
   d. Transmission by an infected pregnant woman to an infant during pregnancy, at birth, and while breast-feeding

Chapter 23

ANSWERS TO MATCHING QUESTIONS

Items 1 Through 5

1. b   2. f   3. d   4. e   5. c

Items 6 Through 11

6. e   7. g   8. b   9. f   10. a   11. d

ANSWERS TO MULTIPLE-CHOICE QUESTIONS

Items 1 Through 14

1. (c) Muscle weakness, atelectasis, and contractures are some of the many problems related to disuse syndrome.
2. (b) Footdrop is a type of contracture that results from prolonged plantar flexion, lack of movement of the ankle joint, and shortening of muscles at the back of the calf.
3. (b) *Posture* refers to the position of the body or the way in which it is held.
4. (b) Keep the feet parallel and about 10 to 20 cm (4 to 8 inches) apart when in a standing position to give the body a wide base of support.
5. (a) Body mechanics is the efficient use of the body as a machine. Using good body mechanics is as important for the nurse as it is for others. Basic principles of body mechanics can be applied regardless of the worker or the task.
6. (c) Use the longest and strongest muscles to provide the energy needed for a task. It is best to use the long and strong muscles in the arms, legs, and hips whenever possible. Small and weaker muscles will strain and injure quickly if forced to work beyond their ability. One of the most common injuries affects the muscles in the lower part of the back. It is a painful injury and usually slow to heal, but it is preventable when proper body mechanics are used.
7. (b) Push, pull, or roll objects whenever possible, rather than lift them. It takes more effort to lift something against the force of gravity. Use body weight as a lever to assist with pushing or pulling an object. This reduces the strain placed on a group of muscles.
8. (a) Stretching and twisting will fatigue muscles quickly. When stretching or twisting, balance will

be poor as the line of gravity falls outside the base of support.

9. (a) An inactive client's position should be changed at least every 2 hours and more frequently if any signs or symptoms of the disuse syndrome have been assessed.

10. (a) A turning sheet is a helpful positioning device. The sheet extends from the upper back to the thighs.

11. (d) Foam acts almost like a layer of subcutaneous tissue. Foam contains channels and cells filled with air. This allows some evaporation of moisture and escape of heat, which reduces the potential for skin breakdown.

12. (c) There are two primary concerns when using the supine position. One concern is pressure on the back of the body where pressure sores commonly develop, especially in the area at the end of the spine. The second is toe pressure from linens, which, when combined with gravity, forces the feet into the footdrop position.

13. (b) The primary concern when using the lateral position is if the upper shoulder and arm are allowed to rotate forward and out of alignment. This tends to interfere with proper breathing.

14. (b) High Fowler's position is especially helpful to clients with dyspnea. It causes abdominal organs to drop away from the diaphragm, relieving pressure on the chest cavity.

ANSWERS TO ALTERNATIVE FORMAT QUESTIONS

1. **Answer: 45**
Rationale: By definition, the semi-Fowler's position elevates the head and torso of a bedridden client 45 degrees. The knees may or may not be elevated, but doing so relieves strain on the lower spine.

Nursing Process:	Implementation
Client Needs Category:	Physiological integrity
Cognitive Level:	Application

2. **Answer: 1, 2, 3, 4, 5**
Rationale: Mechanical lifts are used primarily for clients who cannot help themselves or are too heavy for others to lift safely. Both electric and hydraulic lifts are available for use, with a lifting capacity of 350 to 600 pounds. Agency policy usually recommends that two nurses operate the lift. The seat of a lift is a one- or two-piece canvas sling that supports the back, hips, and thighs during movement. Nurses should also be aware of the anxiety a client may experience while being transferred in this manner and take appropriate steps to reassure the client. Nurses are also responsible for ensuring that the lift and its parts are in good working order prior to each use.

Nursing Process:	Planning
Client Needs Category:	Safe, effective care environment
Cognitive Level:	Application

3. **Answer: 1, 3, 4**
Rationale: The prone position places the client on the abdomen. It provides an alternative for the person with skin breakdown from pressure ulcers. The prone position also provides good drainage from the bronchioles, stretches the trunk and extremities, and keeps the hips in the extended position. The prone position improves arterial oxygenation in critically ill clients with adult respiratory distress syndrome and others who are mechanically ventilated. The prone position poses a challenge for assessing and communicating with clients and is uncomfortable for clients with recent abdominal surgery or back pain. The supine position creates a potential for footdrop. The lateral oblique position produces less pressure on the hip.

Nursing Process:	Application
Client Needs Category:	Physiological integrity
Cognitive Level:	Analysis

ANSWERS TO TRUE OR FALSE QUESTIONS
Items 1 Through 10

1. *False.* Good posture when in the standing position includes holding the head erect with the face forward and with the chin slightly tucked.

2. *False.* It is important to have good posture when lying down. The muscles are in a state of relaxation when resting or sleeping. Unless the parts of the body are properly supported, the body will respond to gravity and fall out of alignment. Poor alignment makes it difficult for the body to function effectively.

3. *True.*

4. *False.* Egg-crate mattresses provide minimal pressure reduction and are often used for comfort only. Thicker waffle-shaped foams offer greater pressure reduction and can be used for preventing skin breakdown.

5. *False.* Trochanter rolls are placed along the outside of the client's thighs at the trochanter region of the femur to prevent outward rotation of the legs.

6. *True.*

7. *False.* When transferring a client from the bed to the chair, the nurse should place the chair alongside the bed on the client's stronger side.

8. *True.*

9. *True.*

10. *True.*

ANSWERS TO SHORT ANSWER QUESTIONS

Items 1 Through 5

1. Characteristics of good posture are:
   a. Standing:
      1. Keep the feet parallel.
      2. Distribute weight equally on both feet to provide a broad base of support.
   b. Sitting:
      1. The buttocks and upper thighs are the base of support.
      2. Both feet rest on the floor.
   c. Lying:
      1. Lying looks the same as standing but in a horizontal position.
      2. Body parts are in a neutral position.
2. Principles of correct body mechanics are:
   a. Distribute gravity through the center of body over a wide base of support.
   b. Push, pull, or roll objects rather than lift them.
   c. Hold objects close to the body.
3. Five positioning devices and the purpose of each are as follows:
   a. Adjustable beds allow the position of the head and knees to be changed.
   b. Pillows provide support and elevate body parts.
   c. Trochanter rolls prevent legs from turning outward.
   d. Hand rolls maintain functional use of the hand and prevent contractures.
   e. Foot boards keep the feet in a normal walking position.
4. Three pressure-relieving devices and an advantage of each are as follows:
   a. Side rails aid clients in changing their own positions.
   b. Mattress overlays reduce pressure and restore skin integrity.
   c. Foot cradles keep linens off the client's feet or legs.
5. Five measures to prevent inactivity in older adults include the following:
   a. Balance periods of activity with periods of rest.
   b. Allow adequate time for performing activities.
   c. Develop hobbies or recreational interests.
   d. Investigate local support groups.
   e. Prevent injury by removing any objects that pose a safety hazard.

Chapter 24

ANSWERS TO MATCHING QUESTIONS

Items 1 Through 11

1. f	2. k	3. h	4. c	5. j	6. i
7. b	8. e	9. a	10. g	11. d	

ANSWERS TO MULTIPLE-CHOICE QUESTIONS

Items 1 Through 10

1. (c) Exercise is the movement intended to increase strength, stamina, and overall body tone.
2. (a) The preferred type of exercise is *active exercise*. People who are ill may need the assistance of another to move. This type of exercise is known as *passive exercise*.
3. (c) *Isometric exercises* involve contracting and relaxing muscle groups with little, if any, movement. These exercises increase the mass and definition of skeletal muscles, but they do not increase the capacity of the heart and lungs to perform.
4. (c) The formula for computing the target heart rate is 220 minus the person's age multiplied by 60% = target heart rate.
5. (a) *Isotonic exercise* is that which involves movement and work. One of the best examples is aerobic exercise. *Aerobic exercise* involves rhythmically moving all parts of the body at a moderate to slow speed without impeding the ability to breathe.
6. (c) Isometric exercise refers to stationary exercises that tend to be performed against a resistive force.
7. (c) The nursing diagnosis Unilateral Neglect is defined by NANDA as a state in which an individual is perceptually unaware of and inattentive to one side of the body.
8. (b) A submaximal fitness test is an exercise test that does not stress a person to exhaustion.
9. (c) The term *body composition* refers to the amount of body tissue that is lean versus that which is fat.
10. (d) Range-of-motion exercises describe therapeutic activity in which joints are moved in the positions that the joints normally permit.

ANSWERS TO ALTERNATIVE FORMAT QUESTIONS

1. **Answer: 99**
   Rationale: Target heart means the goal for heart rate during exercise. It is calculated by first calculating the person's maximum heart rate (the highest limit for heart rate during exercise). The target heart rate is 60% to 90% of the maximum heart rate. Beginners should not exceed 60%.

   Maximum heart rate is calculated by subtracting the person's age from 220.

   Maximum heart rate = 220 − 55

   Maximum heart rate = 165

   Then   Target heart rate = 165 × .60

              Target heart rate = 99

Nursing Process:	Planning
Client Needs Category:	Health promotion and maintenance
Cognitive Level:	Application

2. **Answer: 75**
Rationale: Use the following formulate:

$$\text{Recovery index} = \frac{(100 \times \text{test duration in seconds})}{2(p1 + p2 + p3)}$$

$$= \frac{100 \times 180}{2 \times (45 + 40 + 35)}$$

$$= \frac{18000}{2 \times (120)}$$

$$= \frac{18000}{480}$$

$$= 75$$

Nursing Process:	Evaluation
Client Needs Category:	Physiologic integrity
Cognitive Level:	Analysis

3. **Answer: 2**
Rationale: The walk-a-mile test measures the time it takes a person to walk 1 mile. The person is instructed to walk 1 mile on a flat surface as fast as possible. The examiner then calculates the time from start to finish and interprets the results in terms of fitness level and energy used. A female who walks 1 mile on a flat surface in 10 minutes has a good fitness level. The value of activity (MET) for this test is 2.

Nursing Process:	Assessment
Client Needs Category:	Health promotion and maintenance
Cognitive Level:	Application

ANSWERS TO TRUE OR FALSE QUESTIONS

Items 1 Through 15

1. *True.*
2. *True.*
3. *True.*
4. *True.*
5. *False.* Athletes generally have low pulse rates, but their cells are adequately oxygenated. Any muscle that is exercised increases in tone. Therefore, because the heart is a muscle, exercise increases its tone and it will be able to pump more blood with less effort.
6. *False.* The amount of movement that is possible in a joint is known as *range of motion*. The range that is available in each joint is referred to as its flexibility.
7. *False.* One of the chief minerals that allows bones to be strong and compact is calcium.
8. *True.*
9. *True.*
10. *False.* A stress electrocardiogram is done during exercise and records the activity of the heart while the client walks on a treadmill that moves at a progressively faster pace.
11. *True.*
12. *True.*
13. *False.* According to the National Strategies for Improving Physical Fitness, children should be involved in activities that may be readily carried into adulthood.

14. *True.*
15. *True.*

ANSWERS TO SHORT ANSWER QUESTIONS
Items 1 Through 3

1. Guidelines for assisting with range-of-motion exercises are:
   a. Use good body mechanics.
   b. Remove pillows and other positioning devices.
   c. Position the client to facilitate moving a joint through all of its usual positions.
   d. Follow a pattern; for example, begin at the head and move toward the feet.
   e. Perform similar movements with each extremity.
   f. Support the joint being exercised.
   g. Move each joint until there is resistance but not pain.
   h. Watch for nonverbal communication.
   i. Avoid exercising a painful joint.
   j. Stop if spasticity develops.
   k. Apply gentle pressure to the muscle or move the joint more slowly.
   l. Expect that the client's vital signs will increase during exercise but return to resting rate.
   m. Teach the family to perform range-of-motion exercises.
2. Five benefits of physical exercise are:
   a. Improved cardiopulmonary function
   b. Reduced blood pressure
   c. Increased muscle tone and strength
   d. Greater physical endurance
   e. Increased lean mass and weight loss
   f. Reduced glucose levels
   g. Decreased low-density blood lipids
   h. Improved physical appearance
   i. Increased bone density
   j. Regularity of bowel elimination
   k. Promotion of sleep
   l. Reduced tension and depression
3. Activities necessary for client teaching in order to develop a safe exercise program are:
   a. Seek a preexercise fitness evaluation.
   b. Identify activities within the prescribed level of METs.
   c. Choose a form of exercise that seems pleasurable and involves as many muscle groups as possible.
   d. Plan 3 days of exercise per week at a convenient time of day.
   e. Exercise with a partner for safety and motivational purposes.
   f. Avoid exercising in extreme weather conditions, such as during high humidity or smog.
   g. Dress in layers according to the temperature and weather conditions.
   h. Purchase supportive footwear.
   i. Wear reflective clothing when on the roadside.
   j. Walk or jog against traffic; cycle in the same direction as traffic.

k. Eat complex carbohydrates (pasta, rice, cooked cereal) rather than fasting or eating simple sugars (cookies, chocolate, sweetened drinks).
l. Avoid drinking alcohol, which dilates the blood vessels, promotes heat loss, and interferes with good judgment.
m. Calculate the target heart rate (maximum heart rate multiplied by 60%).
n. Warm up for 5 minutes by stretching muscle groups or doing light calisthenics.
o. Monitor the heart rate two or three times while exercising.
p. Slow down the pace if the heart rate exceeds the preestablished target.
q. Try to sustain the target heart rate for at least 20 minutes.
r. Never stop exercising abruptly.
s. Cool down for at least 5 minutes in a manner similar to the warm-up.

Chapter 25

ANSWERS TO MATCHING QUESTIONS
Items 1 through 6

1. c   2. e   3. f   4. b   5. a   6. d

ANSWERS TO MULTIPLE-CHOICE QUESTIONS
Items 1 Through 10

1. (d) Orthoses are orthopedic devices that support or align a body part and prevent or correct deformities.
2. (c) A cervical collar is a foam or rigid splint around the neck. It is used to treat athletic neck injuries or other trauma that results in a neck strain or sprain.
3. (c) Apply the splinting device so that it spans the injured area from the joint above the injury to beyond the joint below the injury. For instance, if the lower leg has been injured, the splint should be long enough to restrict movement of the knee and ankle.
4. (c) A triangular sling used to support the arm is applied as follows:
   Place the open triangle on the client's chest with the base of the triangle along the length of the client's chest on the unaffected side.
   Place the upper end of the base of the triangle around the back of the neck on the unaffected side.
   Place the apex or point of the triangle under the affected elbow.
   Place the lower end of the base of the triangle across the affected arm.
   Tie the two ends of the base of a triangle in a knot at the side of the neck.
   Be sure the hand is higher than the elbow in the sling to prevent swelling in the hand.
   Fold and secure the material on the affected side neatly. A pin may be used, behind the sling so that it is out of sight, to secure the material.
5. (a) Plaster casts may remain wet for 24 to 48 hours, depending on the level of humidity in the air.
6. (d) Ordinarily, the air circulation in the room is adequate for drying the layers of plaster.
7. (b) Because most casts are applied after an injury and surgical procedure, the nurse may expect that the area will swell and bleed. The extent of swelling and bleeding are the two immediate problems with which the nurse must be concerned. Swelling is especially serious because the cast is rigid and will not expand as the area within the cast becomes larger. The cast can create a tourniquet effect.
8. (c) One assessment technique for determining the extent and effects of swelling and circulation involves performing the blanching test. Swelling affects blood flow. The nurse compares the data on the appearance and sensation in the fingernails or toes to determine if circulation is impaired. A radial or pedal pulse may or may not be palpated, depending on the length of the cast.
9. (c) Examination and treatment should take place within 30-45 minutes after a pneumatic splint has been applied, or circulation may be affected.
10. (a) Braces are custom-made devices designed to support weakened structures during periods of activity.

ANSWERS TO ALTERNATIVE FORMAT QUESTIONS

1. **Answer: 3, 4, 5, 6**
   Rationale: Leave a freshly applied cast uncovered until it is dry. Air circulation aids in the drying. Alcohol and acetone are chemical solvents used to swab fiberglass resin from the skin. Plaster casts are not cleaned with this or any other substance. Circulation and sensation in the exposed toes provide data about vascular and neurologic function. In order to reduce swelling and bleeding, elevate the cast on a pillow or other supportive device and apply ice to the cast over the injured area. To reduce the risk of skin irritation and breakdown, pad the edges of the cast.

Nursing Process:	Implementation
Client Needs Category:	Physiological integrity
Cognitive Level:	Application

2. **Answer: 1, 2, 3, 5**
   Rationale: Providing the client with a trapeze and over-bed frame facilitates mobility and participation in self-care. Positioning the client's body in a line opposite the pull of traction maintains effective traction. Apply traction continuously unless there are medical orders to the contrary. To maintain effective traction, do not allow the weights to rest on the floor. When making the bed, apply clean linens from the bottom toward the top of the bed to maintain client alignment with the traction. Avoid tucking the top sheets, blankets, and

bed spreads beneath the mattress because this will interfere with the pull of the traction.

Nursing Process:	Planning
Client Needs Category:	Physiologic integrity
Cognitive Level:	Application

3. **Answer: 1, 3, 5**

Rationale: During recovery from a neck injury, the nurse must assess the client's neuromuscular status by having the client perform movements that correlate with muscular functions controlled by the cervical spine and peripheral nerve roots. If neuromuscular function is intact, the client can elevate both shoulders, flex and extend elbows and wrists, generate a strong handgrip, spread his or her fingers, and touch his or her thumb to the little fingers on each hand.

Nursing Process:	Assessment
Client Needs Category:	Physiological integrity
Cognitive Level:	Application

ANSWERS TO TRUE OR FALSE QUESTIONS

Items 1 Through 12

1. *False.* A *brace* is designed to support weakened body structures during weight bearing. A *splint* is a device that immobilizes and protects an injured part of the body.
2. *True.*
3. *False.* Inflate a pneumatic splint to the point that it can be indented only 1.3 cm (½ inch) with the fingertips.
4. *False.* Casts made of the newer synthetic materials dry quickly. These casts become rigid so quickly that weight bearing may occur within 15 to 30 minutes of application. On the other hand, plaster casts may remain wet for 24 to 48 hours, depending on the level of humidity in the air.
5. *True.*
6. *False.* Expose the cast directly to the air. A cast produces heat as it dries. If the cast is covered, moisture accumulates and evaporation is delayed.
7. *False.* The blanching test is done to determine the extent and effects of swelling and circulation.
8. *False.* Venous and capillary bleeding under a cast are characterized by a reddish-brown stain on the cast.
9. *True.*
10. *False.* The physician usually uses an electric cast cutter to separate and remove the cast. A cast cutter is a noisy instrument that can be frightening to a client. There is a natural expectation that an instrument sharp enough to cut a cast would be sharp enough to lacerate several layers of tissue. However, when used properly, an electric cast cutter should leave the skin intact.
11. *False.* After the removal of a cast, the skin may be washed as usual with soapy warm water but the semiattached areas of loose skin should not be forcibly removed. Lotion applied to the skin may add moisture and prevent rough edges from catching on clothing.

12. *False.* For clients in skeletal traction, active range of motion along with isometric and isotonic exercise should be encouraged. Body areas that are unrestricted by traction should be kept flexible and in good tone. Isometric exercises may be performed on the areas where motion is restricted.

ANSWERS TO SHORT ANSWER QUESTIONS

Items 1 Through 4

1. General purposes of mechanical immobilization are to:
    a. Relieve pain and muscle spasm.
    b. Support and align skeletal injuries.
    c. Restrict movement while injuries heal.
    d. Maintain functional positions until healing is complete.
    e. Allow activity while restricting movement of an injured area.
    f. Prevent further structural damage and deformity.
2. Important techniques that should be followed when applying an emergency splint are:
    a. Avoid changing the position of an injured part of the body, even if it appears grossly deformed.
    b. Leave a high-top shoe or a ski boot in place if an injured ankle is suspected.
    c. Select a splint or substitute splint material that will not permit movement of the body part once it is applied.
    d. Apply the splinting device so that it spans the injured area from the joint above the injury to beyond the joint below the injury.
    e. Inflate a pneumatic splint to the point that it can be indented only 1.3 centimeters (½ inch) with the fingertips. Avoid inflation longer than 30 to 45 minutes, or circulation in the area may be affected.
    f. Use an uninjured area of the body adjacent to the injured part if no other sturdy material is available.
    g. Cover any open wounds with clean material to absorb blood and prevent the entrance of dirt and additional pathogens.
    h. Apply soft material over any area of the body that may be subject to pressure or rubbing by areas on an inflexible splint.
    i. Use tape or wide strips of fabric in several areas to confine the injured part to the splint so that it cannot be moved. Narrow cord can create a tourniquet effect, especially if it encircles swelling tissue.
    j. Assess the color and temperature of fingers or toes to evaluate if blood flow is adequate. Loosen the attached device if the fingers or toes appear pale, blue, or cold.
    k. Elevate the entire length of the immobilized part so that the lowest point is higher than the heart.
    l. Provide for warmth and safety and seek assistance in transporting the injured person to a health agency.

3. Types of casts are:
   a. Cylinder casts
   b. Body casts
   c. Spica casts
4. Principles for maintaining effective traction are:
   a. Traction must produce a pulling effect on the body.
   b. Countertraction (counterpull) must be maintained.
   c. The pull of traction and the counterpull must be in exactly opposite directions.
   d. Splints and slings must be suspended without interference.
   e. Ropes must move freely through each pulley.
   f. The prescribed amount of weight must be applied.
   g. The weights must hang free.

Chapter 26

ANSWERS TO MATCHING QUESTIONS

Items 1 Through 4

1. c   2. d   3. a   4. b

ANSWERS TO MULTIPLE-CHOICE QUESTIONS

Items 1 Through 10

1. (a) Muscle tone refers to the ability of muscles to respond when stimulated. Strength is the power to perform.
2. (c) Quadriceps setting, sometimes shortened to quad setting, is a form of isometric exercise in which the quadriceps group of muscles are alternately tensed and relaxed.
3. (b) For optimum use, a cane must be adjusted to an appropriate height for the client. When fitted correctly, the cane's handle is parallel with the client's hip, which should provide approximately a 30° angle of elbow flexion.
4. (d) Platform crutches are designed to support the forearm. They are especially useful for clients unable to bear weight with their hands and wrists. Many persons with arthritis use them.
5. (d) The most stable form of ambulatory aid is the walker; straight canes are the least stable.
6. (d) Quadriceps setting is an isometric exercise in which muscles on the front of the thigh are alternatively tensed and relaxed. The client contracts the quadriceps femoris muscles by pulling the kneecaps toward his hips. The client will feel that he is pushing his knee down into the mattress and pulling his foot forward.
7. (b) The cane should be placed about 10 cm (4 inches) to the side of the foot. It should be held in the hand on the uninvolved side.
8. (b) The individual should use the three-point gait for crutch walking when weight bearing is allowed on one leg. The other foot cannot bear weight or can only bear limited weight.
9. (c) When using a cane on stairs, use the stair rail rather than the cane to go up or down. Take each step up with the stronger leg, followed by the weaker one. Reverse the pattern for descending the stairs. If there is no stair rail, advance the cane just before rising or descending with the weaker leg.
10. (a) When using a walker, clients are instructed to stand within the walker.

ANSWERS TO ALTERNATIVE FORMAT QUESTIONS

1. **Answer: 1, 3, 4, 5**
   Rationale: The client should be taught to care for the special requirements of the amputated extremity. Wash, rinse and dry the stump every evening. This will allow sufficient time for the skin to air-dry to avoid skin irritation and impairment. Regular weight checks help detect fluctuations that may alter the size of the stump and the fit of the prosthesis. Periodically lying supine during the day promotes venous circulation, reduces stump edema, and avoids joint contractures. Starting slowly and increasing wearing time prevents overexertion and impaired skin integrity. Covering the prosthetic foot with a sock and shoe coordinates apparel and helps to conceal the appearance of the prosthesis. Never remove water from the nylon sheath by twisting it. It should be stretched and air-dried after washing to maintain its shape.

Nursing Process:	Implementation
Client Needs Category:	Psychosocial integrity
Cognitive Level:	Application

2. **Answer: 30**
   Rationale: The entire horizontal table is tilted in increments of 15° to 30° until the client is in a vertical position. If symptoms such as dizziness and hypotension develop, the table is lowered or returned to the horizontal position.

Nursing Process:	Implementation
Client Needs Category:	Physiological integrity
Cognitive Level:	Application

3. **Answer: 3**
   Rationale: Continual pressure on the axilla can injure the radial nerve and eventually cause crutch palsy, a weakness of the muscles of the forearm, wrist, and hand.

Nursing Process:	Assessment
Client Needs Category:	Physiological integrity
Cognitive Level:	Analysis

ANSWERS TO TRUE OR FALSE QUESTIONS

Items 1 Through 10

1. *True.*
2. *True.*
3. *False.* There should be room for two fingers in the space between the top of the axillary bar of the crutch and the fold of the axilla when the client stands. This prevents injury to the tissues and the nerves in the axilla.

4. *True.*

5. *False.* The nurse should hold on to the handles of the walking belt and walk alongside the client.

6. *True.*

7. *True.*

8. *False.* When walking downstairs while using a cane, take each step with the weaker leg first followed by the stronger one. The reverse is true when going up the stairs.

9. *True.*

10. *False.* Just before the client is placed on a tilt table, the nurse applies elastic stockings. These stockings help to compress vein walls, thus preventing pooling of blood in the extremities, which may trigger fainting.

ANSWERS TO SHORT ANSWER QUESTIONS

Items 1 Through 4

1. Devices and techniques that provide support and assistance with walking are:
   a. Parallel bars
   b. Stable pieces of furniture
   c. Walking belts
   d. The nurse

2. Three common aids for ambulation are:
   a. Cane
   b. Walker
   c. Crutches

3. Three characteristics of appropriately fitted crutches are:
   a. They permit the client to stand upright with the shoulders relaxed.
   b. They provide space for two fingers between the axilla and the axillary bar.
   c. They facilitate approximately 30° of elbow flexion and slight hyperextension of the wrist.

4. The tilt table is used to help clients get acclimatized to being upright and bearing weight on their own feet.

Chapter 27

ANSWERS TO MATCHING QUESTIONS

Items 1 Through 5

1. d   2. c   3. a   4. e   5. b

Items 6 Through 12

6. c   7. g   8. f   9. a   10. d   11. e
12. h

ANSWERS TO MULTIPLE-CHOICE QUESTIONS

Items 1 Through 10

1. (d) The primary disadvantage of outpatient surgery is that it reduces the time for establishing a nurse-client relationship. Considering the client does not come into the hospital until the morning of surgery, there is often little time for the nurses to work with him or her prior to the time of the operative procedure.

2. (b) Regional anesthesia produces loss of feeling in a large area of the body, such as the pelvis and lower extremities, by instilling an anesthetic agent into the spinal canal.

3. (b) Directed donors must meet all the criteria of a public donor.

4. (d) Emotional care continues during the postoperative period in a manner similar to that in preoperative care. The nurse should be alert to feelings and worries that clients may not be able to specifically express. For example, the client may ask, "How am I doing?" when he or she really means, "Do you think I'll make it?" The nurse may need to interpret the underlying question and explain what is happening to the extent to which individuals are interested or able to understand.

5. (c) Deep breathing and, in some cases, coughing are important measures to prevent the possibility of hypostatic pneumonia and atelectasis.

6. (d) The client should be taught forced coughing. Forced coughing is most appropriate for clients who have diminished or moist lung sounds.

7. (d) Inactivity and gravity cause blood to pool and settle in lower areas of the body. The temporarily inactive surgical client can perform leg exercises to promote circulation and prevent the formation of blood clots.

8. (c) Psychological support not only involves providing information, it includes observing and taking the time to listen to the client and others who are concerned about the client. It is usually of no help simply to say that everything will be all right and that there is no cause for worry. The helpful nurse will be available to provide an opportunity for individuals to talk about their problems and express feelings.

9. (c) The smell, nausea, burning, and watering of the eyes, although uncomfortable, are not hazardous. It is the potential inhalation of airborne cells and viruses that is. A conventional mask, even doubled, is not sufficient in filtering substances that measure less than 0.30 micron. Viruses can be as small as 0.12 micron. Thus it is possible, but not proven, that the HIV virus could be transmitted by inhaling the laser plume.

10. (a) Assure a child that he will not be left alone. Encourage him to talk about his fears as much as he is able. Tell him it is all right to cry, answer his questions, and correct the misconceptions most children have of surgery.

ANSWERS TO ALTERNATIVE FORMAT QUESTIONS

1. **Answer: 40**
   Rationale: A pneumatic compression device provides intermittent compression at an appropriate pressure to promote venous circulation. Most medical orders range

from 35 to 55 mm Hg, with a common average of 40 mm Hg.

Nursing Process:	Implementation
Client Needs Category:	Physiological integrity
Cognitive Level:	Application

2. **Answer: 1, 2, 5, 6**

Rationale: It is necessary for the infant to void prior to being sent home to ensure that the urethra is not obstructed. A lubricating ointment is appropriate and is applied with each diaper change. Typically, the penis heals in 2 to 4 days, and circumcision care is necessary during that time. To aid healing and prevent infection, tub baths should not be given until the plastic ring falls off and complete healing has occurred. A small amount of bleeding is expected; a large amount of bleeding should be reported.

Nursing Process:	Implementation
Client Needs Category:	Safe, effective care environment
Cognitive Level:	Application

3. **Answer: 1, 3, 4**

Rationale: The American Society of Anesthesiologists (ASA) developed new guidelines in 1999 so that consumption of clear liquids up to 2 hours before surgery requiring general anesthesia, regional anesthesia, or sedation analgesia is permitted. The client will be expected to do forced coughing postoperatively, accompanied by splinting of the abdomen. Anticoagulants are stopped a few days prior to surgery to prevent excessive bleeding postoperatively. To prevent thrombus development, leg exercises will also be expected. Once nausea and vomiting have passed and bowel sounds resume, the client will be started on a liquid diet and advanced as tolerated.

Nursing Process:	Evaluation
Client Needs Category:	Physiologic integrity
Cognitive Level:	Analysis

ANSWERS TO TRUE OR FALSE QUESTIONS

Items 1 Through 15

1. *False. Evisceration* is the separation of a wound with exposure of body organs. *Dehiscence* is only the separation of a wound.
2. *False.* Clients scheduled for outpatient surgery usually come to the hospital on the day of the operative procedure.
3. *True.*
4. *True.*
5. *False.* Recent studies have shown controversy about the traditional approach used to prepare the surgical site. This included shaving the body in a wide area surrounding the eventual incision. Shaving is done to remove microorganisms attached to the hair. The theory is valid. However, it has been found that a razor causes microabrasions. When skin is abraded, it allows an entry site for microorganisms. These

microbes tend to grow even more vigorously in the plasma-rich environment of the impaired skin. Their growth compounds during the time between shaving and the actual surgery.

6. *False.* The individual who is donating blood as a directed donor must weigh at least 110 pounds.
7. *False.* The directed donor may donate one unit every 56 days.
8. *False.* It is generally agreed that, unless moist secretions can be heard in the lungs, forced coughing should not be routinely performed postoperatively.
9. *True.*
10. *False.* The skin cannot be sterilized, but measures can be taken to reduce the chances of introducing organisms into the operative site.
11. *True.*
12. *False.* Family members appreciate knowing where they may wait and how long the client is expected to be in the operating and recovery rooms. It is better not to predict specific times. Delays sometimes occur, causing relatives unnecessary worry.
13. *False.* When teaching deep-breathing exercises, emphasize that the breathing should be done slowly.
14. *False.* Apply antiembolism stockings in the morning before the client is out of bed or after elevating the feet for at least 15 minutes. Before the feet are lowered, there is a minimal amount of pooled blood in the lower legs and feet. Elevation helps gravity move blood toward the heart.
15. *True.*

ANSWERS TO SHORT ANSWER QUESTIONS

Items 1 Through 4

1. The equipment and supplies needed in the postoperative client's room are:
   a. Blood pressure equipment
   b. Extra tissue wipes
   c. Emesis basin
   d. IV pole
2. The advantages of laser surgery, besides cost effectiveness, are:
   a. Reduced need for anesthesia
   b. Smaller incisions
   c. Minimal blood loss
   d. Reduced swelling around the incision
   e. Less pain following the procedure
   f. Decreased incidence of wound infection
   g. Reduced scarring
   h. Less time recuperating
3. Areas commonly addressed in discharge instructions include:
   a. How to care for the incision site
   b. Signs of complications to report
   c. What drugs to use for relieving pain
   d. How to self-administer prescribed drugs
   e. When usual activities can be resumed
   f. If and how much weight can be lifted
   g. Which foods to consume or avoid

h. When and where to return for a medical appointment
4. General types of measures included in postoperative care are:
   a. The frequency with which vital signs are taken
   b. Assessment of level of consciousness
   c. Effectiveness of respiratory effort
   d. Assessment of need for supplemental oxygen
   e. Observation of wound and dressing
   f. Location of drains, if any
   g. Characteristics of drainage
   h. Location of IV site, type of fluid, and rate of flow
   i. Level of pain and need for medication
   j. Presence of urinary catheter and characteristics and volume of urine

Chapter 28

ANSWERS TO MATCHING QUESTIONS
Items 1 Through 6

1. g   2. c   3. f   4. a   5. e   6. b

Items 7 Through 9

7. d   8. c   9. a

ANSWERS TO MULTIPLE-CHOICE QUESTIONS
Items 1 Through 15

1. (d) The sequence of activities associated with the inflammatory process is swelling, pain, decreased functioning, redness, and warmth.
2. (a) The components of a scar are cells called fibroblasts and a substance called collagen. These two act as building blocks and "glue" to temporarily repair the area that was damaged.
3. (c) Wound healing involves the body's efforts to restore the structure and function of cells in the injured area. This is done either by recovery of injured cells, called *resolution;* by replacement of damaged cells with identical new cells, called *regeneration;* or by the production of a nonfunctioning substitute for the destroyed cells, called *scar formation.*
4. (c) *Granulation tissue* is pinkish-red tissue containing new projections of capillaries.
5. (d) Careful hand washing before caring for the wound probably is the *single most* effective method of preventing infections.
6. (d) The primary cause of a pressure sore is unrelieved compression of capillaries bringing blood to the skin and its underlying tissue. The mechanism for destruction is as follows: The body weight compresses the tissue and blood vessels against the hard surface of a bed, chair, bedpan, and so on. As a result, the cells supplied through the vascular network lack oxygen and a means for carrying away waste products of metabolism. Cells

eventually die if these conditions are prolonged and unrelieved.
7. (d) The earliest sign of excessive pressure is a red appearance to the skin over a bony area of the body. The color is caused by cellular damage in the area.
8. (c) Older adults are most prone to pressure ulcers because they have limited mobility, little fat deposits, and often a lack of good nutrition because of loose-fitting dentures, insufficient money for food, or lack of interest in eating.
9. (a) One of the common purposes of dressing a wound is to absorb drainage.
10. (c) If changing a dressing is likely to be a painful experience for the client, the nurse should give a prescribed medication about 15 to 30 minutes before a dressing change to reduce discomfort.
11. (b) Staples have an advantage in that they are less likely to compress tissue if a wound swells. This is prevented because staples do not encircle the wound; they merely form a bridge that holds the two sides together.
12. (b) The wound heals toward the center; pulling the wound edge could reinjure healing tissue.
13. (a) A solution for an eye irrigation should be approximately body temperature.
14. (d) Older adults are often insensitive to hot and cold applications. Consequently, they are at great risk for sustaining thermal injuries.
15. (c) The purpose of the spiral-reverse turn method of bandaging is to bandage a cone-shaped body part, such as the thigh or leg.

ANSWERS TO ALTERNATIVE FORMAT QUESTIONS
1. **Answer: 1**
   Rationale: Hydrocolloid dressings are self-adhesive, opaque, air- and water-occlusive wound coverings. They keep wounds moist. Moist wounds heal more quickly because new cells grow more rapidly in a moist environment. If the hydrocolloid dressing remains intact, it can be left in place for up to 1 week. It must allow at least a 1-inch margin of healthy skin around the wound. Its occlusive nature repels body substances such as urine and stool.

Nursing Process:	Planning
Client Needs Category:	Safe, effective care environment
Cognitive Level:	Application

2. **Answer: III**
   Rationale: A stage III pressure ulcer has a shallow skin crater that extends to the subcutaneous tissue. It may be accompanied by serous or purulent drainage. The area is relatively painless despite the severity of the ulcer.

Nursing Process:	Assessment
Client Needs Assessment:	Physiological integrity
Cognitive Level:	Analysis

3. **Answer: 110°**
Rationale: Water for the sitz bath should be no hotter than 110°F (43.3°C) to provide comfort without danger of burning the skin.

Nursing Process: Implementation

Client Needs Category: Safe, effective care
                             environment

Cognitive Level: Application

ANSWERS TO TRUE OR FALSE QUESTIONS

Items 1 Through 12

1. *False.* Second intention is a type of wound healing in which widely separated edges of a wound must heal inward toward the center. First intention healing is when the wound edges are directly next to one another.
2. *False.* Third intention is a type of wound healing in which temporarily separated wound edges are eventually brought together at a later time.
3. *True.*
4. *False.* Shearing force is the damaging effect that occurs when compressed layers of tissue move upon each other.
5. *True.*
6. *False.* During the prevention and treatment of a closed pressure sore, the focus is on keeping the area dry. When the skin is broken, the nurse must maintain a moist environment. Moisture promotes the movement of epidermal cells to the surface of the wound, causing it to seal over and heal.
7. *False.* Prevention of additional injury and the promotion of healing are two principal goals of wound care.
8. *False.* Perhaps the best feature of transparent dressings is that they allow assessment without removing the dressing.
9. *True.*
10. *False.* Any wound irrigation that is performed in a body area that contains intact tissue will not necessarily need to follow principles of sterile technique. However, when an irrigation is required for an incision or other open wound, surgical asepsis should be followed.
11. *False.* The drainage basin used to collect the solution from an irrigation need not be sterile, considering it will receive solution contaminated with organisms and debris from the irrigated area.
12. *False.* If the item is a bean, pea, or similar dehydrated substance, irrigation is contraindicated. The solution can cause the object to swell and become fixed even more tightly than before. Solid objects are likely to require removal with an instrument. An exception would be in the case of a live insect. The insect can be suffocated by instilling and briefly retaining water or oil within the auditory canal. The dead insect will usually be flushed out as the fluid drains from the ear.

ANSWERS TO SHORT ANSWER QUESTIONS

Items 1 Through 6

1. The sequence of events that are associated with the inflammatory process is:
   a. The injured cells release chemical substances that set the inflammation in motion.
   b. White blood cells, called neutrophils and monocytes, are drawn to the injured area and begin to engulf dead cells and debris.
   c. Once the area has been cleaned, cells called fibroblasts and a substance called collagen fill the injured area.
   d. The body begins to send new projections of capillaries into the area to supply replacement cells with oxygen and nutrients.
2. Common purposes of dressing a wound are:
   a. To help keep a wound clean and restrict entry of organisms
   b. To absorb drainage
   c. To control edema and bleeding when applied with pressure
   d. To protect the healing area from further injury
   e. To help hold antiseptic medication next to the wound
   f. To maintain a moist environment
3. Equipment and supplies suggested for a dressing change are:
   a. A waterproof bag to receive the soiled dressing
   b. A new sterile dressing
   c. Tape for securing the dressing
   d. Clean gloves for removing the soiled dressing
   e. Sterile gloves
   f. Sterile normal saline for moistening the soiled dressing if it adheres to the wound
   g. An antimicrobial agent for cleaning the wound
   h. Sterile swabs for applying the antimicrobial agent
4. Nursing measures when caring for a wound with a drain are:
   a. Assess the characteristics and amount of the drainage.
   b. Cleanse the area around the drain.
   c. Clean the skin around the drain using circular motions.
   d. Shorten the drain by using a gentle twisting motion. Cut the excess length and replace the safety pin or clamp near the end of the drain.
   e. Remove the drain using the same twisting motion as in shortening.
5. Recommended techniques for securing a dressing are:
   a. Plan to use adhesive or paper tape for most dressings.
   b. Consider shaving the area if necessary.
   c. Remove adhesive remnants before applying new tape.
   d. Fold under each end of an adhesive strip to create a tab.
   e. Apply a protective coating to the skin.
   f. Try using liquid adhesive for small areas.

g. Do not cover the entire surface of the dressing with tape.

h. Observe the client for sensitivity to tape.

i. Use Montgomery straps for large areas that may need changing often.

j. Exert pressure on the wound from the edges toward the center of the wound when securing a dressing.

k. Secure the dressing snugly so that it does not slip.

l. Consider using a binder or bandage when adhesive tape is impractical.

6. Purposes of bandages and binders are:

a. They can be used to hold dressings in place.

b. They prevent tension on sutures when properly applied.

c. They limit movement in order to promote healing.

d. They can be used to provide support for a body part.

e. They provide comfort and a sense of security for the client.

Chapter 29

ANSWERS TO MATCHING QUESTIONS

Items 1 Through 6

1. c   2. e   3. b   4. d   5. f   6. a

Items 7 Through 10

7. b   8. d   9. a   10. c

Items 11 Through 20

11. d   12. i   13. a   14. f   15. h   16. g

17. j   18. e   19. b   20. c

ANSWERS TO MULTIPLE-CHOICE QUESTIONS

Items 1 Through 15

1. (d) One of the common causes of diarrhea associated with tube feedings is a formula that is highly concentrated.

2. (a) Constipation is often a problem associated with tube feedings that lack fiber.

3. (b) To maintain tube patency, it is best to flush feeding tubes with 30 to 60 mL of water immediately before and after administering a feeding or medication; every 4 hours if the client has continuous feedings; and after refeeding the gastric residual.

4. (d) Other than being inserted into the nose, a tube can be inserted through the skin and tissue of the abdomen and secured with gastrointestinal sutures. This method, called a transabdominal tube, is used in lieu of nasogastric or nasointestinal tubes when an alternative to oral feeding is required for longer than a month.

5. (c) The process of removing a poisonous substance through gastric intubation is called lavage.

6. (b) A common cause of feeding-tube obstruction is administering formula at rates that are less than 50 mL/hr.

7. (a) One of the advantages of the nasogastric tube is that it has a low incidence of obstruction.

8. (d) An advantage of the gastrostomy over other feeding tubes is that it can accommodate long-term tube feedings.

9. (c) The Ewald orogastric tube has a diameter of 36 to 40 French, the largest of the gastrointestinal tubes.

10. (a) A bolus feeding is the instillation of a large volume of liquid nourishment into the stomach in a fairly short amount of time.

11. (c) Most formulas used for tube feedings provide 0.5 to 2.0 kcal/mL of formula.

12. (d) Bolus feedings are the least desirable because they distend the stomach rapidly, causing gastric discomfort and the risk for reflux and aspiration to occur.

13. (b) Gastric residual is the volume of liquid within the stomach after allowing a compensatory time for stomach emptying.

14. (a) Despite the fact that tube feedings are approximately 80% water, clients generally require additional water. Adults require 30 mL/kg of weight or 1 mL/kcal of additional water on a daily basis.

15. (a) Instilling a tube feeding too rapidly can result in nausea and vomiting.

ANSWERS TO ALTERNATIVE FORMAT QUESTIONS

1. **Answer: 1, 2, 3, 4**

Rationale: Ambulation helps the tube move through the pyloric valve into the small intestine. When the radiograph confirms that the intestinal tube has advanced beyond the stomach, position the client on his or her right side for 2 hours, on his back for 2 hours, and on his left side for 2 hours. Gravity and positioning promote movement through intestinal curves. Excess tubing is coiled and attached to the client's pajamas to prevent accidental extubation. The tubing is not clamped; it is connected to a wall or portable suction source.

Nursing Process:	Implementation
Client Needs Category:	Physiological integrity
Cognitive Level:	Application

2. **Answer: 9**

Rationale: The nurse determines the length of the nasointestinal tube by obtaining the length from the nose to the earlobe to the xiphoid process (NEX) measurement and marks the tube appropriately. The length from the nose to the earlobe indicates the distance to the back of the throat above the point where the gag reflex is stimulated. The length from the earlobe to the xiphoid process indicates the length required to reach the stomach. The additional 9 inches estimates the length required for the tube to enter the upper small intestine. Distance may vary from individual to individual.

Nursing Process:	Planning
Client Needs Category:	Physiological integrity
Cognitive Level:	Analysis

3. **Answer: 24**

   Rationale: Changing the feeding bag and tubing every 24 hours reduces the risk of contamination.

Nursing Process:	Planning
Client Needs Category:	Safe, effective care environment
Cognitive Level:	Application

ANSWERS TO TRUE OR FALSE QUESTIONS

Items 1 Through 10

1. *True.*
2. *True.*
3. *False.* Transabdominal tubes are used in lieu of nasogastric or nasointestinal tubes when the client requires an alternative to oral feeding for longer than a month.
4. *True.*
5. *False.* Place the tip of the nasogastric tube at the end of the nose, then to the earlobe, and finally to the xiphoid process of the sternum. This is referred to as the NEX (nose-earlobe-xiphoid) measurement. It approximates the length of tubing required to reach the stomach.
6. *True.*
7. *False.* Never reinsert the stylet while the tube is in the client. The stylet can puncture the flexible tube and injure the body structures where it protrudes.
8. *True.*
9. *False.* Intestinal decompression refers to the removal of gas and fluids from the small bowel.
10. *False.* If the gastrostomy becomes accidentally extubated, the nurse may insert a Foley catheter 5 to 10 cm into the opening and inflate the balloon to maintain patency until reintubation can be accomplished.

ANSWERS TO SHORT ANSWER QUESTIONS

Items 1 Through 4

1. Methods for determining if a nasogastric tube is in the stomach are:
   a. Aspirating fluid—fluid appears clear, brownish-yellow, or green
   b. Auscultating the abdomen—instill 10 mL or more of air; listen with a stethoscope over the abdomen. You will hear a swooshing sound as air enters the stomach.
   c. Testing the pH of aspirated fluid—the most definitive method. Stomach fluid is acid with a pH of 1 to 3.
2. Steps to follow for administering an intermittent feeding are:
   a. Wash hands.
   b. Assess bowel sounds.
   c. Measure gastric residual and recheck in 30 minutes if it is more than 100 mL.
   d. Assemble equipment.
   e. Warm refrigerated nourishment to room temperature in a basin of warm water.
   f. Place the client in a 30° to 90° sitting position.
   g. Refeed the gastric residual.
   h. Pinch the tube just before all the residual has been instilled.
   i. Add fresh formula and adjust the height to slow the gravity flow until the desired amount has been administered.
   j. Flush the tubing with 30 to 60 mL of water after the feeding is finished.
   k. Plug or clamp the tube when the water is finished.
   l. Keep the head of the bed elevated for at least 30 to 60 minutes after a feeding.
   m. Record the volume of formula and water administered on the intake and output record.
   n. Provide oral hygiene at least twice daily.
3. Four schedules for administering tube feedings are:
   a. A bolus feeding is the instillation of a large volume of liquid nourishment in a fairly short amount of time. Approximately 250 to 400 mL of formula are given over a few minutes. They are repeated four to six times a day.
   b. An intermittent feeding is the instillation of liquid nourishment into the stomach in the time most people would spend eating a meal. Usually the volume is 250 to 400 mL. They are usually given by gravity drip over 30 to 60 minutes. Feedings are repeated four to six times a day.
   c. A cyclic feeding is one that is given continuously for 8 to 12 hours followed by a 1- to 12-hour pause. This routine is often used to wean clients while providing adequate nutrition. The feeding is given during the late evening hours and during sleep.
   d. A continuous feeding is the instillation of a small volume of liquid nourishment without any interruption. Approximately 1.5 mL/minute is administered. An electric feeding pump is used to regulate the infusion. This type of feeding may be administered directly into the small intestine.
4. Purposes for gastrointestinal intubation are:
   a. Provide nourishment.
   b. Administer oral medications that cannot be swallowed.
   c. Obtain samples of secretions for diagnostic testing.
   d. Remove poisonous substances.
   e. Remove gas and secretions from the stomach or bowel.
   f. Control gastric bleeding.

Chapter 30

ANSWERS TO MATCHING QUESTIONS

Items 1 Through 5

1. e	2. d	3. f	4. a	5. c

Items 6 Through 10

6. b	7. f	8. a	9. e	10. c

ANSWERS TO MULTIPLE-CHOICE QUESTIONS
Items 1 Through 12

1. (c) The kidneys perform the major responsibility for maintaining the balance of water and other chemicals in blood and cells. The blood delivers these substances to microscopic structures called nephrons in the kidneys. The nephrons selectively remove excess water and substances for which the body has no need, forming urine.

2. (b) As the volume of urine increases, the bladder expands and pressure increases within it. When the pressure becomes sufficient to stimulate stretch receptors located in the bladder wall, the desire to empty the bladder becomes noticeable. Usually, this occurs in adults when about 150 to 300 mL of urine collects in the bladder.

3. (a) *Anuria* refers to the absence of urine.

4. (d) *Urinary suppression* indicates that the kidneys are not forming urine. *Oliguria* is the production of a small volume of urine, usually less than 400 mL of urine in 24 hours when oral intake has been adequate and no other excessive amount of fluid has been lost. *Anuria* refers to the absence of urine. Because the kidneys are not producing urine, the bladder remains empty.

5. (b) Residual urine is urine retained in the bladder after a voiding. *Urinary retention* means that urine is being produced but is not being emptied from the bladder. *Urinary incontinence* is the inability to control the release of urine from the bladder.

6. (b) Stress incontinence is a condition in which small amounts of urine are released from the bladder only at times when there is increased abdominal pressure, such as when coughing or sneezing.

7. (a) A healthy adult excretes approximately 500 mL to 2500 mL of urine in each 24-hour period. The average is about 1200 mL.

8. (c) The term for pus in the urine is *pyuria*.

9. (c) Strengthening pelvic floor muscles is one method for controlling some types of incontinence. It is especially helpful for stress incontinence and may extend the time needed for control in urge incontinence. The pelvic floor muscle exercises, also called Kegel exercises, increase the tone of the pubococcygeus muscles.

10. (b) The procedure of catheterization is used as infrequently as possible because of the hazards involved. Only when the benefits outweigh the risks should the nurse propose to insert a catheter. The nurse should also advocate for its early removal.

11. (c) A *straight catheter* is a hollow tube that is intended to be inserted and withdrawn following its use for a temporary measure. An *indwelling catheter* is one that is placed into the bladder and secured there for a period of time. It is sometimes called a retention catheter. The most commonly used indwelling catheter is called a *Foley catheter*.

12. (a) When an external catheter is used, there are certain potential problems that may occur. First, and perhaps the most hazardous, is that the appliance may be applied too tightly and restrict blood flow to the skin and tissues of the penis. Second, moisture accumulates beneath the appliance and this can lead to breakdown of the skin covering the penis. Third, the catheter may not fit well or for some other reason lead to the leaking of urine.

ANSWERS TO ALTERNATIVE FORMAT QUESTIONS

1. **Answer: 1**
Rationale: An unrefrigerated urine specimen is an excellent growth medium. Bacteria may grow and multiply rapidly, thus affecting the results.

Nursing Process:	Planning
Client Needs Category:	Safe, effective care environment
Cognitive Level:	Analysis

2. **Answer: 2, 3, 4, 5**
Rationale: The penis and condom should be checked ½ hour after application to ensure that the condom is not so tight that it impairs circulation. A 1-inch space should be left between the tip of the penis and the end of the condom. The condom is changed every 24 hours, and skin care is provided. The condom is secured to the base of the penis firmly but not tightly. The tubing is taped to the leg or attached to the leg bag.

Nursing Process:	Implementation
Client Needs Category:	Physiological integrity
Cognitive Level:	Application

3. **Answer: 3000**
Rationale: Large amounts of fluid each day ensure a large urine output, which keeps the bladder flushed out and decreases the likelihood of urinary stasis and subsequent infection. Large volumes of urine also minimize the risk of sediment or other particles obstructing the drainage tubing.

Nursing Process:	Planning
Client Needs Category:	Physiological integrity
Cognitive Level:	Analysis

ANSWERS TO TRUE OR FALSE QUESTIONS
Items 1 Through 12

1. *False.* The urethra is the final passageway for urine as it is released from the bladder. The urine is transported from the kidneys through the ureters to the urinary bladder.

2. *True.*

3. *False. Oliguria* refers to the production of only small amounts of urine. *Anuria* refers to the absence of urine.

4. *False. Polyuria* means an excessive production and excretion of urine. The term for blood in the urine is *hematuria*.

5. *False.* A catheter that drains well does not need irrigating, except on rare occasions when irrigation is used to instill medications.
6. *False. Ensuring* that the client with an indwelling catheter has a generous fluid intake increases urine production and dilutes particles that may form in the urine.
7. *True.*
8. *False.* Catheterizations that are performed in health agencies follow principles of surgical asepsis. Self-catheterization is done following principles of medical asepsis.
9. *True.*
10. *False.* A clean-catch midstream specimen is a voided specimen collected under conditions of thorough cleanliness and after a small amount of urine is voided into the toilet.
11. *True.*
12. *False.* Incontinent individuals should be instructed that limiting fluid intake is a dangerous method to control urination.

ANSWERS TO SHORT ANSWER QUESTIONS

Items 1 Through 4

1. Actions that are helpful when a male uses the urinal are:
   a. Make sure the urinal is empty before handing it to the client.
   b. Warm the metal urinal with water.
   c. Instruct the client to spread his legs if he cannot place the urinal himself.
   d. While holding the handle of the urinal, direct it at an angle between the client's legs so that the bottom rests on the bed.
   e. Lift the penis and place it well within the inside of the urinal.
2. Bladder retraining plans could include the following:
   a. Assess for any patterns of dryness versus incontinence.
   b. Set realistic, short-term goals.
   c. Plan a specific trial schedule and be sure all personnel carry it out.
   d. Discourage strict limitation of liquid intake.
   e. Be sure all personnel, family, and any others know the planned schedule.
   f. Teach the client to note any sensation that precedes voiding.
   g. Encourage a relaxed atmosphere and as-near-to-normal circumstances as possible.
   h. Suggest that the client bend forward and apply pressure over the bladder (the Credé maneuver).
   i. Experiment with the success of measures to stimulate urination, such as listening to running water or placing the hands in water.
3. Factors that influence the amount, contents, and characteristics of urine or its elimination are:
   a. The amount of urine normally produced varies with the fluid intake. The greater the intake, the larger the output and vice versa.
   b. Contents and character are related to the individual's diet and the chemical composition of body fluids.
   c. Frequency depends on the amount of urine produced.
   d. The intervals of voiding are generally caused by habit.
   e. Increased abdominal pressure can increase the urge to void.
   f. Stress, embarrassment, and even the occasional need for a urine specimen can cause difficulty in relaxing enough to void.
   g. Women void most easily in a semisitting or sitting position, and men find it easiest to void in the standing position.
4. The following nursing measures should be kept in mind when the client needs assistance with urination:
   a. Provide privacy. Voiding may not occur if the client is tense or worried about being observed or interrupted.
   b. Help females to assume a sitting position. Sitting is the natural position women assume for elimination.
   c. Assist males to stand in front of a toilet or stand at the bedside when using a urinal. Standing is the natural position men assume when urinating.
   d. Maintain an adequate intake of oral fluids. The urge to urinate is dependent on the pressure exerted against stretch receptors as the bladder fills.

Chapter 31

ANSWERS TO MATCHING QUESTIONS

Items 1 Through 8

1. b   2. c   3. a   4. b   5. a   6. c
7. c   8. a

ANSWERS TO MULTIPLE-CHOICE QUESTIONS

Items 1 Through 20

1. (b) The volume of the stool is affected by the amount of food that is consumed. A diet high in fiber and roughage produces a larger stool and promotes quicker passage through the intestinal tract. A diet low in roughage produces a smaller stool and tends to increase the time it remains within the bowel.
2. (c) Constipation is a condition in which the stool becomes dry and hard and requires straining in order to eliminate it. The frequency of stool passage is not always a factor. Some persons may be constipated and yet have a daily bowel movement.
3. (b) A client with a fecal impaction may expel liquid stool around the impacted mass. This symptom in combination with a lack of normal defecation is almost a sure indication of an impaction.
4. (c) Several measures may relieve a fecal impaction. The stool may be passed if sufficient moisture and

lubrication are instilled into the rectum in the area of the stool. An oil retention enema is often prescribed to first provide lubrication to the mass and the mucous membrane that lines the rectum.

5. (d) Digital removal of stool may become necessary if the administration of enemas fails to produce results for the client with a fecal impaction. Digital removal involves inserting a gloved and well-lubricated finger into the rectum in order to break up and remove the fecal mass.

6. (b) An excessive amount of gas within the intestinal tract is known as *flatulence*. Expelled intestinal gas is called *flatus*. When gas is not expelled and accumulates, the condition is called *intestinal distention* or *tympanites*.

7. (c) The largest percentage of gas accumulated in the bowel comes from swallowed air and the air that is present in food. Other minor sources include gas that diffuses from the bloodstream and bacterial fermentation.

8. (c) Insert a rectal tube to help gas escape. Gas will usually follow the path of least resistance. The rectal tube provides a channel through which the gas can travel. An intestinal tube inserted through the nose may be used as a last resort.

9. (d) Diarrhea is the passage of watery, unformed stools accompanied by abdominal cramping. Although frequent bowel movements do not necessarily mean that diarrhea is present, persons with diarrhea usually have stools frequently.

10. (c) To help the client who has diarrhea, the nurse should temporarily limit the consumption of food. Provide clear liquids until the number of stools and the consistency improve and then follow with bananas, applesauce, and light foods. Avoid fried foods, highly seasoned foods, or foods high in roughage.

11. (b) Anal control is dependent ultimately on proper functioning of the anal sphincters. For some clients, functioning of impaired sphincters can be improved. One way is to consult with the physician about using a suppository or an enema every 2 to 3 days. If a pattern can be established by stimulating peristalsis and emptying the lower bowel with these aids, fecal incontinence may become controllable.

12. (a) Defecation usually occurs within 5 to 15 minutes after administration of a large-volume enema.

13. (c) Tap water or normal saline are preferred for their nonirritating effect on clients. However, tap water can be absorbed through the bowel. Tap water enemas that are repeated one after another can result in fluid imbalances.

14. (d) A hypertonic solution is one in which there is a higher amount of dissolved substances than that found in the blood. Hypertonic enema solutions act by increasing fluid volume in the intestine and by acting as a local irritant.

15. (c) The recommended position for the client receiving a hypertonic enema is the knee-chest position. This position allows for distribution of solution to the lower large intestine.

16. (a) The primary purpose of an oil retention enema is to lubricate and soften the stool so that it can be expelled more easily.

17. (d) Prevention of skin breakdown is one of the biggest challenges in ostomy care. Enzymes in stool can quickly cause excoriation.

18. (d) When the client is elderly, intestinal elimination patterns should be assessed with care. Many elderly persons become very bowel conscious and report a problem with constipation erroneously because they lack accurate information concerning elimination.

19. (b) Although laxatives and enemas sometimes play a proper role in intestinal elimination, they are also often abused. Teaching their proper use and the dangers of abuse is a nursing responsibility.

20. (a) The gastrocolic reflex generally precedes defecation.

ANSWERS TO ALTERNATIVE FORMAT QUESTIONS

1. **Answer: 1, 2, 3, 4, 5**
   Rationale: Diarrhea is the urgent passage of watery stools commonly accompanied by abdominal cramping. Blood or mucus in the stool often accompanies diarrhea. Resting the bowel temporarily may relieve simple diarrhea. This means taking in a clear liquid diet and avoiding solid foods for 12 to 24 hours. Resumed eating begins with bland, low-residue foods such as bananas, applesauce, and cottage cheese. It is necessary to rule out fecal impaction because some clients with an impaction pass liquid stool, which may be misinterpreted as diarrhea.

Nursing Process:	Planning
Client Needs Category:	Physiological integrity
Cognitive Level:	Application

2. **Answer: 2, 3, 4**
   Rationale: Overdependence on laxatives and enemas can cause rather than relieve constipation. Oral fluids promote hydration and avoid dry stool. Consuming high-fiber foods adds bulk to stool and pulls water into stool. Bulky, soft stool distends the rectum and promotes the urge to defecate. Not having sufficient time for elimination prevents relaxation and contributes to constipation.

Nursing Process:	Implementation
Client Needs Category:	Health promotion and maintenance
Cognitive Level:	Application

3. **Answer: 60**
   Rationale: Sixty seconds is the length of time required for the chemical reagent to interact with the stool when testing for occult blood.

Nursing Process:	Implementation
Client Needs Category:	Safe, effective care environment
Cognitive Level:	Application

ANSWERS TO TRUE OR FALSE QUESTIONS

Items 1 Through 12

1. *False.* The *external* anal sphincter is under voluntary control.
2. *True.*
3. *False.* Constipation is a condition in which the stool becomes hard and dry and requires straining to eliminate it. The frequency of stool passage is not always a factor.
4. *True.*
5. *True.*
6. *True.*
7. *False.* Consuming gas-forming foods increases the volume of gas in the intestinal tract.
8. *False.* Diarrhea is the passage of watery, unformed stools accompanied by abdominal cramping. Although frequent bowel movements do not necessarily mean that diarrhea is present, persons with diarrhea usually have stools frequently.
9. *False.* A hypertonic enema solution will cause fluid to be drawn from body tissues into the bowel, eventually increasing the fluid volume in the intestine to more than the original amount that was instilled.
10. *False.* An ileostomy is an opening into the ileum, a portion of the small intestine.
11. *True.*
12. *True.*

ANSWERS TO SHORT ANSWER QUESTIONS

Items 1 Through 5

1. The conditions that predispose a person to form greater amounts of gas or interfere with its absorption include:
   a. Swallowing larger than usual amounts of air while eating and drinking
   b. Experiencing bacterial fermentation
   c. Consuming gas-forming foods, which increases the volume of gas in the intestinal tract
   d. Remaining inactive, which tends to impair the movement of gas through the intestinal tract
   e. Having surgery in which the bowel is handled
   f. Taking drugs such as morphine, which tends to decrease peristalsis and thus cause distention as well as constipation
   g. Experiencing the presence of a mass that obstructs the passage of stool, which may also interfere with the ability of the intestine to eliminate gas
2. The chief characteristics of constipation include:
   a. Abdominal distention or bloating
   b. Change in the amount of gas passed rectally
   c. Less-frequent bowel movements
   d. Oozing liquid stool
   e. Rectal fullness or pressure
   f. Rectal pain with bowel movement
   g. Small amount of stool
   h. Inability to pass stool
3. Causes of diarrhea are:
   a. The response of the body to try and rid itself of some allergic substance or the natural defense for eliminating an irritating substance such as tainted food or intestinal pathogens
   b. The response to stress
   c. Certain dietary indiscretions
   d. Intentional or accidental abuse of laxatives
   e. Many intestinal and digestive diseases
4. Nursing measures suggested to help relieve diarrhea are:
   a. Remembering that diarrhea is often an embarrassing situation
   b. Reducing the cause if possible
   c. Temporarily limiting food and then starting by providing clear liquids. Give nonirritating foods and avoid fried foods and foods high in roughage.
   d. Investigating the relationship between the side effects of medications and the occurrence of diarrhea
   e. Remembering that individuals with diarrhea find it very difficult to delay the urge to defecate
   f. Using hygienic measures to clean the perineum following each stool
   g. Counting the number of bowel movements the client is having
   h. Consulting with the physician concerning the possible use of medications to control the diarrhea
5. Causes of fecal incontinence are:
   a. A result of disease or injury
   b. A fecal impaction
   c. A temporary loss of control
   d. A result of waiting for the bedpan or the use of a toilet, which causes some individuals to have a loss of control
   e. An extremely harsh or large dosage of a laxative that may result in rapid peristalsis

Chapter 32

ANSWERS TO MATCHING QUESTIONS

Items 1 Through 6

| 1. d | 2. c | 3. f | 4. h | 5. g | 6. b |

Items 7 Through 10

| 7. c | 8. d | 9. b | 10. a |

ANSWERS TO MULTIPLE-CHOICE QUESTIONS

Items 1 Through 12

1. (b) The trade, or proprietary, name is the name used by the manufacturer for the drug it sells. The generic, or nonproprietary, name is a name that is usually descriptive of the chemical structure and is not protected by a trademark.
2. (c) Medication errors are serious! A medication order should *never* be implemented if the nurse has a question about it until after consulting the physician or another authorized person.
3. (c) Most health care agencies check narcotic supplies at the change of shifts. A nurse completing one shift checks the narcotic count with a nurse beginning the next shift.

4. (b) For many years, nurses have followed five criteria for ensuring that medications are prepared and administered correctly. These criteria have been described as the five rights for administering medication. The five rights are:
   1. The right drug
   2. The right dose
   3. The right route
   4. The right time
   5. The right person

5. (b) The nurse should check the label of the drug container *three* times to ensure safety and accuracy: (1) when reaching for the medication, (2) immediately prior to pouring the medication, and (3) when returning the container to its storage place.

6. (d) When administering medications, the nurse should remain with the client while he or she takes the medication. Do not leave medications at the bedside for the client to take at a later time. The client may forget to take the medication or someone else may take it.

7. (a) Do not give a medication without further checking if the client indicates that the drug appears different from what she has been receiving. A mistake may have been made when supplying the medication or when preparing the medication. Withholding it while checking further may avoid an error.

8. (d) If a medication error occurs, the client's condition is checked and the error is reported to the physician and the supervising nurse.

9. (c) Certain tablets are covered with a substance that does not dissolve until the medication reaches the small intestine. These tablets are enteric coated. If the coating is destroyed, the medication is released in the stomach, where it is irritating to the gastric mucosa. Enteric-coated tablets should never be crushed or chewed.

ERIC FTING

10. (c) One of the main reasons the nurse should stay with the client until the oral medication is swallowed is that the nurse is responsible for documenting that the drug was taken by the correct person. It is possible that a client could discard a drug, misplace it, or accumulate many in order to harm himself or herself.

11. (b) If the nasogastric tube is used for suctioning rather than nourishment, the tube must be clamped for at least a half hour after instilling medication. If that is not done, the drugs are removed from the stomach before they can be absorbed.

12. (c) Monitor the elderly person's medication carefully while taking into account the effects of aging. As a result of aging, the risk of adverse side effects and toxicity to drugs increases. Decreased gastrointestinal motility and decreased ability to absorb drugs tend to reduce the drug action because the drugs are not being taken into the bloodstream as well.

PROPRIETARY NAME = TRADE NAME

ANSWERS TO ALTERNATIVE FORMAT QUESTIONS

1. **Answer: 5**
   Rationale: Drawing a liquid oral medication of less than 5 mL per dose into a sterile syringe allows for accurate measurement of small amounts of medication and greater control over administration, especially if the client is a child.

Nursing Process:	Implementation
Client Needs Category:	Safe, effective care environment
Cognitive Level:	Application

2. **Answer: 6**
   Rationale: In a 24-hour period, a medication given every 4 hours would be given 6 times. Use the following formula:

   Total time in hours divided by frequency of administration = total number of doses

   Then   24 divided by 4 = 6

Nursing Process:	Planning
Client Needs Category:	Physiological integrity
Cognitive Level:	Analysis

3. **Answer: 3**
   Rationale: Use this formula:

   $$\frac{\text{Desired dose}}{\text{Dose on hand}} \times \text{quantity} = \text{Amount to administer}$$

   Then: $\dfrac{60 \text{ mg}}{20 \text{ mg}} \times 1 = 3$

   $$3 \times 1 = 3$$

Nursing Process:	Implementation
Client Needs Category:	Physiological integrity
Cognitive Level:	Analysis

ANSWERS TO TRUE OR FALSE QUESTIONS

Items 1 Through 12

1. *True.*
2. *False.* Clerical activities may be delegated, but the nurse is the one responsible within a health agency for checking, transcribing, and carrying out the medication order.
3. *False.* The trade or proprietary name is the name used by the manufacturer for the drug it sells. The generic or nonproprietary name is a name that is usually descriptive of the drug's chemical structure and is not protected by a trademark.
4. *True.*
5. *False.* A drug that is ordered to be given four times a day may be scheduled in a variety of patterns. For example, it may be given at: 8 A.M., 12 noon, 4 P.M., and 8 P.M.; or 10 A.M., 2 P.M., 6 P.M., and 10 P.M.; or 6 A.M., 12 noon, 6 P.M., and 12 midnight.
6. *False.* Federal law requires that a record be kept for each narcotic that is administered.
7. *True.*
8. *False.* There is a sixth right some nurses have added to the list. It is the client's right to refuse medication. The

right of a rational adult to consent to or refuse therapy is a legal right.

9. *False.* Health care agencies have a special form for reporting medication errors, called an *incident sheet* or *accident report*. In this report, a full explanation of the situation is provided. The report serves as a method for preventing future errors by examining the practices that contributed to the error. The incident sheet is *not* a part of the permanent record, nor should any reference be made in the chart that an incident sheet has been completed.

10. *False.* A notation should be made stating why the medication was not given as scheduled. This is not considered a medication error in most instances.

11. *False.* Medications should not be added to the formula being administered for continuous tube feedings.

12. *False.* Enteric-coated tablets or those designed for sustained release should never be crushed and administered. This interferes with their absorption and the desired therapeutic effects.

ANSWERS TO SHORT ANSWER QUESTIONS

Items 1 Through 5

1. The seven parts of a complete medication order are:
   a. The name of the client
   b. The date and time the order is written
   c. The name of the medication
   d. The dosage to be administered
   e. The route for administering medication
   f. The frequency of administering the medication
   g. The signature of the person who has written the order

2. The five items of information the nurse should know about the client before administering medications are:
   a. Nonprescription medications the client uses and the reason, frequency, and length of time he or she has been using them
   b. Prescription medications that the client has been using and the reason, frequency, and length of time he or she has been using them
   c. The client's pattern for following the directions for medication use
   d. Any allergies the client has to medications
   e. Habits of daily living that may influence drug therapy, such as alcohol and drug consumption

3. The five rights pertaining to administering medications are:
   a. The right drug
   b. The right dose
   c. The right route
   d. The right time
   e. The right person

4. The five steps that the nurse should carry out prior to preparing drugs that will be administered are:
   a. Check the client's medication record with the original medication orders prior to preparing the drugs.

b. Question any part of a drug order that appears inappropriate before proceeding.
c. Be alert to any unusual changes, such as new additions or deletions, of entries on the medication record. Errors can occur when forms are recopied or when transcribing a new medication order.
d. Question any unusual abbreviations that may have been used when transcribing a medication order. Errors have occurred when the person writing the order or transcribing it has used unacceptable abbreviations. This practice can cause misinterpretation when administering the medication.
e. Organize the nursing care so that medications are given as near to the scheduled routine as possible. It is common policy to give the drug no earlier or later than 30 minutes from the time specified. A medication given outside this range of time is considered a drug error.

5. Guidelines the nurse should follow when preparing medications for administration are:
   a. Prepare medications while using a good light, and work alone without interruptions or distractions. Also, allow sufficient time so that all the drugs may be prepared without having to leave and return to complete the task.
   b. Check the label of the drug container *three* times to ensure safety and accuracy: (1) when reaching for the medication, (2) immediately prior to pouring the medication, and (3) when returning the container to its storage place.
   c. Do not use medications from containers on which the label is difficult to read or has come off.
   d. Do not return medications to a container or transfer medications from one container to another.
   e. Check expiration dates on medications, especially those that are in solution. Do not use a medication that has a sediment at the bottom of the container unless the medication is to be shaken well before using. Do not use one that appears cloudy or has changed color.
   f. Prepare medications in the order in which they will be delivered to the client.
   g. Transport drugs from the area of preparation to the client carefully and safely. Use the method of transporting provided by the agency. Identify the drugs in some manner to avoid confusing which drugs are for which clients.
   h. Protect needles for injecting drugs according to the method of the agency's choice to prevent contamination.
   i. Use an individual medicine dropper for each liquid medication dispensed in this manner.

Chapter 33

ANSWERS TO MATCHING QUESTIONS
Items 1 Through 5

1. e   2. c   3. a   4. b   5. d

ANSWERS TO MULTIPLE-CHOICE QUESTIONS
Items 1 Through 10

1. (a) To ensure good absorption when applying an inunction, the nurse should first cleanse the area with soap or detergent and water before applying the oil, lotion, cream, or ointment. This frees the skin of debris and body oil, both of which retard absorption.
2. (c) Do not touch the ointment. The medication can be absorbed through any skin surface.
3. (b) When administering eardrops to an adult, gently pull the ear upward and backward.
4. (d) When administering eardrops to a child, gently pull the ear downward and backward.
5. (b) Some medications are intended to become absorbed through the blood vessels within the mouth rather than be delivered to the gastrointestinal tract. A sublingual administration involves placing a drug under the tongue. A buccal administration involves placing a drug against the mucous membranes of the cheek.
6. (c) The position of choice when inserting a vaginal medication is the dorsal recumbent position with the knees flexed and slightly spread upon the bed.
7. (a) The mucous membrane of the eye is called the conjunctiva.
8. (c) If medication is to be instilled in both ears, it is appropriate to wait 15 minutes before instilling the medication in the other ear.
9. (d) Chewing, swallowing, smoking, eating, and drinking are all contraindicated when a buccal medication has been given.
10. (b) When inserting medications vaginally with an applicator, one should follow the package directions, which usually recommend inserting the applicator about 2 to 4 inches into the vagina.

ANSWERS TO ALTERNATIVE FORMAT QUESTIONS

1. **Answer: 2.5**
   Rationale: At this height (2.5 cm), the pressure of the solution will not damage the eye tissue, and the irrigating device will not touch the eye.

Nursing Process:	Implementation
Client Needs Category:	Safe, effective care environment
Cognitive Level:	Analysis

2. **Answer: 6.2**
   Rationale: At 6 hours, 50% of the drug remains. Every 6 hours, the amount remaining is reduced by $\frac{1}{2}$. Then 6 hours = 50%; 12 hours = 25%; 18 hours = 12.5%; and at 24 hours, 6.25% remains.

Nursing Process:	Planning
Client Needs Category:	Physiological integrity
Cognitive Level:	Analysis

3. **Answer: 3, 4, 5**
   Rationale: The orders for Humulin L (Lente), codeine, and nitropaste are questionable because no exact dose is given. Lasix and ampicillin include the medication name, dosage, route, and frequency.

Nursing Process:	Implementation
Client Needs Category:	Physiological integrity
Cognitive Level:	Analysis

ANSWERS TO TRUE OR FALSE QUESTIONS
Items 1 Through 9

1. *False.* Topically applied drugs may have a local or systemic effect.
2. *False.* Clip, but do not shave, body hair that will be covered by the patch. Shaving creates microabrasions that could increase the rate of drug absorption. Clipping reduces the discomfort during patch removal.
3. *True.*
4. *True.*
5. *False.* It is important to monitor the heart rate and blood pressure of older adults who use inhalers containing bronchodilating drugs. These types of medications often cause tachycardia and hypotension.
6. *True.*
7. *True.*
8. *True.*
9. *False.* Cutaneous applications are those in which topical drugs are applied to the skin. An *inunction* is a medication that is incorporated into a transporting agent. All inunctions are cutaneous applications, but not all cutaneous applications are inunctions.

ANSWERS TO SHORT ANSWER QUESTIONS
Items 1 Through 4

1. The seven guidelines for giving an inunction are:
   a. Cleanse the skin and hands with soap or detergent and water before applying the oil, lotion, cream, or ointment.
   b. Shake the contents of mixtures that may have become separated.
   c. Apply most inunctions with the fingers and hands or use a cotton ball or gauze square.
   d. Wear gloves if there is a contagious skin condition or there are breaks in the skin of the fingers or hands.
   e. Warm the inunction if it will be applied to a sensitive area such as the face or back.
   f. Apply local heat to the area as ordered.
   g. Keep powders away from the nose and mouth. If they are applied near the face, do so as the client exhales.
2. Guidelines for applying nitroglycerin ointment are:
   a. Remove any previous application from the client's skin.

b. Squeeze a ribbon of ointment from the tube onto the application paper. The dosage is prescribed in centimeters or inches. The typical dosage is a 2.5- to 5-cm (1- to 2-inch) ribbon of ointment.

c. Place the application paper containing the ribbon of ointment on a clean, nonhairy surface of the skin. The chest wall and the upper arm are usual sites.

d. Cover the application paper with a square piece of plastic and secure with tape on four sides.

e. Check vital signs approximately 30 minutes after the application to determine the response.

f. Rotate the sites on which the ointment is placed each day to prevent skin irritation.

g. *Do not* touch the ointment. The medication can be absorbed through any skin surface.

h. Inform the physician if the client develops a severe headache or if there is a significant lowering of the blood pressure.

3. Common routes of topical administration for drugs are:

a. Cutaneous—to the skin

b. Sublingual—under the tongue

c. Buccal—between the cheek and gum

d. Vaginal—within the vagina

e. Rectal—within the rectum

f. Otic—within the ear

g. Ophthalmic—within the eye

h. Nasal—within the nose

4. For self-administration of vaginal medications, tell the client to do the following:

a. Obtain a form of medication that meets your personal preference; all come with a vaginal applicator.

b. Plan to instill the medication before retiring for sleep to facilitate retention of the medication for a prolonged period of time.

c. Empty your bladder just before inserting the medication.

d. Place the drug within the applicator.

e. Lubricate the applicator tip with a water-soluble lubricant, such as K-Y Jelly.

f. Lie down, bend your knees, and spread your legs.

g. Separate the labia and insert the applicator within the vagina to the length recommended in the package directions, which is usually 2 to 4 inches (5 to 10 centimeters).

h. Depress the plunger to insert the medication.

i. Remove the applicator and place it on a clean tissue; discard the applicator if it is disposable.

j. Apply a sanitary pad if you prefer.

k. Remain recumbent for at least 10 to 30 minutes.

l. Wash a reusable applicator when hand washing and hygiene are performed.

m. Consult a physician if, after following the package directions, symptoms persist.

Chapter 34

ANSWERS TO MATCHING QUESTIONS
Items 1 Through 4

1. d   2. b   3. a   4. c

ANSWERS TO MULTIPLE-CHOICE QUESTIONS
Items 1 Through 12

1. (a) To ensure that the second vial will not be contaminated when combining drugs from two multiple-dose vials, the nurse should change the needle after drawing out the first medication and before inserting it into the second vial of medication.

2. (c) The common site for intramuscular injections into the gluteus maximus muscle is the dorsogluteal site.

3. (a) The common site for intramuscular injections into the anterior aspect of the thigh is the rectus femoris muscle.

4. (b) The preferred site for intramuscular injections for infants is the rectus femoris muscle. The gluteal muscles of infants are poorly developed.

5. (c) Intramuscular injections into the deltoid muscle should be limited to 1 mL of solution and should be used only for adults.

6. (b) One of the accepted methods for determining the dorsogluteal site to give intramuscular medications is to palpate the posterior iliac spine and the greater trochanter and draw an imaginary diagonal line between the two landmarks. The other accepted method is to divide the buttock into imaginary quadrants by drawing an imaginary vertical line through the bony ridge of the posterior superior iliac spine and an imaginary horizontal line from the upper cleft in the fold of the buttock.

7. (b) The reason for using the Z-track technique when giving intramuscular medication is to seal the medication within the muscle so that it cannot leak back through the layers of tissue following the path of the needle.

8. (d) A shorter needle, usually ½ to ⅝ inch, may be selected when giving subcutaneous injections because the tissue into which the medication will be injected is not as deep as muscular tissue. A 25-gauge needle is most often used because the medications administered by the subcutaneous route are generally not viscous.

9. (b) Insulin is supplied in a dosage strength called a unit. The equivalent now commonly used for measuring insulin is referred to as U-100. This means that when insulin is prepared by pharmaceutical companies, the standard strength is 100 units of insulin per 1 mL.

10. (a) Heparin is an anticoagulant. Various techniques are recommended to prevent bruising and bleeding when heparin is given via subcutaneous injection. Because heparin is also given intravenously, the

nurse should not aspirate the plunger. Drawing back on the plunger of the syringe may cause bruising or bleeding in the area of the injection.

11. (d) The angle of the syringe and needle for intradermal injections is 10° to 15° because the medication is placed within the layers of the skin.

12. (b) Humulin N insulin is an intermediate-acting insulin.

ANSWERS TO ALTERNATIVE FORMAT QUESTIONS

1. **Answer: 0.75**

   Rationale: Calculate as follows:

   $$1 \text{ mL} = 1,000 \text{ mg}$$
   $$x \text{ mL} = 750 \text{ mg}$$

   $$\frac{\text{Dose on hand}}{\text{Quantity on hand}} = \frac{\text{Desired dose}}{\text{Quantity desired (x)}}$$

   $$\frac{1000 \text{ mg}}{1 \text{ mL}} = \frac{750 \text{ mg}}{x}$$

   $$x = \frac{750}{1000}$$

   $$x = .75 \text{ mL}$$

Nursing Process:	Planning
Client Needs Category:	Physiological integrity
Cognitive Level:	Analysis

2. **Answer: 15**

   Rationale: When preparing medications for administration, the nurse may need to convert volume from one system of measurement to another. By learning some basic equivalent measures, the nurse is able to make many conversions easily.

Nursing Process:	Planning
Client Needs Category:	Safe, effective care environment
Cognitive Level:	Application

3. **Answer: 2, 3, 4, 5**

   Rationale: The ventrogluteal site is in the gluteus medius muscle that overlays the gluteus minimus, thus providing the greatest thickness of gluteal muscle for injection. This area is also consistently less fatty than the buttock area and is usually free of fecal contamination. It is safer than other areas because it contains no large nerves, blood vessels, or bone. The area may or may not be free of irritation or infection. The radial artery is a major artery in the forearm.

Nursing Process:	Planning
Client Needs Category:	Physiological integrity
Cognitive Level:	Analysis

ANSWERS TO TRUE OR FALSE QUESTIONS

Items 1 Through 11

1. *False.* The term *parenteral* refers to all routes of administration *other* than oral.

2. *True.*

3. *False.* When combining medications from single-dose and multiple-dose vials, the medication should be withdrawn from the multiple-dose vial first.

4. *False.* An *ampule* is a glass container holding a single dose of a parenteral medication. A *vial* is a glass container of parenteral medication with a self-sealing stopper. A vial may contain one or more doses of a medication.

5. *False.* When giving an intramuscular injection, the needle should be inserted without hesitation. Instill the medication slowly and remove the needle rapidly to decrease the amount of medication that may spread into surrounding tissue.

6. *False.* One advantage of using prefilled cartridges is that they eliminate the time involved in transferring the drug from a medication container, such as an ampule or vial, into a syringe. If the prescribed dosage is less than that contained in the cartridge, the unneeded portion is expelled before its administration.

7. *False.* Most prefilled cartridges are intended for a single-unit dose of drug.

8. *False.* When planning to administer medication via the Z-track method, the original needle used to aspirate medication into the syringe must be changed. This prevents tissue contact with residue of the drug that could be clinging to the outside of the needle.

9. *True.*

10. *True.*

11. *False.* Do not aspirate the plunger when giving heparin via the subcutaneous route.

ANSWERS TO SHORT ANSWER QUESTIONS

Items 1 Through 2

1. Criteria for selecting the appropriate syringe and needle are:
   a. The *route* of administration—a longer needle is required for reaching deeper layers of tissue
   b. The *viscosity,* or thickness, of the solution. Some medications are more viscous than others and require a larger lumen through which to inject the drug
   c. The *quantity* to be administered—the larger the volume of medication to be injected, the greater the holding capacity must be within the syringe
   d. The *body size* of the client. An obese person may require a longer needle to reach various layers of tissue than a thin or pediatric client
   e. The *type of medication.* Some drugs should be measured or administered using specific equipment

2. Recommendations after a needlestick are:
   a. Report the injury to the supervisor.
   b. Document the injury in writing.
   c. Identify the client.
   d. Obtain HIV and HBV status, if it is legal to do so.
   e. Obtain counseling on the potential for infection.
   f. Receive the most appropriate postexposure prophylaxis.

g. Be tested for the presence of antibodies at appropriate intervals.

h. Receive instructions on monitoring potential symptoms and medical follow-up.

Chapter 35

ANSWERS TO MATCHING QUESTIONS

Items 1 Through 5

1. e   2. b   3. c   4. d   5. a

ANSWERS TO MULTIPLE-CHOICE QUESTIONS

Items 1 Through 10

1. (d) Medications can be added to a large volume of intravenous solution and administered slowly over a number of hours. The medication can be added to the solution by the nurse.

2. (c) Tunneled catheters are inserted into a central vein with a portion of the catheter secured within the subcutaneous tissue. The end of the catheter exits from the skin lateral to the xiphoid process. Tunneled catheters are used when extended therapy is required.

3. (d) Antineoplastic drugs are toxic to both normal and abnormal cells. It has been found that these drugs can even cause adverse effects in the pharmacists who mix them and the nurses who administer them. They can be absorbed by health care professionals through inhalation of tiny droplets or dust particles. Long-term, unprotected exposure to small amounts of these drugs can lead to changes in body cells, including sperm, ova, or fetal tissue.

4. (c) There are three types of central venous catheters: percutaneous, tunneled, and implanted. The Hickman is an example of a tunneled catheter.

5. (c) An intermittent infusion is one in which IV medication is given within a relatively short period of time.

6. (a) Because the entire dose of medication is administered so fast, bolus administration has the greatest potential for causing life-threatening changes should a drug reaction occur.

7. (d) One of the best features of a medication lock is that it eliminates the need for continuous, sometimes unnecessary, administration of IV fluid.

8. (d) A secondary infusion involves administering a drug that has been diluted in a small volume of IV solution, usually 50 to 100 cc, over a period of 30 to 60 minutes.

9. (a) A volume-control set may be used for two purposes: to administer IV medication in a small volume at intermittent intervals and to avoid overloading the circulatory system.

10. (c) Central venous catheters may have single or multiple lumens. The advantage of multiple lumens is that incompatible substances, or more than one solution or drug, can be given simultaneously. Each infuses through a separate channel and exits the catheter at a different location near the heart. Thus, the drugs or solutions never interact with one another.

ANSWERS TO ALTERNATIVE FORMAT QUESTIONS

1. **Answer: 2, 6, 3, 4, 5, 1**

Rationale: Identify the client to ensure that the right client receives the medication. Assess the client to ensure that there are no unusual signs or symptoms present to prevent administration of the medication. Washing your hands reduces the transmission of microorganisms, and putting on gloves reduces the likelihood that the nurse's hands will come in contact with the client's blood. Swabbing the port prevents microorganisms from entering the circulatory system during needle insertion. Flushing with normal saline first prepares the lock for receiving the medication by removing blood, debris, and heparin. The second flush with normal saline forces all of the medication out of the lock and readies the lock for the heparin flush, which prevents coagulation within the lock system. Instill the medication at the recommended rate of infusion between saline flushes. Place a new sterile cap over the lock.

Nursing Process:	Implementation
Client Needs Category:	Physiological integrity
Cognitive Level:	Analysis

2. **Answer: 8**

Rationale: The following formula is used to calculate the dose:

$$\frac{\text{Dose on hand}}{\text{Quantity on hand}} = \frac{\text{Dose desired}}{x}$$

$$\frac{25{,}000\ U}{250} = \frac{800\ U/\text{hour}}{\text{mL } x}$$

$$x = 8\ \text{mL/hour}$$

Nursing:	Implementation
Client Needs Category:	Physiological integrity
Cognitive Level:	Application

3. **Answer: 50**

Rationale: Use the following equation:

100 mL / 30 minutes × 15 gtt / 1 mL = 49.9 gtt/minute = 50 gtt per minute

Nursing Process:	Implementation
Client Needs Category:	Physiological integrity
Cognitive Level:	Application

ANSWERS TO TRUE OR FALSE QUESTIONS

Items 1 Through 9

1. *False.* A bolus is a single dose of medication injected directly into an intravenous line.

2. *False.* A heparin lock is a device that facilitates access to the bloodstream without requiring the continuous infusion of fluids.

3. *True.*

4. *True.*
5. *True.*
6. *False.* Tunneled catheters are inserted into central veins and secured within subcutaneous tissue.
7. *False.* A portion of many drugs is bound to protein in the blood. Drugs that are protein bound are basically inactive. The portion that is not bound is called "free drug"; it is the free drug that is physiologically active. Older adults tend to have more free drug in proportion to bound drug. Therefore, they are more likely to experience adverse drug effects.
8. *True.*
9. *True.*

ANSWERS TO SHORT ANSWER QUESTIONS

Items 1 Through 3

1. The four steps (SASH) a nurse should follow when giving medication through a heparin lock are
   a. S = Saline irrigation
   b. A = Administer medication
   c. S = Saline irrigation
   d. H = Heparin instillation
2. The advantages for using a central venous catheter over a peripheral one include the following:
   a. It avoids the necessity for multiple or frequent venipunctures when drug and fluid therapy may involve an extended length of administration.
   b. Because the catheter deposits drugs into a large blood vessel with a high volume of blood, it allows irritating or highly concentrated drugs and solutions to be instilled without traumatizing the vein wall.
   c. Some have a dual use in that venous blood can be withdrawn from the catheter rather than puncturing a peripheral vein when blood tests are ordered.
   d. A central venous catheter reduces the potential for infiltration.
   e. It frees the client's hands for movement and self-care.
3. Intravenous administration is the route chosen when:
   a. A quick response is needed during an emergency.
   b. Clients have disorders that affect absorption or metabolism of drugs, such as a seriously burned client.
   c. Blood levels of drugs need to be maintained at a consistent therapeutic level, such as when treating infections caused by drug-resistant pathogens or when providing pain relief postoperatively.
   d. It is in the client's best interests to avoid the discomfort of repeated intramuscular injections.
   e. A mechanism is needed to administer drug therapy over a prolonged period of time, as in cancer care.

Chapter 36

ANSWERS TO MATCHING QUESTIONS

Items 1 Through 5

1. e   2. a   3. b   4. d   5. c

ANSWERS TO MULTIPLE-CHOICE QUESTIONS

Items 1 Through 12

1. (c) The respiratory tract is lined with mucous membranes. This tissue keeps the passageways moist and sticky so that nongaseous particles are trapped before falling into delicate smaller structures within the lungs. Dry air or reduced volumes of water can alter the moist condition within the air passages.

   The mucous membranes can become dehydrated, causing mucus to become thicker than usual. To avoid this, the nurse may keep the client well hydrated. This is done by encouraging an adequate fluid intake.
2. (d) *Aerosolization* is the process of suspending droplets of water in a gas. *Humidification* is adding moisture to air; the production of rather large droplets is known as *atomization;* and *nebulization* is the production of a mist or fog.
3. (b) Postural drainage should be performed before meals and before bedtime. Some positions for postural drainage are uncomfortable and may produce nausea and vomiting when therapy is carried out soon after eating.
4. (a) *Percussion* is the technique of striking the chest with rhythmic gentle blows using a cupped hand. *Vibration* is the technique of using firm, strong, circular movements on the chest with open hands, producing wavelike tremors.
5. (c) Percussion and vibration are intended to cause thick secretions to break loose from their location within the airway. The client may cough up these secretions after the treatment. Collapse of the lungs may be prevented by using percussion and vibration.
6. (a) To determine the appropriate size of oral airway to use, place the airway on the outside of the client's cheek; the front should be parallel with the front teeth and the back of the airway should reach the angle of the jaw.
7. (c) A sputum specimen is best obtained early in the morning because a higher volume of secretions is likely to have accumulated throughout the night. Another time that may provide a better opportunity for collecting specimens would be following respiratory therapy treatments, postural drainage, and percussion and vibration.
8. (d) When a client has an oral airway in place, it should be removed briefly every 4 hours.
9. (b) The inner cannula of a tracheostomy should be cleaned regularly to help prevent infection. Most agencies specify that cleansing should be performed at least once every 8 hours.

10. (a) When suctioning a tracheostomy, the catheter should be inserted carefully and slowly about 10 to 12.5 cm (4 to 5 inches) into the inner cannula and into the respiratory passage without covering the vent on the tubing.
11. (b) Clients suffering from insufficient oxygen often feel as though they are suffocating. They are usually restless and anxious.
12. (a) The epiglottis protects the airway by sealing the tube when swallowing food and fluids.

ANSWERS TO ALTERNATIVE FORMAT QUESTIONS

1. **Answer: 3**
   Rationale: This quantity is sufficient for analysis.

Nursing Process:	Implementation
Client Needs Category:	Physiological integrity
Cognitive Level:	Application

2. **Answer: 2, 3, 4, 5**
   Rationale: A change in rate and depth of respiration and abnormal breath sounds, are among the defining characteristics for this diagnosis. The muscular structures of the larynx tend to atrophy with age, which can affect the ability to clear the airway. Diminished strength of accessory muscles for respiration, increased rigidity of the chest wall, and diminished cough reflex make it difficult for older adults to cough productively and effectively.

Nursing Process:	Assessment
Client Needs Category:	Physiological integrity
Cognitive Level:	Analysis

3. **Answer: 4**
   Rationale: Removing the oral airway every 4 hours allows an opportunity for providing oral hygiene. Hygiene and cleansing remove transient bacteria and promote the integrity of the oral mucosa.

Nursing Process:	Implementation
Client Needs Category:	Physiological integrity
Cognitive Level:	Application

ANSWERS TO TRUE OR FALSE QUESTIONS

Items 1 Through 9

1. *True.*
2. *False.* The source of suction may be through a wall unit or a separate portable machine. Usually a pressure of 100 to 140 mm Hg using a wall unit or a setting of 10 to 15 mm Hg using a portable suction machine is sufficient to remove secretions from an adult without damaging tissue severely.
3. *True.*
4. *True.*
5. *False.* Sterile technique must be followed when suctioning is performed for a client with a tracheostomy.
6. *False.* Collect at least a 1- to 3-mL specimen to ensure a sufficient quantity of sputum for study.
7. *True.*
8. *True.*
9. *False.* Because the tracheostomy tube is below the larynx, clients are usually unable to speak or call for help. This is frightening for most clients. Therefore, it is important that the nurse check these clients frequently and respond immediately when they signal.

ANSWERS TO SHORT ANSWER QUESTIONS

Items 1 Through 2

1. The steps to follow when inserting an oral airway are:
   a. Gather necessary supplies.
   b. Determine the appropriate size of airway to use.
   c. Wash your hands; put on clean gloves.
   d. Explain what you are going to do.
   e. Perform oral suctioning if needed.
   f. Place the client supine; hyperextend the neck.
   g. Open the client's mouth.
   h. Insert the airway halfway.
   i. Rotate the airway over the tongue and insert it until the front is flush with lips.
   j. Assess breathing.
   k. Remove the airway every 4 hours, provide oral hygiene, and clean and reinsert the airway.
2. Five approaches for airway suctioning:
   a. Nasopharyngeal
   b. Nasotracheal
   c. Oropharyngeal
   d. Oral
   e. Tracheal

Chapter 37

ANSWERS TO MULTIPLE-CHOICE QUESTIONS

Items 1 Through 10

1. (c) The carotid artery is recommended for checking the pulse of an adult during CPR. The carotid artery is a large vessel and is likely to produce more obvious pulsations than could be felt at other peripheral sites on an adult. It is also the most accessible artery.
2. (b) Before starting cardiac compressions, it is particularly important to be sure the victim is without a pulse. If a pulse is present and compressions are given, the victim may develop a potentially fatal cardiac arrhythmia.
3. (c) Rescue breathing for an adult should be done every 5 seconds, each lasting 1 to 1½ seconds.
4. (d) When performing CPR, the ratio of compressions to ventilations should be 15 compressions to two ventilations.
5. (c) The depth of chest compressions for an adult should be 1½ to 2 inches.
6. (a) Inability to Sustain Spontaneous Ventilation is described as a state in which the response pattern of decreased energy reserves results in the inability to maintain breathing adequate to support life.

7. (b) For an unconscious victim, the American Heart Association recommends the use of basic cardiopulmonary resuscitation (CPR). Chest compressions in CPR create enough pressure in unconscious victims to eject a foreign body from the airway.

8. (c) In the presence of complete airway obstruction, the victim will be unable to speak, cough, or breathe.

9. (a) The method of choice for opening the airway is the head tilt-chin lift technique.

10. (b) A breathing victim is placed in the recovery position. The recovery position is a side-lying position, which helps to maintain an open airway and prevent aspiration.

ANSWERS TO ALTERNATIVE FORMAT QUESTIONS

1. **Answer: 20**
   Rationale: Rescue breaths provide essential support for an individual who is not breathing. Current recommended respiratory rates are derived from normal respiratory rate for age, with some adjustment for the time needed to coordinate rescue breathing with chest compressions to ensure that ventilation is adequate. The recommended rate for infants is 20 breaths per minute.

Nursing Process:	Planning
Client Needs Category:	Physiological integrity
Cognitive Level:	Analysis

2. **Answer: 6, 1, 4, 3, 5, 2**
   Rationale: If a person's unresponsiveness is the result of cardiac arrest, rescuers implement a process known as the chain of survival. The steps involve early recognition, early access of emergency services, and placement of the victim on a firm, flat surface in preparation for beginning CPR. It also requires the use of the AED to enhance survival and effectiveness of CPR efforts. Emergency medical support personnel can provide intubation, supplemental oxygenation, and medications to improve the potential for resuscitation during transport of the victim to a hospital.

Nursing Process:	Application
Client Needs Category:	Physiological integrity
Cognitive Level:	Analysis

3. **Answer: 2, 3, 4**
   Rationale: The conditions under which CPR may be interrupted are when there is written evidence that the victim does not want CPR, the rescuer becomes too exhausted to continue, there is a pulse and the victim resumes breathing, the victim's condition deteriorates in spite of resuscitative efforts; or advanced life-support measures are administered. If the victim has no pulse, resuscitation should be begun or continued. Victims who have a communicable disease should be resuscitated using a one-way valve mask or other protective face shield. If these devices are not available, chest compressions without rescue breathing are begun.

Nursing Process:	Application
Client Needs Category:	Physiological integrity
Cognitive Level:	Analysis

ANSWERS TO TRUE OR FALSE QUESTIONS
Items 1 Through 10

1. *False.* Use a brachial artery to check for a pulse in an infant. The carotid artery is recommended for use when doing CPR on an adult.
2. *False.* Two rescue breaths are recommended when starting CPR on individuals of any age.
3. *True.*
4. *True.*
5. *False.* It is possible to identify in an advance directive exactly the type of resuscitation the victim will allow.
6. *True.*
7. *True.*
8. *False.* To dislodge an object from an infant's airway, a series of back blows are delivered followed by a series of chest thrusts.
9. *True.*
10. *False.* The decision to cease is a medical judgment made by the physician leading the code.

ANSWERS TO SHORT ANSWER QUESTIONS
Items 1 Through 3

1. The signs of choking are:
   a. Grasping the throat
   b. Spontaneous efforts to cough and breathe
   c. Producing a high-pitched sound while inhaling
   d. Turning pale and then blue
   e. An inability to speak, breathe, or cough
   f. Collapse followed by a state of unconsciousness
2. The ABCs of basic life support are:
   a. A is for airway
   b. B is for breathing
   c. C is for circulation
3. Criteria for interrupting CPR are:
   a. There is a pulse, and the victim resumes breathing.
   b. Advanced cardiac life-support measures are administered.
   c. Exhaustion of the rescuer occurs.
   d. Deterioration progresses despite resuscitation efforts.
   e. There is written evidence that resuscitation is contrary to the victim's wishes.

Chapter 38

ANSWERS TO MATCHING QUESTIONS
Items 1 Through 5

1. c   2. e   3. a   4. d   5. b

ANSWERS TO MULTIPLE-CHOICE QUESTIONS
Items 1 Through 10

1. (c) An advance directive is a written statement describing the wishes of the writer concerning his or her medical care when his or her death is near.
2. (c) The third stage of dying according to Dr. Elisabeth Kübler-Ross is the bargaining stage.
3. (b) Anger is considered to be the second stage of dying.
4. (c) The nurse realizes that in some instances, the care needed by dying clients is too complex or demanding for family members. Families may have neither the physical nor the emotional strength to deal with the terminally ill person in the home. Care must be taken that the family is not made to feel guilty about not having the ill person at home.
5. (a) Hospice care emphasizes helping the client live until he or she dies, with his or her family with him or her, and helping the family return to normal living after the client's death.
6. (d) Fears are as varied as attitudes toward death. Both may change from time to time as a terminal illness progresses. Most people fear death because it represents a force over which there is no control. Generally, by relieving an individual's fears concerning death, the nurse can facilitate moving to the stage of acceptance wherein the person can die in peace and with dignity.
7. (a) The client may suck on gauze soaked in water or on ice chips wrapped in gauze without difficulty because sucking is one of the last reflexes to disappear as death approaches.
8. (c) When pain is intense, relief is more difficult to obtain with the irregular administration of drugs. Therefore, it is better to try to control pain when it is minimal rather than wait until it is excruciating. Peaks and valleys of pain can be reduced by administering pain-relieving drugs on a routine schedule throughout the 24-hour period rather than only when necessary.
9. (d) The client must be pronounced dead by the physician. At one time the client was pronounced dead when there was no evidence of pulse, respiration, or blood pressure. In the case of extensive use of artificial means for maintaining life support, other criteria have been adopted in order to redefine death. New assessments are now used to declare individuals *brain dead*. Brain wave recordings are taken over a period of 24 hours to validate the death.
10. (c) A coroner has the right to order that an autopsy be performed if the death involved a crime, was of a suspicious nature, or occurred without any medical consultation prior to the death.

ANSWERS TO ALTERNATIVE FORMAT QUESTIONS

1. **Answer: 6**
   Rationale: Virtually anyone, from the very young to older adults, may have the potential to be an organ donor. If the donor is younger than 18 years of age and is able, he or she must sign a donor card along with the parents or legal guardian. Age requirements and organ acceptance are determined on an individual basis at the time of organ procurement. Guidelines established by the Organ Procurement Agency of Michigan recommend age criteria for kidney donation to be from 6 months to 55 years of age.

Nursing Process:	Planning
Client Needs Category:	Safe, effective care environment
Cognitive Level:	Application

2. **Answer: 4, 2, 5, 1, 3**
   Rationale: Dr. Elisabeth Kübler-Ross, an authority on dying, has described stages through which many terminally ill clients progress. They are denial, anger, bargaining, depression, and acceptance. These stages may occur in a progressive fashion, or a person can move back and forth through the stages. There is no specific time period for the rate of progression, duration, or completion of the stages.

Nursing Process:	Planning
Client Needs Category:	Psychosocial integrity
Cognitive Level:	Application

3. **Answer: II**
   Rationale: According to Dr. Kübler-Ross, the five stages experienced by terminally ill clients are Stage I—denial; Stage II—anger; Stage III—bargaining; Stage IV—depression, and Stage V—acceptance. Feeling victimized and the desire to retaliate are characteristic of Stage II—anger. Clients often displace their anger toward nurses, physicians, family members, or even God. They may also express anger by complaining about their care or overreacting to even the slightest annoyances.

Nursing Process:	Planning
Client Needs Category:	Psychosocial integrity
Cognitive Level:	Application

ANSWERS TO TRUE OR FALSE QUESTIONS
Items 1 Through 12

1. *False. Denial* is a psychological technique in which an individual does not believe certain information to be true. *Avoidance* is a technique used to separate oneself from situations that are threatening or unpleasant.
2. *True.*
3. *True.*
4. *False.* Although every person provided with the knowledge of impending death responds in his own distinctive way, studies have shown that there is a pattern. Dr. Elisabeth Kübler-Ross has described stages that a dying person experiences. Not all persons go through the stages in the precise order as described.
5. *False.* Not all persons go through the stages in the precise order as described by Dr. Elisabeth Kübler-Ross. A person may skip one stage or fall back a stage. Stages may overlap. The length of any stage may range from a few hours to months.

6. *False*. Any competent adult has the right to request aggressive treatment or refuse therapy and all variations in between.
7. *True*.
8. *False*. As death approaches, the body temperature usually is elevated, but as the circulatory system fails, the skin usually feels cold to the touch.
9. *True*.
10. *True*.
11. *False*. Pain, if it has been present, subsides. As the level of consciousness changes, the brain may no longer perceive pain.
12. *False*. The physician is required to sign the death certificate. The laws of this country require that a death certificate be issued for each person who has died.

ANSWERS TO SHORT ANSWER QUESTIONS

Items 1 Through 4

1. Signs of imminent death are:
   a. Paranormal experiences may be described.
   b. Motion and sensation are gradually lost.
   c. The temperature is usually elevated, but the skin becomes cold and clammy.
   d. Respirations become noisy (the death rattle).
   e. Circulation fails and blood pressure drops.
   f. Pain, if it has been present, subsides.
   g. The mental condition usually deteriorates.
2. Suggestions the nurse should use when summoning the family are:
   a. Give your name, title, and indicate from where the call is being made.
   b. Determine the identity of the person who has answered the phone.
   c. Explain that you are calling because the client's condition has worsened.
   d. Speak in a calm and controlled voice.
   e. Use short sentences to provide small pieces of information.
   f. Pause to allow the family member to comprehend.
   g. Inform the family member of the care that is being provided at the moment.
   h. Urge the individual to come at once to the health care agency.
   i. Document the time and the individual to whom the information was communicated.
3. Common physical reactions of a grieving individual are:
   a. Anorexia
   b. Tightness in the chest and throat
   c. Difficulty breathing
   d. Lack of strength
   e. Sleep pattern disturbances
4. Examples of pathological grief are:
   a. Retaining all of the deceased individual's possessions as if ready for use
   b. Attempting to make contact with the deceased through various forms of spiritualism
   c. Keeping the dead body within a residence for an extended period after death